LASER TREATMENT for NAEVI

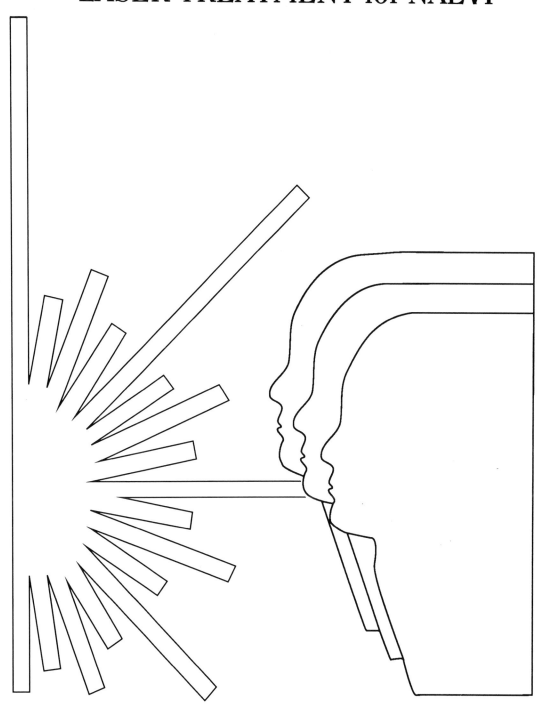

LASER TREATMENT for NAEVI

TOSHIO OHSHIRO
Keio University School of Medicine and Japan
Medical Laser Laboratory, Tokyo, Japan

with contributions from

R. Glen Calderhead
Eiji Itoh
Takashi Maeda
Katsumi Sasaki
Yoshinori Shirono
Minoru Yamada

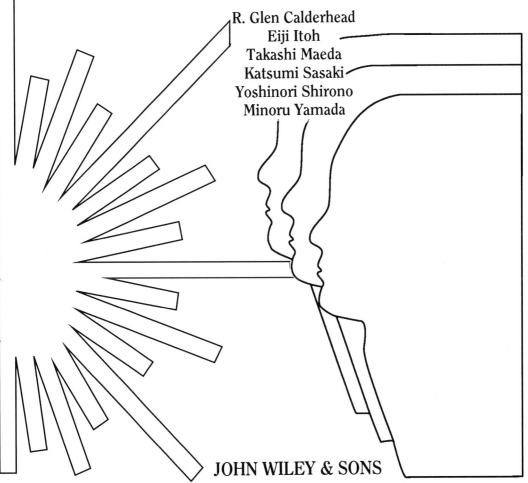

JOHN WILEY & SONS
Chichester • New York • Brisbane • Toronto • Singapore

Copyright © 1995 by John Wiley & Sons Ltd,
Baffins Lane, Chichester,
West Sussex PO19 1UD, England

Telephone: National   Chichester (01243) 779777
              International   (+44) 1243 779777

Other Wiley Editorial Offices

John Wiley & Sons. Inc., 605 Third Avenue,
New York, NY 10158-0012, USA

Jacaranda Wiley Ltd, 33 Park Road, Milton,
Queensland 4064, Australia

John Wiley & Sons (Canada) Ltd, 22 Worcester Road,
Rexdale, Ontario M9W 1L1, Canada

John Wiley & Sons (SEA) Pte Ltd, 37 Jalan Pemimpin #05-04,
Block B, Union Industrial Building, Singapore 2057

British Library Cataloguing in Publication Data

A catalogue record for this book is available from the British Library

ISBN 0 471 95243 5

Produced from camera-ready copy typeset and supplied by
IMELIS Medical Publications, Tochigi, Japan and Fife, Scotland
Printed and bound in Great Britain by Cambridge University Press

Dedication

I should like humbly to dedicate this book to a very important group of people in my life and in my life's work:

To Eiji Itoh MD, for his inspiration while I was his student in the Department of Plastic and Reconstructive Surgery of Keio University School of Medicine, and whose influence really started me off in my life's work with abnormal skin colour;

To Seiji Makoto MD, whose vast knowledge of melanogenesis and melanin abnormalities inspired me, and encouraged me to learn under him in the Tokyo Medical and Dental University;

To Leon Goldman MD, The recognized 'Godfather' of the surgical laser, whose pioneering work with laser treatment of haemangioma simplex lesions inspired me to go to the U.S.A. in 1974 and study lasers under Dr Goldman at the University of Cincinnati, and who is mostly responsible for igniting my continuing passion with this remarkable form of light energy;

And last, but by no means least, to all of my family, who have stood by me, encouraged and supported me during these past two turbulent and light-filled decades. However, my special thanks go to my late father, Asataro, and my mother, Fujiko, who passed on to me their love of Medicine: my mother still sustains it as our family's Matriarch in Okinawa; and my wife, Yoshiko, who has worked faithfully beside me both in the home and in the office and whose calming influence and enduring support have contributed greatly to my continued efforts in my life's work.

Table of Contents

CHAPTER 1: THE NAEVUS

CHAPTER 2: THE LASER

CHAPTER 3: LASER TREATMENT FOR NAEVI

CONTRIBUTORS

Principal Author

Toshio Ohshiro MD

Visiting Associate Professor
Department of Plastic and Reconstructive Surgery
Keio University School of Medicine:
Executive Director
Japan Medical Laser Laboratory:
Executive Clinical Director
Ohshiro Clinic
Tokyo, Japan.

Contributing Authors

(In Alphabetical Order)

R Glen Calderhead MA DrMSc

Executive Director
IMELIS (International Consultants in Medicine and Science)
Tochigi, Japan and Fife, Scotland.

Eiji Itoh MD

Visiting Professor
Department of Plastic and Reconstructive Surgery
Keio University School of Medicine
Tokyo, Japan

Takashi Maeda MD

Deputy Director
Japan Medical Laser Laboratory
Tokyo, Japan.

Katsumi Sasaki MD

Deputy Clinical Director
Ohshiro Clinic
Tokyo, Japan.

Yoshinori Shirono MD

Chief, Pain Clinic
Ohshiro Clinic
Tokyo, Japan.

Minoru Yamada MD

Former Assistant Professor
Department of Dermatology
Tokyo Medical and Dental University School of Medicine
Tokyo, Japan.

FOREWORDS

Leon Goldman MD

In 1980, the first beautiful and important book on nevi from my friend Dr Ohshiro, "Laser Treatment for Nevi", (MEL, Ltd, Tokyo, 1980) stood proudly on the laser library shelf. Fourteen years later I am privileged to offer a FOREWORD again to a great work as I was happy to do for that first one. Now a greater, more detailed and even more colorful review of long experience with nevi appears from a master of lasers.

New photons are now available for the operating surgeon. New techniques are now possible for plastic surgeons and for dermatologists, as well as for general surgeons. Both patients and doctors will now understand the significance of many common and uncommon naevi from this great laser surgical art work. This is also a great reference source for the many naevi.

I wish the author and his book a very well deserved success.

Laser Consultant, US Naval Hospital,
San Diego, California:
Professor Emeritus,
Department of Dermatology,
College of Medicine, The University of Cincinnati,
Ohio, USA.

Francis A. L'Esperance, Jr, MD

It is a great honor and a privilege to have the opportunity to show my appreciation to Dr. Toshio Ohshiro, an outstanding plastic and reconstructive surgeon, who has been, along with Goldman, Apfelberg and others, one of the leading pioneers in the diagnosis and treatment of nevi of the skin by laser interaction.

In the first chapter of this magnificently illustrated book, Dr. Ohshiro proceeds from an extensive classification of nevi, through a detailed explanation of the histology and physiology of the skin. For dealing with the actual treatment of the nevi, the second chapter thoroughly takes the reader through a comprehensive and clear section on basic laser theory, the characteristics of various laser devices, usual and unusual optical elements and their various effects, and even to the mechanics of the generation of a pulsed laser beam with modalities such as the mechanical, ultrasonic, or electro-optical Q-Switch devices. This is followed closely by an excellent section dealing with various types of laser-tissue interactions which can occur, particularly with the treatment of skin nevi.

The most exceptional part of the book is Chapter 3, which is dedicated to the actual laser treatment for nevi, and which deals with the various diagnostic criteria which are considered to be important by Dr. Ohshiro. The mechanisms of wound healing after laser surgery and therapy are discussed in detail, as well as the very important subject of wound management. The multitude of various types of laser treatments, the relationship of the doctor to the patient during these treatment sessions, and comparison of laser therapy to other types of dermatologic treatment of these disfiguring malformations is compared. The Total Treatment Concept as devised by Dr. Ohshiro is reviewed excellently, and even delves in detail into the laser safety issues, as well as the future applications of other types of lasers.

There is no doubt that physicians operating in this field of plastic and reconstructive surgery must have a far reaching range of interdisciplinary skills. They must have excellent pathophysiologic knowledge of birthmarks, as well as to be well-versed in the fields of laser physics and colorimetry. Of course, they must also be skillful in the basic tenets of plastic and reconstructive surgery.

Dr. Ohshiro's textbook adds immeasurably to setting a clear, well-defined and brilliant view of the entire subject of skin nevi and their treatment by laser technology. Dr. Ohshiro must be congratulated for creating one of the finest textbooks concerned with the use of lasers in medicine, and certainly the definitive book in the world literature concerned with the diagnosis and treatment of nevi by the interaction of this congenital abnormality with laser radiation.

Francis A l'Esperance

Clinical Professor of Ophthalmology,
Columbia University,
New York,
New York, U.S.A.

Toyomi Fujino MD FACS DrMedSci

The naevus has long been a problematic physiological and psychological blemish. In the past, naevi were associated with witchcraft and the devil, and surgical methods of the time could not help the sufferers. Now, in the 20th century, we understand more and more about these cutaneous abnormalities: their physiology and their aetiology. As our understanding of naevi has increased, so has the development of one of the most important surgical tools to treat naevi: the laser. Many departments of plastic and reconstructive surgery (PRS) now have a laser, but too few of them seem to be fully used: perhaps with the aid of this book that will change.

In 1980, Dr Toshio Ohshiro published a first-class text book, "Laser Treatment for Nevi". This book was actually well ahead of its time, and even now some of Dr Ohshiro's early ideas are appearing in the literature from other workers in the field as 'new' methods.

The present book, "Laser Treatment for Naevi" is an even more complete reference volume for the dermatologist and plastic surgeon who are treating naevi. The book gives a thorough grounding in all of the basics necessary in a clear and well-ordered way: the anatomy and physiology of the different classes of naevi, and the skin itself; the basics of the physics on which laser energy is based and from which it is generated the photobiological considerations of laser-tissue interaction; and, of course, a strong section on laser safety. 'People skills' are also covered, including the important issue of public relations, and the 3-way human interaction between the clinician, his or her staff and the patient and family. All of the above elements are then drawn together in what Dr Ohshiro calls his 'Total Treatment Concept' (TTC), a wide-ranging and complex combination of all of the above factors, enabling the surgeon to select the correct treatment for each naevus patient on a truly individual basis.

In the third chapter, examples are given which clearly show how the Total Treatment Concept really works: Dr Ohshiro's results speak for themselves. At times when other clinicians were quick to condemn the laser because of 'inappropriate indications' resulting in unacceptable scarring, Dr Ohshiro has persisted with his TTC, in which scarring is minimized. I think it is true to say that for these other surgeons, it was not the indication of the laser that was inappropriate at all: it was the way in which they were applying the laser to their patients that was inappropriate. With the TTC in action, all aspects behind laser treatment for naevi form a solid but flexible basis from which a surgeon can achieve consistently good results. Dr Ohshiro does, and his busy practice is a living testimonial to how his patients feel about their treatment.

It is my pleasure and honour to write this Foreword to this new volume of "Laser Treatment for Naevi" by my colleague, Dr Toshio Ohshiro. In addition to holding the post of Visiting Associate Professor in my department Dr Ohshiro is also a Keio PRS 'Old Boy', so we are all proud of, and happy for him. In December of 1992, I had the honour of presiding at the inaugural congress of the International Society for Simulation Surgery, recently renamed to the International Society for Computer Aided Surgery. An important aspect of the practical aspect of 'simulation surgery' is colour and configurational simulation in patients with skin and soft tissue defects, including naevi. Dr Ohshiro has shown in this book some excellent examples of this simulation surgery from the standpoint of PRS. I am sure that laser treatment for naevi will advance strongly into the 21st century, and that a lot of this advance will be due to the ideas and concepts expounded in this book. I wish both the book and its author a very deserved success.

Professor and Chairman,
Department of Plastic and Reconstructive Surgery,
Keio University School of Medicine,
Tokyo,
Japan.

PREFACE

Once upon a time, as all good stories start, in the early 1960's when the laser was in its infancy, I was a student in the Department of Plastic and Reconstructive Surgery (PRS) at Tokyo's Keio University School of Medicine. I did not realize then that I was really embarking on just a single aspect of the huge field of medicine which would become both my life's work and my passion. In this Preface I would like to share with the reader the development of that passion, and acknowledge some of the principal figures who helped fan it and increase my small clinical knowledge so that the passion could be transformed into a vocation.

My Professor at Keio was **Dr Eiji Itoh**, who encouraged me very much to make a special study of abnormally coloured skin lesions and that was, as they say, the beginning of it all. From my graduation from Keio in 1965 until the present, for almost 30 years, my life's work has been the study and treatment of naevi, those physically disfiguring and mentally disturbing manifestations of some abnormality in the development of skin cells.

I studied first at Keio University for a yea, then I continued my skin colour studies under **Dr Seiji Makoto**, who was then Professor of Dermatology at the Tokyo Medical and Dental University. Dr Makoto's speciality was melanogenesis in both its histological and histochemical aspects, normal and abnormal, and in which he is now recognized as the world's foremost authority.

I spent two years studying in this field, then studied general surgery for two years at Ogikubo Hospital, Tokyo. Following that I returned to Keio University, Department of PRS and founded my first Colour Clinic in 1972. At that period, interesting news of the laser as a clinical tool was reaching Japan from the USA and this sparked off (or even illuminated) another stage in the development of my work. I went to The States in 1974 where I had the honour and pleasure of studying under and working with Professor **Leon Goldman** of the Department of Dermatology at the University of Cincinnati and the main pioneer in the applications of the laser for the treatment of haemangioma simplex, or port-wine stain. His influence and teachings really fired my imagination, and I arranged on my return from the USA to import the first ruby laser system for clinical use in Japan. **Dr Yasushi Sakamoto**, one of my class-mates, was with the Japanese Ministry of Health and Welfare, and his assistance in the importation of the laser system to Japan was invaluable, as was the **Far East Trading Company** which handled the actual import procedures. During this time I was lucky enough to get involved with the *Shizuoka Red Cross Hospital,* and its President, **Dr Ichiro Hosokawa**, was an inspiration for me to continue my studies into naevi aetiology and treatment. I used my connections with the Shizuoka Red Cross Hospital and founded near there in 1975 the *Japan*

Medical Laser Laboratory (JMLL) whose first task was to turn the commercial Korad ruby laser from an industrial unit into one which could be used safely, efficiently and consistently in the medical field for the treatment of naevi.

In 1976 I was accepted into Keio University as an Assistant Professor in the Department of PRS, and in 1977 opened the *Ohshiro Clinic of Plastic and Reconstructive Surgery* in Tokyo, which is alive and well today under the abbreviated name of the Ohshiro Clinic. At the same time I moved the JMLL from Shizuoka to Tokyo. I would like to acknowledge here the help I received in these early days from Professor Itoh, and Associate Professor **Toyomi Fujino,** who is now Professor of the PRS Department and was also good enough to write one of the Forewords to this volume.

By 1980 I had treated over 3,500 patients in the Ohshiro Clinic using the laser alone, in combination with other lasers (Combined Laser Treatment), or in combination with conventional methods (Combination Treatment Method): that was the genesis of my Total Treatment Concept or TTC, which underpins all my treatment methods in the clinic and forms the backbone round which the skeleton and body of this book were evolved. I published the first version of *"Laser Treatment for Nevi"* in 1980, which was I am happy to say well-received by those working in the field. Now, 14 years later, and with over 19,000 cases of naevi treated and recorded in the Ohshiro Clinic records, I felt it was time humbly to share some of the results of my life's work with you, the readers. I have gone on to add nondestructive laser therapy to laser surgery in my Total Treatment Concept, but the aim remains the same as it did when I opened my first Colour Clinic all these years ago in Keio Hospital: to give the optimum treatment to each and every patient on a truly individual basis, a concept which is supported and shared by all my colleagues in the Ohshiro Clinic and backed up by research and development by my colleagues in the Japan Medical Laser Laboratory. It is interesting to note that, of the 19,000-plus group of cases, the melanin anomaly and blood anomaly groups account for more than 86%, so those first in-depth studies under Professors Makoto and Goldman really formed the strongest possible basis for my continued research and clinical application of the laser for the treatment of naevi. These 19,000-plus cases were treated by laser surgery. As I said above I have added laser therapy to my armamentarium, and with low reactive-level laser therapy (LLLT) I have treated over 10,000 further cases involving naevi, in LLLT for both colour and wound healing applications.

In this volume I would like to present with great humility the sum total of the knowledge and experience of my contributors and myself in the form of an introductory volume, covering the basics of the skin and its naevi, light and the laser, and finally bringing it all together in an introduction as to how the laser can be used in the treatment of naevi. This is however only a basis on which to build, and I am at present in the process of putting together a much more practically-based compilation of specific laser and other treatments for conditions in the dermatological field, in which I am being joined by contributors of international fame and status. It is hoped that this will be published by John Wiley and Sons, as is this introductory volume, and I would like here to record my sincere gratitude to **Verity Waite**, the Editor in Medicine at Wiley's Chichester, UK, office, for her continued patience, advice and cooperation.

In addition to the people I have already mentioned in my dedication and this Preface, I would now like to acknowledge the help and support of the following friends and colleagues, without whom neither this book nor the continuation of my life's work would be possible.

First of all, thank you to the contributors for this volume: Drs R Glen Calderhead, Eiji Itoh, Minoru Yamada, Takeshi Maeda, Katsumi Sasaki and Yoshinori Shirono. They have generously filled gaps in my knowledge to help make this book as complete an introduction as possible in all its aspects.

To my colleagues in both the JMLL and the Ohshiro Clinic I owe a long debt of gratitude for all advice and support in the development and applications of the surgical laser in the treatment of naevi, what I refer to as HLLT, or high reactive-level laser treatment. In the field of low reactive-level laser therapy, or LLLT, in the late 1970's and early 1980's my JMLL colleagues and I worked to develop the GaAlAs diode semiconductor laser with the strong and active cooperation of the late **Dr Kenjiro Sakurai,** Director of the Optoelectronics Division of the Japanese Ministry of International Trade and Information (MITI) Electrotechnical Laboratory, and **Mr Iwajiro Senbokuya** of Matsushita Electric Company. After the untimely death of Dr Sakurai, **Dr Kazuhiko Atsumi** then Professor, the Department of Medical Engineering of the University of Tokyo, joined the team and together we were able to bring the *Panalas 4000®* system through Japanese Ministry of Health and Welfare approval in 1986. For the LLLT side of my life's work, may I here say a heart-felt thank you to Dr Sakurai, Mr Sembokuya and Dr Atsumi.

I sincerely hope that, by showing the necessary blend of interdisciplinary skills which go to make up the Total Treatment Concept, I can help others achieve the histologically cell-selective treatment of naevi which I have been fortunate enough to attain. Using this true cell-selectivity and the technology we have develped to achieve that in laser treatment for naevi, in the future it may well be possible to apply this in other fields, for example, in the true cell-selective treatment of cancer. Let us go forward into the twenty-first century together with the laser, the curative light of the future which is here with us today.

Tokyo, March 1994

Toshio Ohshiro

Toshio Ohshiro MD

CHAPTER 1:

THE NAEVUS

1-1 THE NAEVUS

This chapter will look at the historical aspect of naevi; will introduce the definition of the naevus; will examine the physiology and psychology of the naevus and its treatment; will discuss the classification of naevi; and will introduce examples of a large range of naevi. The final part of the chapter will examine the structure and physiology of the skin.

1-1-1 Historical Background

"Beauty is bought by judgment of the eye" so wrote Shakespeare (*Love's Labour Lost*) in the 17th century. In more modern times, Margaret Wolfe Hungerford wrote that "Beauty is in the eye of the beholder" (*Molly Bawn*, 1878). From time immemorial, any blemish of the skin, especially on an easily seen region like the face, and which could detract from the concept of 'looking beautiful' has been the cause of much anguish to those unfortunate people so afflicted.

The Ancient Egyptians recorded in their scrolls instances of a depigmented vitiliginous lesion, which, in a particularly brown-skinned race, placed a particularly outstanding stigma on the victim. The Ancient Greeks, well-known for their love of classical beauty and aesthetics, looked on those with birthmarks as somehow incomplete and outside of normality. However, because of their high level of civilization, they were able to temper their abhorrence with understanding, and although they regarded the birthmark as abnormal, they did not force the victim to leave society as some other groups have done during the development of mankind. The Aztecs of Mexico had a human menagerie in the capital city of Miclatan, a large proportion of which were naevus sufferers, sold to the menagerie by their family, there to live the rest of their unhappy lives as an object of, at best, pity and, at worst, fun and ridicule. The American Indians believed that a naevus, especially of the blood vessel anomaly type, was a mark of the Gods: the man or woman thus afflicted would often be chosen to assist the medicine man in his mystic and magical preparations. In their case, the birthmark which was the curse of the Mexican Indian was in its way a blessing. However, the American Indians were more or less alone in that aspect. In mediaeval Europe, the birthmark was not a mark of God, but much more often associated with the Devil, and evil. Men and women marked with haemangioma simplex, in particular large, hemifacial lesions, were denounced as witches. Ostracized socially, many of them died in the so-called 'trials', branded as agents of Satan: the birthmark was in fact their 'deathmark'.

The most damaging birthmark, at least visually if not psychologically, is probably haemangioma simplex, also known as naevus flammeus, port wine stain or mark. Although observed for centuries, it did not actually get the name 'port wine stain' until after the mid 17th century, which was when the fortified wine 'port' first appeared in the taverns and the English language: that dark-red wine in turn derived its name from the city of Oporto in Portugal from which it was shipped to Britain. Medical writing and novels of the late eighteenth and early nineteenth centuries contain many references to port wine marks or port wine stains, typified in the remark by the nineteenth century English physician A.T.J. Squire in his *Essays on the Treatment of Skin*

Diseases: "The hideous disfigurement of the countenance known as port-wine mark which ordinarily colours the greater part of one side of the face of a dark moreen or purple-brown-red colour has long engaged my interest." More superstition surrounded the port wine stain than any other congenital pigmented anomaly. Very often the mother, (strangely enough, never the father), was blamed for subjecting the unborn foetus to some prebirth accident, such as a fall, or even caused by eating too many strawberries, raspberries or blackberries in the latter stages of pregnancy.

"Beauty is but skin deep", claims another saying: many birthmarks by their very nature are also only skin deep, but they have a much more profound and lasting effect on those who are forced to bear them as an unexpected and unasked-for burden. Fortunately, in modern times, the birthmark is recognized as an unfortunate mischance, a haphazard maldevelopment of normal cells, even though it is not yet fully understood how it happens. Unfortunately, until the advent of the medical laser, this understanding did very little by itself to effect a cure for these lesions, and in some cases following surgical intervention the 'after' was actually worse than the 'before'. Indeed, Doctor Squire remarked in 1876 that he truly believed that no one who was afflicted (with a birthmark) ever applied for that particular problem to a hospital for treatment. In addition to conservative treatment for haemangioma simplex such as blood-letting and application of leeches, one particular method called for the injection of 'hospital pus', which one assumes would definitely have a sclerosing effect. The vast range of more modern (and more clinically acceptable) treatment techniques such as skin grafting, excision, flap rotation, dermabrasion, cauterization, irradiation, ligature, injection of sclerosing agents, cryotherapy and tattoo camouflage attest to the difficulty in finding a single consistently successful methodology. However, it became very clear very soon after the laser was first successfully developed, that this beam of pure and special light had a possibly revolutionary role in the selective removal of the disfiguring birthmark. Indeed, dermatology was the first specialty, along with ophthalmology, to apply the laser in clinical practice. Under the principal author's Total Treatment Concept (which is explained in detail below, and forms an important foundation for this book), the reader will see that the laser is by no means a 'cure-all'. However, by understanding its unique properties, it can be added to the arsenal of medical tools available to the dermatologist and plastic and reconstructive surgeon in their quest to restore normality to an abnormal condition or situation. There are certainly times when the laser should be used in preference to other conventional methods: times when it should be used together with these conventional techniques, and times when it must not be used at all: as the principal author's friend and mentor, Dr Leon Goldman is fond of saying often: "If you don't need the laser, don't use it!". However, as we proceed into the tenets of the Total Treatment Concept, the valuable contribution of the laser in the treatment of naevi, and in the postoperative management of wounds, will become clear, and the ability to judge when the laser should be used, and in conjunction with whatever other appropriate methodology, will thus be able to be developed.

1-1-2 Physiology of the Naevus

In the modern literature, the word "naevus" is often principally associated with the brown or black melanin-associated skin lesions. The naevus is known under many other names: pigmented skin lesion; cutaneous lesion; chromatic macula; skin fleck; skin blemish; birthmark, and so on. Of all of these names, the one which is actually nearest to the etymological origins of the word *naevus* is birthmark. *Naevus* is a Latin word, meaning in the original 'a body blemish, especially a birthmark'.'Naevus' has been associated with '*nativus*', Latin for 'birth', and as the majority of these troublesome lesions are often first seen at or just after birth, the association is quite clear. From Dr P.G. Unna's definition a naevus is a localized abnormality, with abnormal colour and configuration peculiar to each case, and which may have been present from birth, or acquired at some stage thereafter (*Histologie der Hautkrankeheiten*, 1894). Most naevi are fairly stable in their colour and configuration, but some may spontaneously regress: others however may equally spontaneously, or as the result of some injury or damage, begin to grow larger, with uneven changes in the colour abnormality.

The word 'pigmented' in connection with skin lesions has become particularly but erroneously associated with naevi of the melanin anomaly group. However, if the reader consults any of the recognized medical dictionaries, for example the most recent edition of Stedman's, they will find that as far as the general classification is concerned, the definition as seen there is basically the same as Unna's, and it has been expanded from that into the one used throughout this book. Both the *Concise Oxford* and *Chambers 20th Century* dictionaries define naevus as: "A birthmark: a pigmented spot or overgrowth of small blood vessels in the skin." The following chapter will examine the classification of naevi by their various etiologic groups, but based on the broader definition of what a naevus is, the author would now like to examine the general physiology of the naevus, and how this physiology determines the optimum treatment methodology.

'Normal' skin colour is due to the combination of a number of pigment cells and materials, the main two being the melanin content in the skin, and the number, density and degree of oxygenation of the haemoglobin of the erythrocytes (red blood cells) in the bloodstream in the area of interest. Other biological pigments which add to the overall impression of 'normal skin colour' are carotene, myoglobin, bilirubin and cholesterin.

The colour abnormality may consist of an excess of normal biological pigment cells or materials, the presence of abnormal biological or exogenous pigment cells or materials, or the absence of normal pigment cells or materials in otherwise normal tissue. In a typical chromatic macula, the coloured materials exist like sawdust in clear water. There are a number of methods of removing the sawdust. The water can be poured away complete with the sawdust, and replaced with fresh clear water: clinically, this represents surgical excision of the affected tissue, and repair of the defect with a skin or tissue transplant, a non-cell-selective procedure. Alternatively, only the water with the sawdust in it can be scooped out, with the remaining clear water moving in to replace the sawdust-containing water: this is an analogy for cut and suture techniques, a tissue-selective procedure. In both the above methods, clear water (normal tissue) is removed along with the sawdust (coloured materials). The ideal method is to remove only the sawdust, leaving the water with its original clarity and volume: this is an analogy for cell-selective treatment, and represents the best possible method for treatment of abnormal coloured naevi. Figure 1.1(a) shows in schematic form a typical abnormal coloured naevus, with the black spots representing the abnormal coloured cells or material. In Figure 1.1(b) the block of tissue containing the coloured materials is completely excised, together with surrounding normal tissue, and replaced with a block of remote tissue in a skin graft or flap procedure. Cut and suture is shown in Figure 1.1(c), where the tissue containing the coloured materials is excised, and by undermining the surrounding normal tissue the edges of the excision can be approximated and sutured closed. According to Ohshiro's definition, a coloured naevus consists of a concentration of coloured materials in normal tissue. It is this surrounding of abnormal coloured materials by normal tissue which has presented

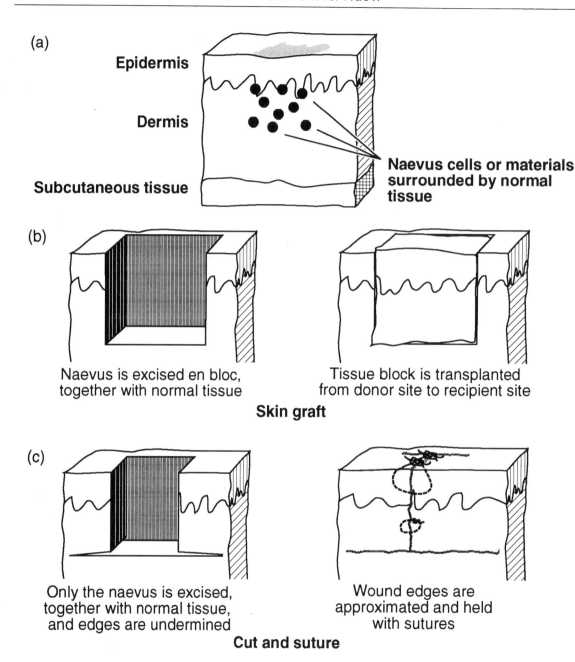

Fig 1.1: *Simple surgical treatment for a naevus.* **a:** *schematic representation of a naevus, with abnormal coloured cells or materials in the epidermis and upper dermis. Light incident on the tissue is reflected from the naevus materials back up through the skin, giving the appearance of an area of abnormal colour surrounded by normal skin colour.* **b:** *Schematic of tissue graft. A block of tissue complete with the naevus materials is excised, and replaced with a block of tissue as similar as possible taken from a donor site elsewhere on the patient. This is an example of tissue selective treatment.* **c:** *Schematic of cut and suture. Only the tissue containing the naevus materials is excised, the wound margins undermined, and the wound edges approximated and held with carefully-placed sutures. This is tissue selective treatment.*

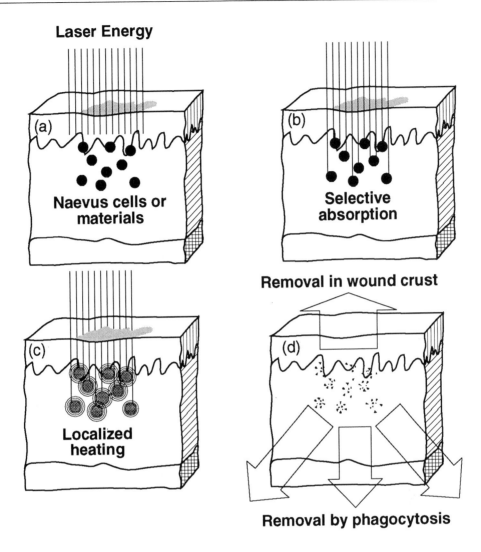

Fig 1.2: *Schematic representation of cell-selective laser treatment for a naevus. **a:** Laser energy penetrates tissue above naevus materials. **b:** Laser energy is selectively absorbed in naevus materials. **c:** Absorbed light energy is converted to heat, destroying or severely damaging naevus materials. **d:** Detritus are removed from the tissue, ether in the wound crust or by phagocytosis, to leave normal tissue.*

the clinical challenge to physicians from ancient times to the present. In order to remove these abnormal materials selectively, some method is required which will remove the coloured materials, while not affecting the surrounding normal tissue. Many children have played the game of placing a lit torch or flashlight in their mouth, in a darkened room, thus transilluminating the oral cavity. From this simple experiment, it is obvious that tissue will allow the light from a torch bulb to pass through to a certain extent, the degree of penetration depending on the type and amount of biological pigments present in the tissue. Certain colours are better absorbers of visible light, or other specific wavebands, than others: for visible light in general, the darker the colour, the better it absorbs the incident light. Fine tuning this concept, a given colour will broadly speaking absorb its complimentary colour much more efficiently than any other colour. This concept is the principle on which laser treatment for naevi is based, and will allow truly selective removal of coloured materials from normal tissue, while causing minimal damage to surrounding normal tissue cells. Figure 1.2 shows schematically and in an extremely simplified form the process discussed above. Laser energy of the chosen wavelength is incident on the target tissue, penetrates into and is propagated on through the tissue. The laser energy is selectively absorbed by the abnormal naevus materials, and the light energy is transformed to heat in these materials by the process of absorption. The heat damages or destroys the target materials, with minimal damage to surrounding normal tissue. The damaged and dead naevus materials are then removed from the normal tissue: the superficial detritus are removed in the wound crust, and those in the deeper tissue are macrophaged and excreted with body waste in the usual manner.

The choice of the wavelength of the laser beam is another important factor. For example, in cases where melanogesic hyperpigmentation is combined with haemangioma simplex (HS), the superficial pigmentation should be treated first with a laser having an appropriate wavelength for the melanin, or with another form of treatment such as snowy dry ice and epithelial peeling. Once that layer has been successfully removed, then the laser of choice for the blood vessels of the HS can be applied, again on a layer-by-layer method depending on the type and depth of the HS.

1-1-3 Psychological Aspects of the Naevus

To quote again from Doctor Squire's comment on haemangioma simplex, he said: "The hideous disfigurement of the countenance known as portwine mark ......" The key words are "hideous disfigurement". In treating naevi the clinician must always bear in mind that they are not only treating the disease, but perhaps even more importantly they are treating the patient, and part of that encompassing treatment must be concerned with the patient's psyche.

The naevus patient, although not often suffering from a physical functional abnormality, is constantly aware in his or her mind of the 'hideous disfigurement' which the naevus has caused, if it is located on an easily-visible part of the anatomy particularly the face. The patient feels 'set apart' from his or her peers, and particularly in their schooldays, the naevus patients' peers, with childish and often but not always unintentional cruelty, are the ones who really torment the patient the most, planting the psychological seeds which can easily in the formative years blossom into deep-seated psychoses. In the case of the average, normal, naevus free person, there is neither physical pain nor mental distress: a state of balance. In the case of a patient suffering from a purely physical ailment, for example a broken limb, there is in the average case a great deal of physical pain and inconvenience, but very little mental distress. In the naevus patient, on the other hand, there is usually no physical pain, and very little actual inconvenience: however, the mental distress ratio can be inordinately high. The Total Treatment Concept (TTC) demands that the clinician take the psychological aspects of each naevus patient into consideration and treat these aspects equally with the removal of the physical colour and configurational abnormality. However, the TTC is not always confined to the patient.

Some naevus patients are presented for treatment in their infancy by their parents. The infant is as yet unable to compare what is normal with abnormal, and has no concept of 'difference' from others. From the stages of new-born through weaning, the young child is not conscious of the 'colour' of his or her lesion, and therefore at that stage has no psychological problem of living in society. The parents, however, and the child's other relatives sometimes have a burden additional to the actual physical lesion, in that there is some guilt concerning the possible genetic and hereditary defect which might have caused the lesion: in this respect, modern society is not so different from that of the Middle Ages, mentioned above. Mothers in particular tend to be very defensive regarding their child's lesion, because of any possible influence the mother might have had on the foetus during pregnancy. This consideration tends to force mothers in particular to bring their children in for treatment before the 'deformity' can be seen by those in the family who are unaware of any problem, but especially before the child itself becomes really aware of the lesion. In the Middle Ages, as already discussed, there was a connection between naevi and the devil, and both parents and child were ostracized from normal society: some children thus born were burned alive, following the concept of returning 'darkness to darkness'.

Surgeons in the Middle Ages did not have the skill to remove naevi without leaving some other visible form of scarring disfigurement in its place. In modern times, treatment methodologies have become more refined, and the aetiology and genesis of naevi has been carefully researched, and is much better understood, so very few educated people believe the old wife's tales about diabolical influence. Some social stigma still persists, however, so parents continue to present children for treatment at an early age. General and local anaesthetic methods have developed in tandem with treatment techniques: there is now a topically-applied anaesthetic cream which is ideal for the younger patient. Infants at under one year of age have not yet developed an understanding of the concept of pain, and so it is possible to treat the very young without anaesthetic. Naturally, general anaesthesia can be indicated, but taking possible side effects, the age and physical condition of the patient into account, it is essential that the treatment be completed in as few sessions as

possible. In those patients where the treatment time is liable to be extremely extended, the author recommends the remaining treatment be postponed until the child is three years old. At that age, awareness of the naevus will have started, and the psychological anxiety about the naevus will more likely take precedence over the possible discomfort of treatment and postoperative wound healing and care. It is imperative that this desire for treatment is there in children over three years old, whether it is because of their own feelings of difference or because of peer pressure from their friends. If the pressure for treatment comes entirely from the parents, without any such need on the part of the patient, then children look at the pain or discomfort of treatment as an unnecessary imposition. Sometimes, parents scold their children when they react to the pain of a laser impact, telling their child that he or she must stand the pain 'like a grown-up' because it is 'for their own good'. First of all, a child is still a child, and secondly, if children have no personal need for the treatment, why force them to undergo it? Good doctor-patient rapport is a fundamental necessity, and cooperative children who want their naevus treated are much more likely to build up that rapport strongly than those who are forced, screaming and kicking (quite often, literally) to have laser treatment. Those children may build up resentment against the parents, the clinic and the treatment itself, leading to an increase in psychological problems and bad distortion of normal behavioural characteristics.

In the case of children with no self-consciousness over their naevus, there is a possible psychological dilemma, in that the patient's desires are placed second to those of the parents and relatives. Accordingly it is the author's advice to wait as long as possible before treatment, provided treatment is not carried out as a very young infant, so that the patient himself or herself will gradually come to *want* the naevus removed, and by understanding what the problem is, will therefore be much more cooperative: however, it sometimes takes time for this understanding to evolve. As children grow older, they will be able to see for themselves, and to hear from their peer group, sometimes not in the kindest way, that they are 'different' from normal children. Thus the cooperation factor increases, and the ability to build up a good, strong doctor-patient and clinic-patient rapport is enhanced. Lack of this rapport can lead to many problems, specially in postoperative wound care, resulting in possible wound infection: or the patient will deliberately pick at the wound, which has the result of enlarging the wound to the point sometimes of ulceration, and a very poor treatment result. Both the young patient and the parents are then the losers in this situation.

The role of the parents, both in and out of the clinic, is therefore extremely important. During treatment, parental support and understanding will go a long way to ensuring full cooperation from the younger patient. In many cases, before bringing the child to the clinic for his or her first consultation, examination and treatment session, the parents, without their child, must attend an educational programme at the colour clinic or naevus clinic. In this programme, the disease itself, and the possible treatments and prognosis of the particular disease are explained in depth. The parents must then go back and explain this to their child in terms the child can understand. When the child then comes for the initial consult-ation, the attending physician goes over the disease and treatment directly with the child: if the child can then understand that what the doctor is saying corresponds with what his or her parents have also explained beforehand, then the founda-tions of a good doctor-patient relationship are laid. Children thus tend to cooperate better during treatment: this does not mean to say they may like it, but at least they can understand why they are having the treatment. Postoperative wound man-agement is also handled with more cooperation and understanding, and then a good treatment result will be much more readily obtained. This

'triangle of forces' involving doctor, parents and the young patient is an essential component of the TTC when dealing with patients who are still young children. In addition, all components of the TTC must be taught to the members of the clinic staff, from receptionists through nurses, laser en-gineers, and laser therapists to the doctors (see Section 3-4 below for a more detailed explana-tion).

Occasionally, adult patients, who are slightly mentally retarded, present for treatment. This retardation may often be a symptom from the main disease which also has the naevus requiring treatment as a symptom. Just as with the child, the retarded adult patient requires a lot of support from parents and relatives to enable the founda-tions of a good doctor-patient relationship, built on trust, mutual respect and good cooperation. Similar to the case of the younger patient, a trian-gular relationship involving doctor, parents or relatives and the mentally retarded adult patient is a fundamental component of the TTC.

A common problem with mentally normal adult patients is seen in those who have been anxious about their naevus over a long period of time, and so their psychological problems be-come chronic. If they have attended other institu-tions for repeated but ineffective treatment ses-sions, such patients tend to have built up a strong feeling of mistrust for all clinics and physicians. It is therefore very difficult to establish any sort of good doctor-patient rapport immediately. As has been said above, this rapport is a fundamental component of the TTC, and so it must somehow be established. Consider the following routine of the author's clinic, which has been de-signed to build up a good doctor/patient rela-tionship. First of all, the clinic is run on an appointment system. Patients come to the clinic through a variety of channels: doctor referral; television or other mass media information and programming; or word-of-mouth referral from friends or acquaintances who have themselves been treated or know someone else who was treated at the clinic. In the first instance, patients or parents must contact the clinic directly by themselves, to make the appointment for the initial consultation. At that time, the patient is sent an information pamphlet about naevi, and laser treatment. When they attend for the initial consultation, they therefore have at least a very basic understanding about what will be involved, including the disease, different possible treatment modalities, and prognosis. Patients are streamed into disease-related groups, so that when they attend, they are together with others with the same or a related naevus type. At the initial consultation, they first watch an AV presentation, involving slides and videos. After that, there is a one-on-one question and answer session followed by an explanation of methodology, time course and possible result, with the clinician in charge. The explanation includes other possible treatment methods in addition to single laser or multi-lasers, the possibility of correction of colour and configurational abnormalities, and the possible differences in the same type of naevus even for each individual patient. This all helps to establish the individuality of the patient in their minds, rather than being treated *en masse*, with a 'cookbook' approach. The concepts of wound management are introduced, and the possible occurrence of side effects: hypertrophy, hyperpigmentation, ulceration, etcetera. However, the control of such side effects, even if they should occur, is also explained, again in detail. This is the beginning of the doctor-patient relationship, and time taken at this stage will be repaid in the laser treatment course by good understanding and careful cooperation with wound management precepts. During this doctor-patient session, the patient's record card is started, which will remain with their treatment details and results up to the end of treatment, and which is referenced in the clinic's computerized system together with every photographic record for ease of location during follow-up.

This explanation and recording all precedes the test treatment, another important component of the TTC in the laser treatment of the naevus. After the explanation, and before the test treatment, the nurse in charge again explains exactly what is going to happen during the treatment session, and goes over the treatment course again, including wound care and management. After the test treatment, the patient is then given a detailed set of instruction, warning and information leaflets, so that they can reinforce at home all the points gone over in the initial consultation and test treatment work-up. Using this method, good wound management is assured, and side effects are kept to a minimum, but can be quickly controlled early on in their appearance, should any appear.

Every week, the clinic holds a free, open instructional course for patients: the subjects for each week's course are posted on an information board in the clinic, and are usually shown up to eight weeks in advance, so that patients can select which ones are of particular interest to them. There is a news letter, published once per two months, *Laser Clinica*, which is distributed free to patients. It contains articles by and on the clinic's staff, useful information on new developments in the laser worlds, and other items of interest to the clinic's patients. Once again, this reinforces the aspect of 'belonging' to a clinic that cares for its patients as individuals, as part of the good doctor/patient relationship.

In the case of severe naevi, if necessary, a biopsy is taken for a histological assessment and report. This, together with 35 mm slides of the patient, are shown each week at the Doctors' Meeting, and diagnosis, treatment and prognosis are discussed. A special clinic for severe naevi is held once a week for the severe naevi patients. The Doctors' group consists of a minimum of six members, and they will meet the more difficult patients as a group and discuss the problems directly with the patient. The group consists of three plastic and reconstructive surgeons, one general surgeon, one dermatologist and one pathologist. If outside specialists are required, which can happen in complicated syndromes with multiple symptoms, then they are consulted, such as experts in neurosurgery, ophthalmology, ENT, paediatrics, and so on. If at any stage it is not possible to get good cooperation between the patient and any of the clinical staff, then the treatment is halted.

The clinic has been set up as an open plan layout, so it very accessible to patients, doctors and the ancillary clinical staff. This all helps to build a good doctor-patient and clinical staff-patient relationship.

A naevus is a physical disease entity, with abnormal colour and configuration, but with a very strong additional psychological component. If the doctor can remove the mental problems that the naevus patient usually has to some degree, then it is certainly an excellent step towards ensuring a good treatment result. On the other hand, achieving a good treatment result will certainly help alleviate psychological problems, so there is a very strong duality built in to the psychological/somatological considerations in the TTC.

In the author's clinic, naevi patient throughput averages 200 per day, including initial treatment, further treatment, and posttreatment consultations. Because treatment sessions are disease-streamed in a similar fashion to the initial consultation, patients tend to find themselves in the waiting room beside others with the same condition as themselves. Tuesday is for HS patients, and Wednesday is the day for Ohta's naevus patients, for example. In such a situation, discussion of treatment experiences is a natural occurrence, and so patients can form a patient-patient relationship, and give each other mutual support, which is very helpful to achieve a good mental attitude. The patient - patient rapport thus also helps the general atmosphere in the clinic and

forms the commitment to mental support which is part of the TTC.

There is no doubt that the clinical and surgical treatment given by the doctors is designed to help the patient and to cure the disease, but healing of naevi can also be helped from within the patients themselves. In all patients, good healing is a complex interaction between external skill (from the clinic and staff) and internal will (from the patient, helped by relatives and friends), but this interaction is not possible without some efforts towards mental stability, which stems directly from the strength and depth of the doctor-patient relationship. Having said that, the author also recognizes that good physical condition helps achieve good mental balance, and so the TTC embraces both the psychosomatic and the somatopsychic approaches with equal consideration.

In short, clinical expertise and sound knowledge of diseases and their treatment methodologies are extremely important to cure any disease. In the treatment of naevi, where there is an extremely strong psychological component inherent in the disease itself, the inclusion of sound psychological care in tandem with the physiological treatment becomes of paramount importance in the successful indication of the Total Treatment Concept.

These considerations are an essential component of the author's TTC. Throughout the book, the reader will come to understand that the TTC involves many multiple factors, including good basic medical and surgical skills and a sound understanding of the following: the anatomy of skin; the physiology and pathology of naevi; the histological differences between normal and affected skin; laser physics; physical characteristics of each laser system to be used; physics of laser/tissue interaction; treatment methodology; wound management; and the wound healing process. Only through this interdisciplinary blend of essential components, knowledge and techniques, applied on an individualized patient by patient basis in the TTC, can the laser clinician

hope to treat these physically disfiguring and mentally disturbing lesions known as naevi.

1-1-4: Classification of Naevi

The root cause for the abnormal colour which characterizes a naevus is usually an excessive amount of a biological pigment or pigment cell, or lack of that pigment. Because of this, naevi can be broadly classified under the heading of their particular biological pigment. Traditionally, naevi are also classified by their histological origin. In general, a naevus is the result of a dysotogenetic process in the foetal stage, and naevi are accordingly subclassified into three distinct types: 1) epithelial naevi; 2) naevi originating from the neural crest; and 3) naevi originating from the mesoderm. Table 1:1 shows the most common naevi broken down by this method of classification.

However, from the consideration of laser treatment, it is very difficult to keep the above origin-based classification because of the many factors involved, such as the interaction between laser and different types of tissue, and the wavelength/pigment reaction or nonreaction. Accordingly, the author has developed his own classification of naevi, broadly based on Unna's

definition, but with the added considerations imposed by the fact that the laser is used to remove the naevi. The author would therefore like to classify naevi from a practical, clinical treatment viewpoint.

1-1-4-(A) Ohshiro's Classification of Naevi

Ohshiro's classification of naevi is shown in Table 1.2. Naevi can be classified into abnormal-coloured naevi (AColN) and abnormal configurational naevi (AConN). AColN contain coloured materials of the skin (CMS) such as melanin, haemoglobin, and so on, in abnormally high concentration: when we consider AConN, on the other hand, the concentration of CMS is within the normal range, and so the colour of this group appears almost normal, because melanin and haemoglobin levels are not elevated, although there may be minor abnormalities.

AColN are subdivided into the moving type and the static type. Consider a laser with an irradiation time of 0.05 -> 1.0 s. When the speed of movement of the CMS or CMS-containing cells

Table 1.1:   *Common naevi classified by origin*

Epithelial Naevi	Neural Crest Origin	Mesodermal Origin
1: Epithelial naevi (hard naevus, verrucous naevus)	1:Naevus cell naevus	1: Mesenchymal naevus
2: Comedo naevus	2: Juvenile melanoma	2: Connective tissue naevus
3: Hair follicle naevus	3: Naevus spilus	3: Vascular naevus (blood vessel & lymphatic)
4: Sebaceous naevus	4: Mongolian fleck	4: Anaemic naevus
5: Eccrine naevus	5: Blue naevus	5: Cartilaginous naevus
6: Apocrine naevus	6: Vitiligo	6: Superficial dermal fatty naevus
7: Accessory mammary naevus	7: Ohta's naevus	7: Smooth muscle naevus

Table 1.2: *Ohshiro's classification of naevi*

Naevi Group	Examples
Abnormal Coloured Naevi, (AColN)	**Moving Group:** haemangioma simplex, strawberry mark, cavernous haemangioma, capillary ectasia, rosacea, keratoangioma, Sturge-Weber syndrome, Klippel-Trenaunay-Weber syndrome, von Hippel-Lindau disease, anaemic naevus, facial papules in Bourneville-Pringle's disease, *etcetera*.
	Static Group: naevus cell naevus, hairy pigmented naevus, naevus spilus, Becker's naevus, Ohta's nevus, cafe au lait spots of von Recklinghausen's disease, miliary spots of skin and mucosa in Peutz-Jeghers syndrome, chloasma, ephelides, lentigo, vitiligo, naevus depigmentosus, xanthoma, tattoo, *etcetera*.
Abnormal Configurational Naevi, (AConN)	cylindroma, seborrhoeic naevus, verrucous naevus, seborrhoeic hyperkeratosis, acrochordon, miliaria, *etcetera*

is less than that range, then the naevus is of the static type: if the rate of movement is greater, then the AColN is of the moving type. From the consideration of laser treatment, The moving type of AColN consists of the blood vessel anomaly group (BVAG) and the static type includes the melanin anomaly group (MAG), the xanthoma of cholesterol and members of the tattoo group.

In any event, the AColN group is characterized by 2 types of abnormality: either a higher or a lower concentration of CMS compared with the level in the surrounding normal skin. The higher CMS in the BVAG includes haemangioma simplex (HS), capillary ectasia, etcetera; a lower CMS concentration is found in anaemic naevus. Higher CMS concentrations in the MAG are found in naevus spilus (NS), naevus cell naevus (NCN), etcetera; lower CMS concentration is found in the hypopigmented group of vitiligo.

When we consider the AConN group, there is usually normal skin colour, but it is often accompanied by abnormal configuration. Syringoma, miliaria, etcetera, are included in the

AConN group. The colour from the outside appears normal, and so it is convenient from the point of laser treatment to include them in the AConN group.

In some cases, examples of the AColN group will have configurational abnormality in addition to the colour abnormality.

The velocity of naevus growth is usually relative to the rate of growth of the body. Thus the shape of the naevus in childhood usually resembles the shape of the mature naevus in the same patient in their adulthood. The rate of growth of a tumour, benign or malignant, is much faster than that of a naevus: thus the shape of a tumour in childhood will not resemble that in adulthood in the same patient. Because the rate of growth of a tumour is much faster than the surrounding normal tissue, the tumour is capable of invading the surrounding normal tissue, rather like the legs and pincers of a crab: hence the term cancer, which is a direct borrowing from the Latin word for 'a crab'. In the case of a malignant tumor, it can spread to distant parts of the body by the process of metastasis, but benign tumours show no such metastatic tendency, similar to the case of naevi.

For treatment of AColN, cell-selective laser treatment is the treatment of choice, usually using the ultra-short acting Q-switch pulsed, high peak power type of laser. In the case of AConN, the longer-acting type of laser is indicated to achieve tissue selective laser treatment. These treatment types are dealt with in detail in the appropriate section later in this book.

1-1-4-(A-1) Abnormal Coloured Naevi

The AColN group of naevi can be subdivided into the moving type of the blood vessel anomaly group and the static type of the melanin anomaly group and others.

1-1-4-(A-1)-(a) The Blood Vessel Anomaly Group (BVAG)

The BVAG group of naevi usually derive their names from the specific abnormality of the affected blood vessels and, at the same time, the abnormal colour is due to the presence of blood itself. The author would therefore like to discuss firstly the characteristics of the various blood vessels and the blood within them; secondly, the composition and function of the blood; and thirdly, the erythrocytes. Following that, each of the main naevi in the BVAG will be examined individually.

The blood vascular system of the skin consists of a network linking the arteries to the veins through the smaller and more intricate subnetworks of the arterioles and capillaries, anastomosing with the venules, and thence to the veins. Therefore, when considering the blood vessel anomaly group naevi, it is important to identify in which part of the vascular system the abnormality exists which is giving the naevus its abnormal colour.

In the venous type of BVAG, capillaries gradually increase in diameter until they form venules or veins, or sometimes make the venous type of lake formation. In advanced cases, they become the varicose type of abnormality. In the arterial BVAG, capillaries or venules sometimes demonstrate an arterial abnormal change, or AV shunt formation.

The author would therefore like to discuss the characteristics of blood vessels themselves, dividing them into 4 groups: (1) arterioles; (2) arterial BVAG; (3) venules; and (4) venous type of BVAG. These characteristics are summarized in Tables 1.3 and 1.4.

Usually, the greater the internal diameter of the blood vessel and the higher the concentration of blood vessels in tissue, the higher the concentration of erythrocytes per volume of tissue. The perceived skin colour is then affected by the colour of the blood. In the Caucasian case, the arterial BVAG colour is pink to fresh red, but in the Oriental case the colour is yellow-red. If pressure is applied to a BVAG naevus using a finger, the

Table 1.3: *Characteristics of blood vessels*

Blood Vessel Type	Inner Diameter of BV Wall (bigger - smaller)	Thickness of BV Wall (thicker - thinner)	Colour of B.V. (as seen through the skin)
Arteriole	4	1	Cannot see
BV in arterial BVAG	2	2	Fresh red (Caucasian) Yellow-red (Oriental)
Venule	3	4	Cannot see
BV in venous BVAG	1	3	Red/purple - cyanotic

Table 1.4:   *Characteristics of blood*

Type of Blood	Type of Hb	Colour	Temperature (Warmer-Cooler)	Blood Flow Rate (Faster-Slower)
Arteriole blood	HbO_2	Fresh red	1	1
Blood in arterial BVAG	HbO_2	Fresh red	2	2
Venule blood	$HbCO_2$	Purple	3	3
Blood in venous BVAG	$HbCO_2$	Deep purple	4	4

surrounding area under the finger blanches out, and with careful observation the blanched area will recolour in a series of pulsations which corresponds to the patient's pulse rate.

The venous types of BVAG include haemangioma simplex, strawberry haemangioma, cavernous haemangioma and so on. Haemangioma simplex and strawberry haemangioma are usually dark red to a cyanotic deep purple. In cavernous haemangioma, which usually contain veins of a large diameter, the colour is usually blue-purple. The nearer the blood vessel to the skin surface, the more effect the colour of the blood itself has on the perceived colour of the lesion. When the effectiveness of laser treatment is considered, the blood vessel types in descending order are: venous BVAG, larger diameter and thinner walled BVAG. Additionally, superficially-located blood vessels with immature endocells are more effectively treated by laser. The cooler the target tissue, the greater the laser effectiveness, so many methods have been devised to cool tissue in the laser treatment of BVAG naevi. The slower the blood flow, the more effective the laser.

One of the two most important biological pigments which accounts for the 'normal' colour of the skin is blood. There are on average 5.4 litres of blood in a normal 60 kg human, which accounts for just over 9% of total body weight. Blood consists of a light yellow or grey-yellow plasma fluid in which are suspended erythrocytes (red blood cells), leukocytes (white blood corpuscles) and thrombocytes (platelets). Plasma is approximately 91% water, and 9% of nutriments, electrolytes, metabolic and waste products. The main function of the blood is to supply the body with the oxygen and nutrients necessary for metabolic processes which enable life itself. The skin is the largest single organ in the body, and demands a large and constant supply of oxygen and nutrients. Blood also acts as an elaborate cooling system and even in a normal metabolic and emotional state, over 20% of the body's blood supply is in the peripheral dermal plexi, bringing oxygen and other nutrients to the skin through the arterioles, and returning waste products from the skin to be filtered out and excreted in the liver and kidneys. At the same time, the blood either carries excess heat to the surface of the skin, and returns cooled to the viscera, in the case of a fever, for example, or is pumped out to the skin to cool the body's protective envelope when it gets overhot as in direct summer sunlight. The amount of blood in the peripheral dermal blood vessel network will thus have an important influence on the perceived skin colour: an excess of blood in the dermal vessels and microvessels, such as after exertion or in embarrassment, carrying with it the red-pigmented erythrocytes, will give a pinkish or frankly red colour; lack of dermal blood, as in shock, where the blood has been shunted to the viscera to ensure a constant supply to the organs and glands, will result in a pale whitish or gray appearance. But these are emotional changes, and are reversible once the metabolic or emotional norm is reestablished.

The erythrocyte is the red blood cell or corpuscle, whose main job is as the carrier of oxygen to the body, via the blood stream. The mature erythrocyte is a yellowish, nonnucleated biconcave disc, measuring from approximately 7.2 to 8.6 mm in diameter, and having a thickness at the centre of 1 mm, and at the outer ring of approximately 2 mm. Erythrocytes are formed in erythroblastic islands in the bone marrow, and in their early stages of formation as normoblasts (erythroblasts) are nucleated cells. On expulsion from the island, the erythroblast extrudes its nucleus, and then becomes a reticulocyte, an immature but free-bodied red blood cell, which gets its name from the net-like formation of its scattered ribosomes on supravital crest blue staining. Approximately 2.5 million erythrocytes are formed every second in the normal mature human adult, with a life span of around 120 days. The mature erythrocyte contains haemoglobin, Hb or Hgb, an oxygen-carrying protein. The colour of the haemoglobin varies from a bright red, when saturated with oxygen, (oxyhaemoglobin), to a deep purple when all the oxygen has been given up (deoxyhaemoglobin). Arterial blood naturally contains the bright red erythrocytes, and venous blood the deep purple ones, thus giving these blood vessels their distinctive colour. The hue (colour) and the value (brightness) and chroma (intensity) of each lesion will depend on both the amount of erythrocytes present and their metabolic state as far as the amount of oxygen left in the haemoglobin.

The author would now like to examine the main members of the BVAG, limiting the discussion to the elements essential for laser treatment.

1-1-4-(A-1)-(a-1) Haemangioma Simplex

A common and psychologically distressing member of the BVAG seen in the plastic and reconstructive and dermatological practice is haemangioma simplex, or HS, also known as port-wine stain. HS is caused by local abnormalities in the dermal capillaries: there is usually no elevation of the skin, they have a clearly-defined margin, and present on average a homogeneous red fleck-like colour, which can range from light pink to deep purple. HS lesions do not regress spontaneously. They may fade with increasing age because of changes in the skin thickness. Some HS may also get darker with aging. As for the frequency of HS per head of the population, the following statistics have been presented by workers in Japan: 56 per 3,257 (1.7%) from Hidano; and 95 per 7,435 (1.4%) from Maruyama; these data are compiled for Japanese native patients. The incidence of HS was greater in females than in males, and the most common site was on the face and neck.

HS consists of five distinct submembers, classified by vessel type and depth, from Ohshiro's classification: (1) spotty type; (2) coarse reticular type; (3) fine reticular type; (4) pinkish type; and (4) the mixed type, with a mixture of two or more of the preceding four types. In some cases, HS exhibits certain characteristics of the arterial and venous types. In the case of elevated lesions, the colour of the venous type is typically dark red, thus occasioning the popularized name of port wine stain. In this type of lesion, the blood vessels are enlarged, with a sluggish blood flow, leading to pooling and stagnation: The concentration of deoxyhaemoglobin is high with a cyanotic tendency, thus giving the deep red/purple colour.

Clinically speaking, HS can be classified into two types: the flat type, in which there is no change in configuration, but with a change of colour in the time course, and in which group most patients are; and the elevated type, in which the elevation usually occurs around the twenty years of age mark, with an increase of both the degree of elevation and the colour with the appearance of some tumours with advancing age. Such cases of elevated HS occasionally demonstrate ulceration with haemorrhage, crusted scars and additional possible complications.

Treatment in pre-laser times consisted of a variety of conventional techniques, including cryotherapy, electrocoagulation, radiotherapy, sclerosing injections, and so on, and for the superficial spotty and rough reticular types these methods were sometimes partially successful: but the deeper-sited fine reticular and pinkish types were extremely difficult to remove successfully without creating some adverse side effects, such as ulceration, hypertrophic scarring and contractures, or bony atrophy, radionecrotic ulcers and basaliomas as late sequalae following radiotherapy.

With the laser now added to the surgeon's armamentarium, the treatment of HS has become much more successfully managed. For colour removal in the flat type, cell-selective treatment using the radiant heat effect is very effective, but for the elevated type, some secondary conducted heat effect helps remove the bulk of the lesion by coagulative tissue shrinkage. From this consideration, it is clear that a combination of lasers must be applied on a case-by-case basis. At the same time, conventional plastic and reconstructive surgical techniques must be used in the Total Treatment Concept, coupled with the use of make-up such as Covermark®.

1-1-4-(A-1)-(a-2) Salmon Patch

Salmon patch appears after birth during the suckling stage, appearing on the midline of the face or neck, most usually on the forehead, glabella, nose, upper lip or nuchal area of the neck. There is no skin elevation, with some capillary ectasia, but presenting a salmon-pinkish red colour with occasional light purple, thus giving the lesion its name. The lesion margins are unclear, with an overall nonhomogeneous appearance to the colour, compared with HS. After bathing, during exertion or crying, the colour becomes darker.

Salmon patch is easily blanched using digital pressure. Spontaneous regression nearly always occurs. After 6 months, the lesion will usually have commenced fading, and be approximately one-sixth the original size: by one year, one-tenth; and by 18 months it will usually have completely regressed. Cases of Unna's naevus with the nuchal type, however, tend to persist to about 50% of the original size. Sometimes this naevus is thought to be the result of friction between the head and pillows.

1-1-4-(A-1)-(a-3) Strawberry Mark

Strawberry mark is characterized by proliferation of both the blood vessel endocells and the capillaries themselves, leading to the occasional term of *naevus vasculosus*. Strawberry mark (SM) appears in about 1% of the population, with a girl:boy ratio of almost 2:1, at least in the Japanese statistics. Based on the prognosis and treatment methodology, Mizutani has divided SM into the localized plateau type, and the tumour type. The localized plateau type tends to involve the surface of the skin along the plane of the surface, and is dark red in colour, with a fine spotty or granular appearance. In 90% of the tumour type, both the dermal and the subdermal area are involved. There is also the subdermal localized type, a subclass of the tumour type, which is slightly elevated, with more of a bluish colour. Occasionally two or more lesions will overlap, but this occurs in less than 10% of this type. In some cases, the platelet count falls in the lesion, and it may evolve into Kasabach-Merrit syndrome, with plateletpenia.

SM commonly appears at seven to ten days after birth, either as an anaemic naevus, or as areas of vascular ectasia, which get larger and fuse together with passage of time. At three-four weeks, the lesion usually becomes elevated, and growth typically continues for several months, exhibiting a tumour-like growth pattern with very little lateral spread, at least at the beginning. The flat type usually reach their maximum growth stage in three-six months, but the tumour type typically take longer, reaching the maximum growth point at around one year. Complete spontaneous regression is reported in the localized flat type by the fifth year of age, but the tumour type may well show 30% - 40% of the lesion persisting after the seventh year.

For the localized flat type, the conventional wisdom is to adopt a 'wait and see' attitude, but the author strongly recommends sessions of LLLT (low reactive-level laser therapy) to promote spontaneous regression. The tumour type needs a more positive approach, especially in the case of pressure symptoms of the orbital zone, or obstruction of the respiratory duct such as the inner surface of the nasal ala, oral cavity and so on. The tumour type often demonstrates spontaneous haemorrhage and ulcer formation.

The argon and dye laser are useful for the tumour type, and the diode laser for the flat type. In cases of the tumour type of SM, the author recommends the application of diode LLLT right from the beginning, which will hasten the spontaneous regression phase. Snowy dry ice has been recommended, but there is a problem with ulcer formation using that modality for this type of lesion. Radiotherapy and sclerotherapy, formerly indicated, are now not used because of the strong possibility of scarring and unwanted sequalae. Locally injected, topically applied or orally administered steroids have been suggested, but again there is a large problem of affecting the infant's kidney function, so that approach is not used in the author's clinic.

1-1-4-(A-1)-(a-4) Cavernous Haemangioma

Cavernous haemangioma (CH) can appear at birth or very soon after. There is mature capillary proliferation in the mid to lower dermal and subdermal regions, giving the lesion its name, *cavernous* meaning 'deep'. CH appears as a soft, bluish tumourous growth, with a palpable subcutaneous volume. It can be easily compressed, and will occasional exist in combination with superficial strawberry haemangioma. There is no tendency to spontaneous regression: the strawberry haemangioma element may well regress, but the CH does not. If multiple lesions can be seen, then there is a strong chance that the CH will involve the body organs, and in such case is referred to as the rubber bleb naevus syndrome, or Maffucci's syndrome.

The treatment of choice is usually electrocoagulation, with a sheath-insulated needle to enable introduction of the active electrode into the CH without electrocoagulation of the overlying tissue. Sclerotherapy is also indicated. After these, a range of standard plastic and reconstructive surgical techniques can be indicated. The Nd:YAG laser has been applied for deep coagulation.

1-1-4-(A-1)-(a-5) Capillary Ectasia

Capillary ectasia occurs at the skin surface, and usually appears on the face, particularly involving the cheek, perioral and nasal zones. Treatment is usually with the focused beam of the CO_2 or argon lasers, depending on the site and the size of the blood vessels. The argon laser is used for the larger vessels. Coagulation must be carried out from the outer branches in to the stem of the capillary. For treatment of the fine reticular type of capillary ectasia, the dye laser is recommended.

Vascular Spider: The vascular spider is a kind of capillary ectasia. It resembles a red spider with its legs spread out on the skin, hence the name. In the case of adults, vascular spiders may occur with chronic hepatic dysfunction or hepatitis. It is considered as a disturbance involving oestrogen inactivity. When the same sort of lesion appears on the face of a child without any general disease, it is termed naevus aranaeus.

1-1-4-(A-1)-(a-6) Rosacea

Rosacea can be found mostly on the middle-aged male, appearing usually on the nose and upper cheeks. At first it has the appearance of capillary ectasia, but that stage is followed with local circulatory disturbances which involve sebaceous oversecretion: at the same time a pus-like secretion is produced with small nodules visible as a result of epitheloidal cell proliferation. In such case, this is a true rosacea.

Treatment is carried out with oral tetracycline and methoronidazole. Razor shaving coupled with LLLT sessions is recommended.

1-1-4-(A-1)-(a-7) Naevus Anaemicus

When a localized anaemic area can be seen surrounded by otherwise normal coloured skin, then that is referred to as naevus anaemicus. Normal capillaries exist in the lesion, but depending on the abnormal function of capillary ectasia, they appear to be anaemic: the lesion architecture resembles capillary ectasia but the blood volume and flow are less than normal. Naevus anaemicus

appears from the neonatal period through childhood, and is clearly seen at puberty. The lesions appear singly and hemilaterally on the lower extremities or upper breast, and appear as a multiple fusion of off-white flecks. The margin is unclear. Even after raising the temperature or rubbing the lesion the lesion will not turn red. The white lesions are best seen clearly after bathing. In about 20% of cases of von Recklinghausen's disease, naevi anaemici can be isolated on the upper breast.

These are the main BVAG members, but this list is by no means exhaustive: however, these are the ones most likely to be seen by the skin spe-

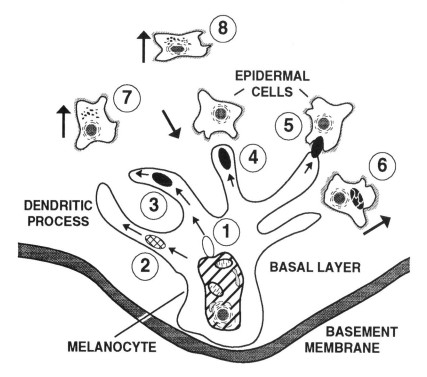

Fig 1.3: *Schematic representation of a normal melanocyte and its functions. **1:** A clear melanosome is excreted from the melanocyte nucleus. **2** and **3:** As it travels out along the dendritic processes, it oxidizes and turns black. **4:** An epidermal cell moves in to the end of a process to receive its melanin package. **5:** The melanin is engulfed by the skin cell. **6:** As the epidermal cell starts its upward mitosis, the melanin fractures into smaller granules. **7:** The granules form a protective cap (nuclear cap) over the cell nucleus, to protect it from harmful radiation (e.g. UV). **8:** As the epidermal cell moves up through the prickle cell layer it gradually flattens, and prepares to discharge its melanin granules on reaching the granular layer.*

cialist, and as the reader proceeds through this volume, the author hopes that their treatment under the Total Treatment Concept will become clear.

1-1-4-(A-1)-(b) The Melanin Anomaly Group (MAG)

The erythrocytes in the bloodstream are one of the two major influences on skin colour: the other single major influence is the biological pigment, melanin. As with the BVAG, the melanin anomaly group (MAG) consists of several members, all having as their root cause an excessive pigmentation, or lack of it, attributable to abnormal synthesis of melanin, either over- or underproduction, or abnormal location of otherwise normal melanin-producing cells.

Melanin, (derived from the Greek *melas*, meaning 'black'), is a black pigment, produced in special factory cells, the melanocytes, located in the basal layer of the epidermis, side-by-side with keratinocytes (skin cell factories) and at an average ratio of 1:40 with them. The melanocyte is a dendritic cell, with the dendritic processes connecting with several newly-formed skin cells. The normal functioning melanocyte produces clear melanosomes, which contain the amino acid tyrosine and the copper-rich enzyme tyrosinase. The tyrosinase catalyses oxidation of tyrosine to dihydroxyphenylalanine (dopa), and to dopa quinone. By further oxidative processes, granules of melanin are synthesized, and are transferred to upward-migrating skin cells (keratinocytes) from the dendritic processes of the melanocyte by a process of phagocytosis. The phagocytosed granules then fragment into a cluster of particles which locate over the nucleus of the cell (nuclear cap formation), as a protective cap against possible harm from ultraviolet (UV) radiation. Tyrosine can be activated by UV radiation to produce more melanin as a protective factor against further cell damage, thereby inducing a 'suntan'. The skin cell then moves upwards towards the surface of the skin, gradually flattening as it does so, and releases its stored melanin in the stratum granulosum, the granular layer. These stages are shown schematically in Figure 1.3. If a melanocyte produces more melanin than usual, or the melanin granules do not fragment or fragment incompletely, the pigmentation of the skin changes, giving an area which is darker than the surrounding normal skin. Likewise, if the melanin production is below normal, or the oxidative process is incomplete or absent, an area lacking normal melanin density is created, and appears depigmented.

The site of the naevus cell may also affect the pigmentation of the skin: melanin exists normally in the epidermis only. A naevus cell is defined as a cell which remains at one of the early stages of cellular differentiation. The melanocyte is a cell in the final stage of differentiation. The existence of any naevus cells is an abnormal condition in the skin, and these naevi also form part of the MAG. The historical overview of the various proposed origins of the naevus cell could be introduced as follows:

HO-1) Epidermal Origin
Unna (1894) classified the naevus cell as being of epidermal origin, where pigment cells migrate spontaneously from the epidermis into the dermis, and thus become abnormal naevus cells.

HO-2) Mesodermal Origin
Virchow proposed the connective tissue cells as being the origin of the naevus cell; the lymphatic vessels as the origin were proposed by Recklinghausen; and Jadassohn proposed the outer tunic of the blood vessels as being the point of naevus cell origin.

HO-3) Non-Malpighian Cell Origin
Friebols suggested that the origin was to be found in a specific cells, which he christened the *Epithelfasermutterzellen*, or epithelial fibre naevus cells.

HO-4) Neural Origin
Soldan in 1899 and Masson in 1926 advanced the possibility of naevus cells being derived from neural tissue.

HO-5) Combined Epithelial and Neural Origin

Ohta proposed the so-called bipolar origin theory in 1940.

HO-6) Melanoblast Origin

Masson in 1951 pointed to a specific melanoblast as the origin of the naevus cell.

HO-7) Neural Crest Origin

In 1954, Kawamura put forward the embryonic neural crest as the origin.

It was Mishima who picked up the neural crest origin theory from Kawamura, and developed his classification table, which was subsequently modified by Ohshiro in 1980, and is shown in Figure 1.4. Deep dermal naevus cells look very much like Schwannian cells, and so Mishima organized them into the categories further adapted by Ohshiro.

Having touched on the historical and histological aspects of the origin of the naevus cell, the

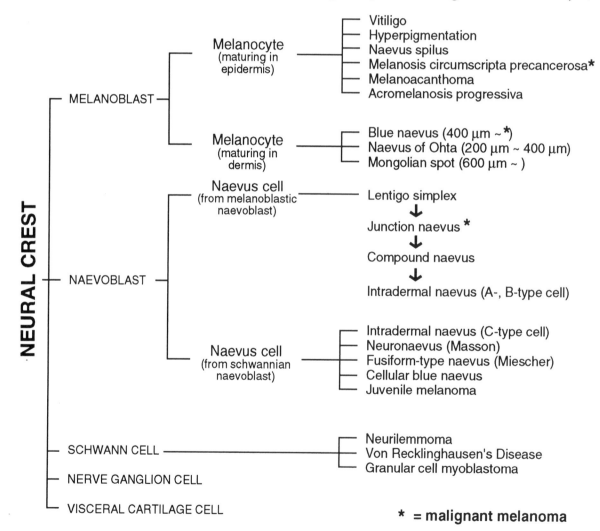

Fig 1.4: *Ohshiro's adaptation of Mishima's classification of cells of neural crest origin.*

Table 1.5:   *Comparison of naevus spilus and naevus spilus tardivus*

Characteristics	Naevus Spilus	Naevus Spilus Tardivus
Time of appearance	Congenital	Around puberty or before
Preferred site	None	Acromiodeltoid - 44.5%*1 Lumbogluteal-thigh - 14.5%*1
Colour	Light brown/dark brown	Dark brown
Size	Fist-sized	Usually extensive from hand-span upwards
Superficial appearance	Normal skin surface	Hair follicle cornification - 9.5%*1 - 13%*2
Hair	Normal	High density hair:- 43%*1- 45%*2 Coarse hair:- 18%*1 - 28.7%*2
Complications	von Recklinghausen's disease, etc. If more than 6 spots together, classified as café au lait spots	None
Histology	Melanocyte density normal, with extra melanin granules seen in keratinocytes	Same as for NS, but with hypertrophy of hair follicles and cornification
Reactivity to treatment	High recurrence rate	Compared with NS, easier to remove completely.

*1: Mizutani - 209 cases
*2: Tsukada - 100 cases

author would now like to examine some members of the MAG in more detail.

1-1-4-(A-1)-(b-1) Naevus Spilus

Naevus spilus (NS) is an abnormality having its origins in the neural crest. The direction of differentiation of the NS blastocyte is considered to be very similar to the normal melanocyte, and the band in the differentiation spectrum is also thought to be narrow. Usually, the ratio of the NS melanocyte to the surrounding skin mother cells is normal, but there is a difference in the number of melanin granules seen in the ascending skin cell, with no naevus cells seen in the dermis or epidermis.

NS can appear anywhere over the entire body surface, with the exception of the plantar and palmar regions. The lesions have a distinctly clear margin, exhibiting a yellow-brown to dark brown homogeneous hyperpigmentation, usually congenital, with a flat surface and no change in the shape of the lesion through life.

Café au lait spots: Café au lait spots are members of the same family as NS, and in general accompany diseases such as von Recklinghausen's disease (see below for a fuller explanation) and Albright's syndrome, usually seen more in females than males, with fibrous dysplasia of bone, endocrine dysfunction, early maturation and some degree of mental retardation: the spots appear in homogeneous profusion over the body surface, although the colour may change spot by spot.

Treatment is recommended in the early stages of the disease, before the age of 3 years, when low reactive-level laser therapy (LLLT) can be indicated alternated with a depigmenting ointment such as hydroquinone. At ages over 3, the dye laser, Q-switched ruby or pulsed ruby laser can be used on a case-by-case basis. For children, anaesthesia is often required, and one of the most effective methods is topically-applied anaesthetic ointment.

NS can be subdivided into the recurrent and nonrecurrent types. The nonrecurrent type responds very well to laser treatment, and is easy to remove completely. The recurrent type is however more of a problem, and will often require many retreatments on the same spot. As the pigment is epidermal, a possible method is epidermal detachment, where the dermo-epidermal junction is somehow ruptured, and the epidermis peeled off the underlying and undamaged dermis. If an ultrashort acting pulsed laser is not available, then the absorption rate of the epidermis can be enhanced by painting the affected area with a black pigment for use with a short acting laser, for example, switched continuous wave lasers.

1-1-4-(A-1)-(b-2) Naevus Spilus Tardivus

Naevus spilus tardivus (NST) is subclassified into Becker's naevus and non-Becker's naevus. NST appears in later years, usually around puberty. Favoured sites of Becker's naevus are the shoulder, sternum, deltoid-upper arm, and the lesion usually appears hemilaterally. The lesions are dark brown in appearance, with coarse, hard hair: the margins tend to be unclear, and the pigment is nonhomogeneously distributed. There may be some elevation at the hair follicles, resembling follicular papules. There is usually no colour change with age.

Histologically, an increase in the number of melanin granules is seen in the epidermal keratinocytes, but the number of epidermal melanocytes remains at the normal ratio. Cases of non-Becker's naevus resemble NS, but appear in puberty. Table 1.5 (previous page) compares the characteristics of NS and NST (NST data from Mizutani and Tsukuda). From that data compiled in the Ohshiro clinic, involving 484 cases of NST, Becker's naevus accounted for 42.8%, of which

34.5% are the acromiodeltoid type, and the remaining 8.3% are the lumbogluteal-thigh type.

1-1-4-(A-1)-(b-3) Naevus Cell Naevus

Naevus Cell Naevus (NCN) also referred to as pigment cell naevus is a congenital abnormality of neoplastic formation of the skin, also of neural crest origin, and consists of large nests of naevus cells.

Miescher and Albertini classified NCN into three types:

CA-1) Epitheloid type: *Structure Globeuse et Cordonale*
Circular in shape, large nests of cells exist in the papillary and subpapillary layer, usually pigmented, but not necessarily always.

CA-2) Lymphocytoid type: *Structure Infiltrative*
Nests of smaller cells exist in the mid-dermis, seldom containing pigment, although they may stain as if they did.

CA-3) Neuroid type: *Structure Neurofibromateuse*
These spindle-shaped cells exist in the deeper portion of the dermis, and never contain any pigment.

This division by depth is commonly followed in modern histology. The naevus cells are spindle shaped in the deeper portions, columnar-shaped in the intermediate area, and square-shaped in the superficial layers. They are usually relatively large polyhedral cells, containing plenty of nuclear chromatin and resembling histiocytes.

From the point of present-day histology, NCN is subdivided into the following three types depending on the location.

CB-1) Junctional Naevi
Naevus cells, round in shape, are found in the epidermo-dermal junction in the area of the basal membrane, and usually the dopa reaction is positive. Palmar and plantar naevi, and naevi of the genital area are usually of the junctional type.

CB-2) Compound Naevi

When naevus cells exhibit both junctional and intradermal area, they are referred to as the compound type. Those in the intradermal area tend to be slightly flattened. Juvenile melanoma is a specific example of a compound naevus.

CB-3) Intradermal Naevi

Naevus cells exist only in the dermis. When naevus cell naevus appears after puberty, it is usually of the intradermal type. This type may also be accompanied with some elevation of the skin surface.

NCN lesions can vary in size from milliary pin-head spots to hand-span areas or larger, and anywhere in between. Congenital NCN lesions are usually larger, whereas acquired NCN lesions tend to be smaller. The smaller lesions tend to exhibit a circular pattern, and the larger lesions have no particular set shape. NCN exhibits many types of elevation: the junctional type is seldom elevated; the intradermal type is usually elevated in a hemispherical shape. The colour of the lesions depends on the volume and number of melanin granules, so the colour can range from light brown to almost pure black. Superficial NCN appears yellowish-brown, and deeper NCN has a bluish tint. Some NCN is accompanied by hard hair, and the lesion is then known as hairy pigmented naevus. Hairy pigmented naevus occurring over very extensive areas of the body is known as Tierfel naevus.

Clinically, NCN can be divided into three types:

CC-1) Lentigo Type

Histologically, this is the intradermal type

CC-2) Average Type

The majority of NCN appear in this type, and exhibit junctional and intradermal histologies.

CC-3) Huge Type

The huge type exists in extensive lesions on the extremities, trunk and face. This type will occasionally involve the central nervous system (CNS), and can exhibit a malignant change:

when the Tierfel naevus involves the CNS and there is hydrocephalus with abnormality in electroencephalograms (EED), the disease is known as melanose neurocutaneosus. Of the three types, this is the most difficult to treat.

There are some special types of the NCN family, which have their own names:

ST-1) Divided Naevus

The NCN naevoblasts appear at 2-3 months in the embryonic stage of development on both the upper and lower eyelids, which are still fused. On division of the eyelids, a developed NCN lesion appears equally distributed on the upper and lower lids, and so on opening of the eye, the black or sometimes brown lesion is divided between the upper and lower eyelids.

ST-2) Ungual Linear Naevus

This takes the form of a black-brown to black lineal band, running along the nail. It arises from NCN in the nail bed. It is important with this lesion to make a differential diagnosis with sub-ungual melanoma.

ST-3) Juvenile Melanoma

This is a special type of compound naevus histologically very similar to malignant melanoma, but clinically belonging to the benign type. It usually appears on the child's face, with a light red colour, sometimes accompanied by capillary ectasia and elevated smooth-surfaced tumours: occasionally the surface may be verrucous in appearance. Juvenile melanoma may appear in multiple sites on the one patient.

ST-4) Sutton's Naevus

If small NCN lesions are surrounded by a halo of vitiligo, which enlarges in a centrifugal pattern, this is referred to as Sutton's naevus. Sometimes the NCN pigmentation will spontaneously resolve. It is believed this is an immunological phenomenon, but it is still unclear exactly what the aetiology is.

ST-5) Spotty NCN

This type of NCN is sometimes found in the hair follicles and sweat glands with or without naevus spilus. The dark brown spotty naevus conglomerates on the light-brown naevus spilus.

As far as treatment for NCN is concerned, because there is a large range of types, sizes and sites and due to the possibility of malignant change, many different treatments are required. For volume control in elevated lesions, a continuous wave laser is required. For colour control and removal, the author recommends a pulsed laser, depending on each individual case. Laser can be combined with laser, or with any other conventional methodology. In those cases where there is a strong possibility of malignant change, or it has already been histologically found, then total excision with the CO_2 laser followed by skin graft or flap to repair the deficit is recommended.

1-1-4-(A-1)-(b-4) Ohta's Naevus

Ohta's naevus (oculodermal melanosis) is characterized by its somewhat speckled appearance, and is composed of brown and/or blue pigments. These colours depend on the depth and concentration of the pigment.

This naevus appears at birth or at puberty. Some examples appear or get darker after birth, at the age of from 3 to 5 years, at puberty, after marriage, at pregnancy, after delivery, after the menopause and so on. Ocular melanosis usually exists congenitally. The lesion tends to inhabit the skin around the eye, innervated by the first and second branches of the trigeminal nerve. Histologically, elongated dendritic naevus cells are seen scattered at various levels of the dermis, subdermal tissue, and occasionally in the periocular muscles. The conjunctiva and the sclera in the eye may also be involved. Although usually associated with the oriental patient as a benign disease, Ohta's naevus has been reported in Caucasians, in whose case the chance of malignant melanoma is much higher.

Treatment has been difficult using conventional surgical methods, with skin grafts or flaps giving less than satisfactory results. Camouflage with cosmetic products such as O'Leary's *Covermark*® has been successful for some patients.

The author, however, has been treating this condition with a great deal of success over the past 18 years, and the basis of the treatment lies in the consideration of the disease as a series of naevi, each of which must be treated in turn, from the superficial to the deeper. For the superficial pigment, the application of snowy dry ice to the affected area causes detachment at the dermo-epidermal junction: the epidermis can then be peeled from the dermis, complete with the hair sheaths which extend down into the dermal hair follicles. This causes inflammation in the superficial and mid dermal layers, which in turn activates damage and removal of the upper and mid-dermal naevus cells and their associated melanin pigment.

There are three stages in hair growth. If the clinician wants to remove the hair sheath from the hair canal, the location of the hair follicle is the most important factor. The degree and depth of pigment damage after one treatment varies from patient to patient, and so the number of treatment sessions must be changed according to the strength of application and the degree of exposure of the snowy dry ice, the concentration of the pigment, the depth of the pigment, the concentration of the hairs and the depth of the hair follicles. The most important factor in carrying out snowy dry ice treatment followed by epithelial peeling is to arrive at the macroscopically intact skin condition. Thus to remove intermediate or deeper pigment, the laser offers a better treatment method compared with snowy dry ice followed by epithelial peeling, because the laser can give cell selective treatment in the deeper regions after successful removal of the superficial pigment.

The focused Nd:YAG laser has proved effective for diffuse layers, and the CO_2 laser used in the microvaporization 'pinhole' technique for the isolated deeper pigment nests, or alternatively the Q-switched ruby or Nd:YAG lasers. At all stages diode LLLT is applied immediately after the other treatment. However, use of the laser from the very first stages of treatment will simultaneously affect the superficial, intermediate and deeper tissues. In this case, such treatment methodology can easily damage the irradiated tissue beyond the upper threshold of the recovering power of the skin, easily producing superficial scarring with possible hypertrophy. The author's staged pigment removal method is a good example of the Total Treatment Concept, combining laser surgery, laser therapy and conventional techniques. The actual treatment methodology will be dealt with in more detail in a future volume dedicated to the practical aspects of the use of the laser in dermatology.

1-1-4-(A-1)-(b-5) Lentigo

Lentigines, (plural form of lentigo, and derived from the Latin word *lens*, meaning 'a lentil') are brown-coloured spots with a sharp margin, usually seen in children, and are slightly elevated. These last two characteristics help distinguish lentigines from ephelides (see below), coupled with the fact that they appear on areas not usually exposed to the sun. Histologically, there is proliferation of the rete ridges, with solitary naevus cells dispersed in the basal layer. Lentigo is classed as a junctional naevus.

1-1-4-(A-1)-(b-6) Chloasma

Chloasma is an acquired naevus, occurring usually on the face. Physiologically, an increase in the number and density of epidermal melanin granules can be seen.

Chloasma usually gets worse after sunbathing, particularly in females over thirty years of age. It can appear bilaterally on the forehead, cheeks and periocular zones. Colour ranges from light brown to dark brown flecks with clear margins but irregular map-like shapes. Chloasma is usually not accompanied by inflammation or itching. Chloasma is considered to be caused by hormonal irregularities, especially connected with pregnancy, the 'mask of pregnancy' or *chloasma gravidarum*. The lesions will usually appear 2-3 months after conception, and may spontaneously fade after delivery, but will often remain, becoming 'normal' chloasma. With ad-

vancing years, it is usually accompanied by hypercornification, and is then known as senile fleck. After chronic hepatic dysfunction, chloasma will sometimes appear on the temporal zone, with a distinctive 'dirty-brown' colour. It may also appear after a regimen of drugs such as EP hormone or Hydantoin. Chloasma may also occur in areas photosensitized by contact with such agents as lemon peel, perfumes containing coumarins, hypercins or porphyrins, and so on.

Histologically, there is an increase in the number of epidermal melanin granules in the keratinocytes, with no melanophage increase seen in the papillary layer.

Differential diagnoses include the following:

DD-1) Riehl's Melanosis

In this case, the lesions are accompanied by itching and inflammation, and occur bilaterally on the face in the female. The colour ranges from a grayish-brown to a purplish-brown, and the spots are irregularly sited in a reticular pattern.

DD-2) Adult Type of Pigmented Urticaria

These lesions appear on the forehead in puberty, and have the appearance of multiple nail-sized flecks

DD-3) Ephelides

These multiple milliary brown spots appear in puberty, especially after solar exposure. Refer to the following section [1-1-4-(A-1)-(b-8)].

DD-4) Addison's Disease

This involves total-body hyperpigmentation, particularly the axillae, nipples and genitalia, and on the bucal mucosa. The condition is associated with fatigue, loss of appetite and hypotension.

Treatment for chloasma involves applications of a UV suncut cream or lotion; good sleep; increased intake of vitamin C, both oral and intravenous; application of a depigmenting ointment, such as hydroquinone; and laser peeling or other forms of epidermal detachment: these may be applied singly or in combination, depending on each patient's requirements.

1-1-4-(A-1)-(b-7) Senile Fleck

As the name suggests, this is a naevus associated with advanced years. It is seen as a light brown to dark brown lesion, sometimes with nonhomogeneous colour distribution, and tends to appear on the forehead, cheek and the back of the hands, ranging from the size of a finger-nail to golf-ball. The shape is irregular, and is usually accompanied by hyperkeratosis. It is popularly known as 'liver spot', although there is no connection with liver dysfunction. Treatment consists of hydroquinone ointment plus LLLT. That has proved very effective. Defocused CO_2 laser or ruby laser epithelial detachment followed by topical application of a UV 'suncut' cream is also effective.

1-1-4-(A-1)-(b-8) Ephelides

These lesions appear on areas exposed to the sun, and so could be called summer sun fleck, or freckles. They tend to appear after 5-6 years of age, and increase with age. Ephelides appear particularly around puberty, but thereafter the margins become unclear. Their density increases in spring and summer, and the colour tends to deepen. There is a very strong relationship between their appearance and solar exposure, and there is also a strong hereditary factor with autosomal dominance.

Macroscopically, they appear as small, smooth surfaced, roughly circular brown spots on the skin, principally over the cheeks and the bridge of the nose. There is no irregularity in the skin architecture, just an increase in the density of the melanin granules in the epidermis, and an increased number of melanophages in the papillary layer.

Differential diagnoses include the following:

DD-1) Lentigo
   Lentigines have a clear margin, but are slightly elevated spots, seen on children; areas need not be exposed to the sun.

DD-2) von Recklinghausen's Disease
   The milliary brown spots associated with this disease are seen all over the body surface, and are accompanied by multiple neurofibroma formation.

DD-3) Chloasma
   Please refer to the previous section.

DD-4) Ohta's Naevus
   In mild cases of Ohta's naevus, it is sometimes very difficult to make a differential diagnosis. Ohta's naevus tends to have a larger fleck, with a less homogeneous pigment distribution than ephelides. There need not be any history of solar exposure.

DD-5) Senile Fleck
   This lesion tends to appear on the forehead and cheek, but is larger than the ephelides lesion, ranging from the size of a finger-nail to golf-ball (see above).

Treatment for ephelides involves the application of a UV suncut cream or lotion; the wearing of a large-brimmed hat; use of a parasol or sunshade; oral ascorbic acid; topical hydroquinone; electrocautery; skin abrasion using abrasive paper; cryosurgery; CO_2 laser peeling; LLLT; or cell-selective treatment with pulsed laser. The above list can also be used singly or in combination, depending on each patient's needs.

1-1-4-(A-1)-(b-9) Mongolian Fleck

Mongolian fleck (or spot) is a lesion which is very much associated with the Mongolian race, as the name suggests. It consists of a smooth-surfaced, blue-blue/gray homogeneously coloured lesion with clear margins. It appears on the buttocks and

Table 1.6: *Relationship between age and disappearance rate of Mongolian fleck*

Age (in years)	Disappearance Rate (%)
1	2.6
5	41.5
10	94
13	97
20	98

upper back. Although mostly found on the Mongol races, it is also found in blacks, but very seldom on Caucasians. The percentage of appearance is 95%-97% in the Oriental, 80%-90% in the Black, about 20% in southern European and approximately 1% in northern European. It is most noticeable at 4-5 months of age, and usually fades spontaneously, 2.6% disappearing by the end of the first year of age. Table 1.6 shows the time course of fading by age.

Histologically, a layer of dermal melanocytes is seen in the mid-layer of the dermis. These melanocytes exist parallel to the collagen fibres, and also tend to surround blood vessels. Collagen and elastin fibres are normal in every other respect. Although usually found on the buttock, lumbar or back regions, Mongolian fleck can also appear on the extremities, abdomen or face: in such cases it is referred to as aberrant Mongolian fleck. Aberrant cases tend not to regress spontaneously. There is no noted tendency to malignant change, so the current wisdom is to adopt a 'wait and see' attitude. However, from the aspect of the Total Treatment Concept the psychological impact of the lesion must be considered, and the author recommends treatment with snowy dry ice followed by epithelial peeling, cryosurgery with liquid nitrogen: for laser treatment, the pulsed or Q-switched ruby lasers are recommended.

1-1-4-(A-1)-(b-10) Blue Naevus

There is a benign type of naevus which exists between the Schwannian cell naevus and naevus cell naevus in the course of embryonic differentiation and which has its origins in the neural crest. Histologically, this naevus is a benign dermal melanocytoma. These naevus cells exist in the intermediate to deeper dermal regions, occasionally in the subdermal fatty tissue, with the melanocytes exhibiting a spindle or dendritic shape and forming conglomerate nests with each other. Histologically, blue naevus is divided into common blue naevus and cellular blue naevus. Clinically, cellular blue naevus usually exists as a larger lesion. The lesion may either be congeni-

tal, or appear in early childhood. In the time course, the lesion may exhibit small changes, but not so noticeable as naevus cell naevus. Lesions range from pin-head to pigeon egg in size. In the smaller lesions, there is not much of a tendency to malignant change, but the malignant potential of the larger lesions is comparatively high. Morphological changes which accompany the malignant change include a large change in shape and partial necrosis appears on the lesion.

For treatment, all traces of blue naevus pigment and cells must be removed, even when they exist in the subdermal fatty tissue. Histological biopsies should be carefully examined to ensure total removal. When we consider the metastasis of malignant cells, laser excision and vaporization is recommended, using the CO_2 or any laser capable of removing tissue rapidly and safely.

1-1-4-(A-1)-(b-11) Vitiligo Vulgaris

Vitiligo vulgaris is an example of dyspigmentation. The lesions are seen as local areas of hypopigmentation or depigmentation. Both the congenital type and acquired type of vitiligo can be found. There is no apparent difference between sexes, and vitiligo tends to appear more frequently in adults and geriatrics than children. The hereditary tendency is also unclear. According to Itoh et al, the frequency in Japan is 1.3% - 1.9%; according to Takeda et al, 2.04%. The frequency in blacks is very high, but it is seldom seen in Caucasians.

Clinically, the lesions usually begin with the size of a small coin, and spread outwards, maintaining their roundish shape. Several lesions exist usually, and gradually their borders merge to form a map-shaped lesion. There is usually hyperpigmentation in the marginal zone.

Lesions are reported on most parts of the body, but preferred sites are the face, head, back and lumbar region and the extremities. When found on the extremities, the lesions are usually symmetrically distributed.

Pigment recovery is usually from the hair follicles, and vitiligo can be divided into the general, localized and the segmented types. The localized type may sometimes spread to form the general type, which usually appears symmetrically. The segmental type is often referred to as 'zosteriform' as it tends to follow dermatomal skin divisions with a unilateral appearance.

Histologically, systemic vitiligo skin demonstrates a lack of melanocytes and melanin granules with corresponding lack of dopa-positive staining: however, in the peripheral zone of the lesion, large melanocytes with bigger dendritic processes can be seen, accompanied by dilatation of the blood vessels, and a large number of lymphocytes can be seen migrating into the area.

Occasionally, after some form of inflammation or injury, pigment loss occurs in the affected area. Contact dermatitis, burns, solar overexposure and herpes zoster may be followed by local depigmentation in the areas affected: the author refers to that as cicatrical vitiligo, as distinct from the systemic type.

Three hypotheses have been advanced for its cause.

Hy-1) Autoimmune Theory

Vitiligo can be regarded as a systemic disease, as it can be linked with hypo- or hyperthyroidism, anacidity and Addison's disease, amongst others. These combinations of diseases are all connected with an immunological origin, and so the autoimmune theory has been advanced. This is the most popular of the theories so far put forward.

Hy-2) Neurogenic Hypothesis

Vitiligo skin has a greater connection with the parasympathetic nervous system, as a higher volume of perspiration is seen in vitiligo lesions compared with surrounding normal skin. Through the observation of the contact area between the melanocyte and the nerve endings at the marginal zone of vitiligo, these contact areas are considered to be the cause of the vitiligo lesion: the aberrant melanocytes are therefore thought to be under parasympathetic abnormal control.

Hy-3) Autocytotoxcicity Hypothesis

This hypothesis holds that the melanocytes in the affected area have some genetic coding abnormality which causes them spontaneously to die: the mechanism has not yet been demonstrated, and nothing has been found in the DNA or messenger RNA to substantiate this hypothesis.

Other hypotheses also exist such as stress hyperpigmentation, genetic hyperpigmentation and so on.

Differential diagnoses include the following:

DD-1) Naevus Depigmentosus

Depigmentation is patchy and incomplete.

DD-2) Piebaldism

Totally depigmented lesions are seen congenitally or from childhood, with no tendency to increase in size: hereditary factor, with autosomal regressive tendency.

DD-3) Vitiligo Syphilitica

Seen in the lower back and inguinal areas only: incomplete depigmentation.

DD-4) Pityriasis Versicolor Alba

Coin-sized lesions, scattered on the trunk, with incomplete depigmentation.

DD-5) Bourneville-Pringle's Disease

In the early stages of this disease, follicular leaf-shaped depigmented zones appear on the back.

DD-6) Sutton's Naevus

Halos of depigmentation surround small naevus cell naevus lesions.

DD-7) Idiopathic Guttate Leukoderma

Incompletely depigmented lesions of less than 1 cm in diameter which appear on the adult male, usually on the back.

Treatment has consisted of a variety of methods, including topical or oral psoralen, followed by UVA irradiation (PUVA therapy); steroid cream and ointment; skin grafting; contour laser treatment, using the argon laser around the periphery of the lesion to encourage inward migration of normal melanocytes, aided by the melanogesic effects of the blue waveband of the argon laser; and diode LLLT sessions alternated with application of steroid ointment, which has proved the most successful and least invasive of all the methods especially for systemic vitiligo.

1-1-4-(A-1)-(b-12) Naevus Depigmentosus

Also known as naevus vitiligoides, naevus depigmentosus (ND) is a congenital disease, with patches of depigmentation following the dermatomes, sometimes zosteriform, with clear but irregular margins. ND will sometimes appear soon after birth (a few months - 1 year), and the depigmentation becomes more distinct with the passage of time.

The depigmented patches have melanocytes, but their function is weak, thus lowering the level of melanin pigment production. This condition can therefore be described as a disturbance in the maturation of the melanosome. Clinically, ND is described as depigmentation of the skin, but incomplete, therefore it cannot be classified as vitiligo. Because of the presence of active melanocytes in the basal layer, tyrosinase activity is positive. The number of melanocytes can be assessed using the positive dopa reaction, and usually the ratio of melanocytes to keratinocytes is not very different from surrounding normal skin.

There are no subjective symptoms, no atrophy and no elevation. When ND first appears, the initial shape remains comparatively unchanged, but in the long-term passage of time, the depigmentation may regress spontaneously to give normal skin colour.

Differential diagnoses include the following:

DD-1) Vitiligo Vulgaris
(See above)

DD-2) Partial Albinism
This hereditary condition appears in the midline of the forehead accompanied by white hair in the parietal area. Areas of normal colour can be seen in the depigmented areas. There are no dopa-positive melanocytes in the basal layer or hair follicles.

DD-3) Depigmentation in Bourneville-Pringle's Syndrome
In this disease, white, leaf-shaped macules can be seen, appearing multiply together with the other usual symptoms of this syndrome.

DD-4) Pityriasis Simplex
In cases of atopic dermatitis, some areas can exhibit depigmentation. In this case the macules are depigmented with unclear margins.

DD-5) Pityriasis Versicolor
These lesions are slightly inflamed, with slight depigmentation, and have redness accompanied by itching on the affected areas.

For treatment of naevus depigmentosus, long-wave UV-A irradiation, natural sun tanning or PUVA therapy are the conventional methods. Diode LLLT can be used to activate the melanocytes, thus shortening the spontaneous regression of the depigmentation to normal skin colour.

1-1-4-(A-2)   Abnormal Configurational Naevi (AConN)

In addition to naevi with abnormal colour, with or without abnormal configuration, there exists a group of lesions with normal colour, but abnormal configuration. The main examples of these will now be given.

1-1-4-(A-2)-(a) Naevus Verrucosus

Naevus verrucosus, or verrucous naevus, is a member of the epidermoid family of naevi. It is also referred to as naevus durus. It can appear at birth, or be acquired in later childhood years. It is an epidermally-located naevus, with a hard dirty brown surface, and is subclassified into the comedo type naevus. Occasionally it will appear unilaterally in zosteriform lines. Because it is in the epidermal naevus syndrome group, it can appear in combination with other epidermal naevi.

Histologically, they demonstrate epidermal hypertrophy, with hypercornification and granular degeneration. Spontaneous regression is not usual. Conventional treatment usually consists of surgical resection, followed by skin graft. For laser treatment, the CO_2 laser is indicated as a laser scalpel, sometimes in addition to the defocused Nd:YAG laser, with black ink or other colouring material applied to the target area to improve the absorption rate. The conventional ruby laser, Q-switched ruby laser, pulsed dye laser, etcetera, can also be used to remove the affected epidermal component by laser epidermal detachment.

1-1-4-(A-2)-(b) Verruca Vulgaris

Verruca vulgaris or the common wart appears after infection with the Papillomavirus types 1, 2, 4, and 7 of the family Papovaviridae. 'Wart' is from the Old English *wearte*, meaning an excrescence of the skin. Common warts can appear on the skin anywhere on the body, but are commonly found on the dorsal aspect of the hand and foot, the fingers and also on the toes. The lesion starts as a soft, lustred and semitransparent exanthoma with a size of 2 ~ 3 mm in diameter. They gradually increase in size and number, and the centre surface of the lesion becomes flat and verrucous in nature. These lesions can reach the size of a thumbnail, and can often merge together to form large multipart verrucae. They are skin-coloured to greyish-brown. In children, when they appear at the end of the digits, they will often fuse together around the body of the nail, maintaining the typical flat verrucous surface.

Histologically, papilloma-like proliferation occurs in the superficial squamous and granular layers, presenting an almost columnar epithelial cross-section. Conventional techniques have involved surgical excision, cryosurgery with liquid nitrogen, electrocautery, bleomycin injection, application of local acidic agents and so on, but the recurrence rate was high, with a high rate of scar formation. The defocused Nd:YAG can be used, after painting the target tissue with black ink, or other pigmented medium, to enhance the absorption rate. The optimum laser technique involves a C/W laser with enough power density to excise or to vaporize the lesion, working from the central portion out towards the periphery. Finally, the roots of the lesion should be vaporized bit by bit until normal tissue architecture is seen. The thermal action of the laser seals blood vessels and lymphatics, preventing viral dissemination and helping to stop recurrence. After laser treatment, if there is recurrence, it is best to wait, as spontaneous detachment usually occurs with the retarding effects of simultaneous LLLT, the virus having perhaps been weakened by the laser energy.

1-1-4-(A-2)-(c) Syringoma

This lesion usually appears in females at puberty, especially in the Japanese, and is a 5 mm - 1 cm in diameter, flat, elevated, yellowish, brownish or pinkish exanthema. The lesions usually appear on the eyelids, the forehead, the neck, the breasts and abdominal regions. There are no especial physiological problems associated with syringoma, it is purely a subjective cosmetic problem. The lesions usually proliferate in the epidermal part of the dermal eccrine duct, so a pathological examination for accurate diagnosis is recommended.

Histologically, the lesions can be seen emanating from the mid-dermal portion of the eccrine duct lumen, resembling a tadpole, with the head at the surface of the skin, and the tail extending down the duct. Conventional treatment is either electrocoagulation, or excising the lesion. Laser treatment is best done with CO_2 vaporization or laser dermabrasion.

1-1-4-(A-2)-(d) Seborrhoeic Naevus

This lesion, known as naevus sebaceus, can appear after birth on the parietal zone of the skull, or face and neck. It has been described as a localized circumscribed verrucous sebaceous hamartoma, and hair is usually absent. At puberty, the lesions get harder, with a more pronounced verrucous and granular surface. Some 5% - 10% of these lesions exhibit malignant differentiation into basal cell carcinomas (basaliomas), with a few rare cases exhibiting squamous cell carcinoma development. If large sebaceous naevi are present, there is a strong possibility that there will also be multiple abnormalities of other body organs.

Histologically, proliferation of the horny layer is seen and thickening of the granular layer. These naevi are better removed at as early a stage as possible because of the possibility of malignant change. The CO_2 laser is recommended in excision or laser vaporization, because of the photothermal sealing of blood vessels and lymphatics which helps to prevent any dissemination of the naevus components into the surrounding normal tissue.

1-1-4-(A-2)-(e) Miliaria

Miliaria is an eruption characterized by small white or yellowish papules of about 2 mm in diameter. The name comes from *milium*, Latin for a millet seed, which the papules resemble in size and colour. The eruption is caused by abnormal retention of fluid in sweat glands, and is seen on both eyelids, especially of middle-aged females, histologically resembling a comedo-type naevus. Treatment is usually conservative, such as expressing the contents of each papule with a manual expressor after pricking the papule with a needle. Laser treatment involves microvaporization with the CO_2 laser in the pinhole technique, which softens the hard deeper component, followed by the manual expressor.

1-1-4-(A-2)-(f) Corns (Clavi)

Corns, which consist of a hard, knotty build-up of the horny layer of the skin, are usually found on the feet, and are the result of constant friction and pressure between the skin and ill-fitting shoes, principally over a bony prominence. The usual treatment is application of a special kind of dressing, or plaster, which encourages the disruption of the epidermo-dermal junction, and the eventual separation of the hard corny tissue from the dermis. Chiropodists will often shave the hard and sometimes painful tissue off with a special knife. In laser treatment, the focused CO_2 laser can be used to make a line of incision around the periphery of the clavus, and then the defocused beam is used on the central portion to detach it from the dermis, and then to vaporize any remaining root formation.

1-1-4-(A-2)-(g) Senile Keratosis

This disease is, as the name suggests, seen generally in patients of advanced years. 20% of these lesions exhibit a malignant change to squamous cell carcinoma. If cancerous change is suspected, then the lesion must be removed. Soft X-ray treatment has been applied. In all cases, patients must be educated about the relationship between solar-related skin damage and the possibility of cancer.

This kind of lesion may also present a cosmetic problem when it is accompanied by abnormal pigmentation, so laser can be used to remove any pigment: the defocused CO_2 laser, pulsed dye, ruby and Q-switched ruby laser are all useful in treating the abnormal coloured component of this lesion, in the laser epidermal detachment method.

1-1-4-(A-2)-(h) Acrochordon

Acrochordon, or skin tags, are small pedunculated lesions, demonstrating a polypoid outgrowth of both epidermis and dermal tissue. Treatment can consist of simple clipping of the stalk of the peduncle, or the CO_2 laser can be used to excise larger stalks. In case of laser excision a damp cotton swab must be used as a 'back-stop' to prevent damage to surrounding tissue from the CO_2 laser beam.

1-1-4-(A-3) Phacomatoses

A phacomatosis is generally used as a generic term describing one of a group of hereditary diseases where some form of tissue abnormality with or without abnormal colour is accompanied by other abnormal conditions elsewhere in the body. When not less than two naevi types exist at the same site of the body, the author would like to include these naevi conditions under the classification of 'local phacomatosis'.

1-1-4-(A-3)-(a) Recklinghausen's Disease

The epidermal part of Recklinghausen's disease, also known as von Recklinghausen's disease, consists of café au lait spots, varying degrees of neurofibromatosis and osteitis with fibrous degeneration and cyst and nodule formation.

For laser treatment of the café au lait spots, refer to 1-1-4-b-ii(a) (naevus spilus). For the fibromas, surgical resection with the CO_2 laser is generally indicated.

1-1-4-(A-3)-(b) Albright's Syndrome

This disease, also known as Albright-McCune Sternberg syndrome, consists of café au lait spots, multiple fibrous bony dysplasia, dysfunction of the endocrine system and precocious puberty. It appears particularly in girls. Café au lait spots appear asymmetrically on the trunk, thighs and so on from birth or several months after birth, and are light to dark brown, non-elevated, with a clearly defined saw-tooth margin. Histologically, an increase in melanin content is seen in the basal membrane. In the case of female children there is an abnormality in the endocrine system, resulting in abnormal growth of the breasts and pubic hair, with early onset of menstruation. The café au lait spots can be treated using the laser, following the treatment techniques for naevus spilus.

1-1-4-(A-3)-(c) Peutz-Jegher's Syndrome

Peutz-Jegher's syndrome is characterized by generalized multiple polyposis of the intestinal tract, accompanied with milliary brown spots appearing on the lips and oral mucosa, occasionally found also on the fingers, toes, elbows and perianal area. It is a hereditary disorder, with autosomal dominant inheritance.

Spotty maculae, with a diameter of from 1 mm to 5 mm, will appear on the red lips and oral mucosa from the age of six months up till two years of age. The maculae may also occasionally appear in the nasal cavity or the periocular area. The intestinal polyposis may be accompanied by bleeding, diarrhoea, invagination and sometimes with abdominal pain. Malignant change in the polyposis appears in about 15% of cases, and is usually delayed until after the appearance of the dermal and mucosal pigment.

The pigmented maculae on the lips and oral mucosa are effectively treated with the ruby and argon lasers. For treatment of the polyposis, laser endoscopic polypectomy is recommended.

1-1-4-(A-3)-(d) Incontinentia Pigmenti

Known as Bloch-Sulzberger disease, incontinentia pigmenti is characterized by pigmented lesions in linear, zebra-stripe or other strange configurations. They may be preceded by vesicles or bullae, and are often followed by verrucous lesions. It is due to an X-linked gene, which is dominant in females but fatal in males, who tend to die *in utero*. The disease may also be accompanied by developmental disorders. Incontinentia pigmenti achromiens (hypomelanosis of Itoh) is characterized by hypopigmented lesions appearing in a 'marble cake' pattern, associated with epidermal naevi, alopoecia, and ocular, skeletal and neural abnormalities.

Conventional wisdom dictates no treatment for the pigmented lesions, as the final stage pigmented areas tend to start to fade by the age of two, and almost completely regress.

1-1-4-(A-3)-(e) Sturge-Weber Syndrome

This syndrome is typified by a unilateral facial haemangioma simplex (HS), involving skin innervated by the ophthalmic branch of the trigeminal nerve. This lesion is accompanied by a range of ipsilateral anomalies including cerebral calcification, mental retardation, retinal detachment and forms of epilepsy.

Treatment of the HS lesions can be carried out with suitable laser treatment and/or split-thickness skin grafts or flaps for more extensive lesions, but the tendency to epilepsy must be ascertained. Treatment under general anaesthesia is recommended. But for treatments under local anaesthesia or no anaesthesia, an intraprocedural epileptic attack must be countered by prophylactic administration of suitable control medication.

1-1-4-(A-3)-(f) Klippel-Trenaunay-Weber Syndrome

This syndrome, known as angio-osteohypertrophy syndrome, is seen by the presence of large haemangioma simplex lesions and deep venous lakes in tandem with bony and soft tissue hypertrophy of one limb. If there is in addition an arteriovenous fistula, then it is termed Klippel-Trenaunay-Parkes-Weber syndrome.

The soft tissue hypertrophy is controlled using elastic bandages or other forms of pressure dressings. The hypertrophy is said to be caused by augmented arterial inflow, so irradiation with diode LLLT is indicated for the purpose of increasing natural blood and lymph return from the affected area and normalizing the blood supply. Laser treatment for the haemangioma simplex, as discussed in the HS section above, can be applied in Ohshiro's layered technique, using ruby, Q-switched ruby, pulsed dye and argon lasers as appropriate in combined laser therapy. Combined laser therapy is the term coined by the author to describe the use of multiple lasers in the treatment of a disease or lesion.

1-1-4-(A-3)-(g) Kasabach-Merrit Syndrome

This syndrome consists of haemangioma and plateletpoenia, (thrombocytepoenia). It appears in the early stages of infancy, during suckling. In the early stages, haemangioma simplex lesions are accompanied by palpable subdermal hard tumours. The HS soon grows to giant proportions, and assumes a dark reddish-purple colour. There is plate-like or huge tumour-like induration. Oedema is clearly visible in the surrounding areas, and small areas of spontaneous haemorrhage. In the time course, areas of HS with spontaneous haemorrhage will involve more and more of the body surface. In the case of a high tendency for spontaneous haemorrhaging in the neonate, disseminated intravascular coagulation (DIC) can be indicated. Although fatal in some cases, the prognosis is better than could be expected.

1-1-4-(A-3)-(h) von Hippel-Lindau Syndrome

This disease is hereditary, with autosomal dominant inheritance. In this syndrome, angioblastoma of the cerebellum, medulla oblongata or retinal membrane is seen, with haemangioma of the liver, kidney, pancreas or spleen. Skin haemangiomas are however rare. In the case of involvement of the ocular region, the change in the blood vessels causes detached retina, secondary glaucoma, cataract, cyclitis and shrinkage of the eyeball. The prognosis is not so good. Radiation therapy and photocoagulation of the retina can be indicated for this condition, but treatment is often ineffective, or, at best, poor.

1-1-4-(A-3)-(i) Bourneville-Pringle's Disease

This disease has three components: adenoma sebacum, epilepsy and mental retardation. Facial adenomata can range from pin-head to bean-sized. The colour ranges from red to dark red, and they have a smooth, lustred appearance.

Skin abrasion has been applied in conventional methodology. The argon laser can be used to treat the facial adenomata. From the cosmetic viewpoint, suitable lasers of the longer-acting type can be used to remove the abnormal configuration in addition to the abnormal colour.

The other symptoms of the disease require specialist consultation.

1-1-4-(A-3)-(j) Combined type of naevus (Local phacomatoses)

As the name suggests, this condition is typified by two or more different types of naevus existing together in the same site. Treatment must therefore be decided by the depth of each type of naevus, and treated using wavelength-specificity of the abnormal colour on a layer-by-layer, colour-by-colour basis. Examples include combinations of haemangioma simplex (HS) and naevus spilus, HS and naevus anaemicus, Ohta's naevus and HS, HS and tattoo, Ohta's naevus and tattoo, and so on. The author classifies these conditions as local phacomatosis.

1-1-4-(A-4) Tattoo

Tattoo is an artificial skin anomaly, and some tattoo recipients wish to have their tattoo removed, for whatever reason. Some tattoos are acquired for artistic purposes, and some are acquired through trauma: explosion, or sudden contact with a gravel surface, for example. All tattoos consist of the tattoo pigments or materials surrounded by normal skin cells, and thus resemble naevi.

1-1-4-(A-4)-(a) Artistic Tattoo

Artistic tattoos, although some people might argue that the name is in itself a contradiction in terms, are applied for punishment, medical use, social reasons and decorative purposes. The tattoo is traditionally applied by using a needle or a bundle of needles tied or held together, which are dipped into the required pigment. The needle or needles are then inserted into the skin at an angle, and drawn out in such a manner as to leave the pigment behind in the skin. The traditional tattooist's needles have been replaced with an electric tattooing machine with which the artist can control the homogeneity of the depth and width of pigment penetration.

The most basic tattoo pigment is carbon, and depending on the depth of the pigment deposition in skin, it can appear anywhere from light blue to black, depending too on the skill of the tattoo artist. Modern tattoo pigments may still have some degree of toxicity. Red is provided by cinnabar, ferric oxide, carmine, and so on. Blue is provided by indigo, azure blue and carbon powder, and so on; cadmium sulfide and curcuma yellow give yellow; and chrome oxide is used for green.

Histologically, in the professional tattoo, pigment particles exist from the superficial to the mid-portion of the dermis, visible light cannot be reflected back from particles at depths greater than 0.7 mm - 0.8 mm. Tattoo particles, once deposited in the skin, are attacked by the body's natural phagocytic macrophage cells as foreign bodies. Some are in fact removed, but many are simply surrounded by cells and encapsulated to keep them 'safe'. Depending on the skill of the artist, professional or amateur, the histological aspect of a tattoo pigment can vary widely from specimen to specimen. In the case of large tattoos, pigment can be found by X-ray even in the deep lymphatic system.

Tribal tattoos were and still employed by American Indians and other tribes for the purpose of identification or for celebration and recognition of rites of passage. Modern aesthetic cosmesis uses tattoo to complement or replace eyelashes and eyebrows, and even the red of the lips.

Moxibustion, chemical injection, chemical abrasion, mechanical abrasion, salabrasion, electrocoagulation, further tattoo camouflage, excision with split-thickness skin graft or flap reconstruction have been reported in the literature. The success rate, sadly, has been very low. Cases are reported where the pigment has been successfully removed, but in place of a brilliant red *"I LOVE MARY"*, the wearer is left with a depigmented, mildly or frankly hypertrophic trace of the original tattoo.

With the advent of lasers, it was hoped that they would provide a solution to the problem of tattoo removal with the ability to match laser wavelength to a specific tattoo pigment. Recently the ultrashort pulse high peak power Q-switched ruby laser has been reported in tattoo removal with some success, but still many factors are required for the really successful removal of tattoos.

1-1-4-(A-4)-(b) Traumatic Tattoo

Traumatic tattoos are the result of some trauma: an explosion near the skin, causing gunpowder burns and carbon particle stippling; a road traffic accident in which particles of paint, plastic and metal are driven into the skin; a bicycle or motor cycle accident where particles of dirt, tarmacadam or concrete are forced into the skin; or an accident with a high pressure paint spray, where the paint pigment is forced deep into the skin by the high pressure in the line.

Histologically, there is no real difference between traumatic tattoos and the artistic tattoo, except the very important fact that the dispersion of the particles is much more random, rather than being limited to the upper dermal layers, and can often reach the deeper layers of the dermis, or even the subdermal fatty layer. In addition, the physical or chemical nature of the particles may induce a secondary reaction in the dermis, so that hyperpigmentation or hypertrophy can occur in the affected site. The only approach for such tattoos is a long-term layered approach under the Total Treatment Concept. Any secondary hyperpigmentation or hypertrophy should be controlled. In the case of the traumatic tattoo, the following procedure should be followed:

As soon as possible after the incident, rub or scrape any surface residue of the tattoo materials from the surface of the skin.

In the case of patients presenting with infection in the affected area some time after the incident, the skin surface and any tattoo particles there must be debrided.

For old, healed cases, the particles can be selectively removed using an ultrashort acting laser (or some other method) in cell- or material-selective treatment. The tissue can be vaporized together with the particles in tissue selective treatment, using the power of the long-acting laser to control damage to the surrounding tissue to below the survival threshold. Laser shaving using the CO_2 laser may also be applied.

After treatment, secondary hyperpigmentation or hypertrophic scarring may occur. In such cases, laser therapy (LLLT) is recommended for the control of any such side effects.

1-1-4-(A-5) Abnormal Coloured Skin Disease

The final consideration in this section involves abnormal pigmentation induced in the skin by aspects other than naevi or tattoos: such pigment induction can be metabolic, endocrinous, nutrition-caused, or chemically induced. Before treatment of the pigment, the disease itself must be removed.

1-1-4-(A-5)-(a) Metabolic Induced Hyperpigmentation

1-1-4-(A-5)-(a-1) Haemochromatosis

This appears in the male face and extremities, lower extremities in particular, and genital region. It consists of a diffuse generalized grey-blue colour, accompanied by epidermal atrophy plus an increase in melanin granules in the basal membrane. Haemosiderin deposits occur in the skin appendages.

1-1-4-(A-5)-(a-2) Wilson's Disease

The Kayser-Fleischer ring is seen to be pigmented greenish yellow in the outer margin of the cornea, and the skin pigment is more brown than usual, especially in the lower extremities. This disease was also known as hepatolenticular disease, and is considered as an abnormality of copper metabolism, indicated by a decrease in ceruloplasmin levels in blood chemistry assays.

1-1-4-(A-5)-(a-3) Gaucher's Disease

Also known as familial splenic anemia, and seen with particular severity in infants, this autosomal recessive inheritable disease is marked by splenomegaly, hepatic hypertrophy, anaemia, lymphadenopathy and bony destructive deformities. At the same time, brown and yellow pigment accumulates on the face and extremities.

1-1-4-(A-5)-(a-4) Nieman-Pick's Disease

In this autosomal recessive inheritable disease, also known as sphingomyelin lipidosis, blue-black pigmentation collects on the upper back to sacral zone. There is cerebral involvement, with hepatomegaly, splenomegaly and anaemia.

1-1-4-(A-5)-(a-5) Porphyria

This group of disorders is subdivided into the hepatic and bone-marrow types. Frequency is very high of porphyria cutanea tarda (PCT, autosomal dominant inheritance) and congenital erythropoieietic porphyria (CEP, autosomal recessive inheritance). Both of these types exhibit photosensitization of the skin, with blistering and bleeding following normal solar exposure, followed by severe postinflammatory hyperpigmentation.

1-1-4-(A-5)-(a-6) Amyloidosis

40 % of the group of general amyloidoses have some kind of skin syndrome as a symptom, especially hyperpigmentation which is wave-like, with unclear margins and a deep brown colour. Mixed types of lichen and macular amyloidoses of the cutis exhibit this hyperpigmentation.

1-1-4-(A-5)-(a-7) Xanthoma

When lipid phagocytosis occurs, and there is a build up of these lipid-laden histiocytes, the resulting lesion is known as xanthoma. Xanthoma is usually followed by familiar hypolipoprotenaemia and acquired hypolipoprotenaemia. These lipid-based hyperpigmented lesions can occur without hypercholesterolaemia, Xanthoma can exist with cholesterol in histiocytosis xanthoma and juvenile xanthoblastoma.

Exp-1) Eruptive Xanthoma

This appears as acute xanthomatous small, raised, red-brown to orange coloured nodules on the trunk, elbow, palmar and plantar regions.

Exp-2) Xanthoma Tuberosum

A variety of sizes of tuberosa appears on the extensor side of the joints, followed by hypercholesterolaemia.

Exp-3) Xanthoma Palpebrarum

This is the most common type of xanthoma, and appears as soft yellow-orange plaques appearing about the eyes; the plaques, which have a clear margin, are not followed by hyperpigmentation.

Exp-4) Tendinous Xanthoma

This takes the form of pale yellow-coloured or almost colourless elevated nodules which appear on the Achilles tendon, and the extensor side of the joints of the fingers, followed by hypercholesterolaemia.

1-1-4-(A-5)-(b) Endocrine-Induced Hyperpigmentation

1-1-4-(A-5)-(b-1) Addison's Disease

Addison's disease is a form of chronic adrenocortical insufficiency, one of the symptoms of which is spotty flecks of hyperpigmentation of the skin and oral mucosa including the hard and soft palate, the gingival area, and the genital mucosa, with a tendency towards obesity and hypertension.

1-1-4-(A-5)-(b-2) Acromegaly

Hypermetabolism of the melanin stimulating hormone (MSH) produces the pigmentation typical of this disease.

1-1-4-(A-5)-(b-3) Cushing's Syndrome

10% of patients with Cushing's syndrome (pituitary basophilism) have pigmentation similar to that of Addison's Disease (see above), sometimes accompanied by hypercornification and striae atrophicae in the skin. Physically, the disease is accompanied by trunkal obesity, moon face, and psychiatric disturbances.

1-1-4-(A-5)-(b-4) Hyperthyroidism

Hyperthyroidism is an abnormality of the thyroid gland, with increased thyroid hormone no longer under control of hypothalamic-pituitary centres. In 10% of these patients, a blue-brown pigmented band appear on upper and lower eyelids.

1-1-4-(A-5)-(b-5) Hyperpigmentation of Pregnancy

(cf chloasma gravidarum, 1-1-4-(A-1)-(b-6) above) In addition to the 'mask of pregnancy', hyperpigmentation may appear around the nipples, on the upper surface of the breasts and on the genital areas. It usually fades spontaneously. If there is a tendency for the hyperpigmentation to remain, it can be treated with diode LLLT.

1-1-4-(A-5)-(c) Malnutrition-Induced Hyperpigmentation

1-1-4-(A-5)-(c-1) Vitamin B_{12} Deficiency

Vitamin B_{12} is the erythrocyte maturation and anti-anaemic factor. In dietary vitamin B_{12} deficiency, dark brown hyperpigmentation is commonly seen in the extremities, on the bucal mucosa and the tongue: this hyperpigmentation may also appear in the form of clusters of brown spots.

1-1-4-(A-5)-(c-2) Sprue

Associated with folate deficiency and primary intestinal malabsorption, sprue has the dermatological symptoms of facial dermatitis and chloasma-like pigmentation.

1-1-4-(A-5)-(c-3) Vitamin A deficiency

In the case of dietary vitamin A deficiency, diffuse and generalized hyperpigmentation can be seen.

1-1-4-(A-5)-(c-4) Pellagra

Pellagra, or Saint Ignatius' itch, is an affliction caused in part by dietary or metabolic lack of niacin (nicotinic acid). It includes such symptoms as gastrointestinal disturbances, accompanied by erythema: the erythema is followed by hyperpigmentation resembling Addison's disease (see 1-1-4-(A-5)-(b-1) above).

1-1-4-(A-5)-(c-5) Riehl's Melanosis

This is classified as one of the diseases associated with malnutrition. It was first recognized by the Austrian dermatologist Gustav Riehl (1855-1943) during WW I and WW II, seen in females in their second and third decades, attributed to the lack of ample food caused by shortages due to the war years. The hyperpigmentation appears usually bilaterally and symmetrically on the forehead, temporal and zygomatic areas, is accompanied by cornification and cornified plaques or comedos seen in the hair follicles.

Typical histology shows melanophages in the papillary layer and surrounding the blood vessels. Melanin may occasionally be found in the dermis, and it is hypothesized that melanosomes have escaped from their keratinocytes, dropped into the dermis, and been absorbed by Schwannian cells or the epidermal melanophages, which then migrate from the dermis into the epidermis. This excess of epidermal melanin

from normal melanocytes is considered as a genetic hormonal anomaly or as a function of endogenous vitamin deficiency.

There is also an exogenous type, associated with activation by contact with materials such as oils or grease during the patient's occupation with the same histologic picture of epidermal pigment found in dermal melanophages.

Treatment consists of hydroquinone or kojic acid depigmenting ointment and other conservative methodologies. Recently, diode LLLT has been successfully used to heighten the skin absorption rate for these ointments.

1-1-4-(A-5)-(d) Inflammation- and Infection-Induced Hyperpigmentation

In most situations involving inflammation of the skin or in cases of many infectious or contagious diseases which have skin symptoms, such as rubella, rubeolla or varicella, there may be some degree of secondary hyperpigmentation. The same applies to burn injuries, psoriasis vulgaris, fungoid infections and other examples. This hyperpigmentation can be treated under the Total Treatment Concept.

1-2 THE SKIN

The skin, or cutis, covers the human body, and acts as protective barrier between the body and the outside world. For a 60 kg male the average skin area is approximately 1.6 m²: the average weight is 3 kg, or 0.5% of the total body weight. When the weight of the subcutaneous fatty tissue is added, the total is approximately 9 kg, 14% of the total body weight.

Not only is the skin a barrier between the living body and the outside world, but it is also a

very important living organ, a complex controlling membrane with many functions: a cooling system; many excretory functions, and so on.

The thickness of the skin varies from 0.6 mm to 4 mm, with the thinnest on the eyelids, and the thickest skin found on the plantar and back regions. The skin of the female is thinner on average than the male, and a child's skin is thinner than adult skin.

1-2-1 Structure of the Skin

1-2-1-(A) The Skin Surface

The skin surface consists of many fine interconnecting furrows, the sulcus cutis, which form a variety of typical patterns, triangular, rhomboid

and polygonal. On palmar skin and the skin of the palmar aspect of the fingers, the furrows run in parallel, to help give grip, forming the distinctive loops and whorls on the ungual phalanx of the

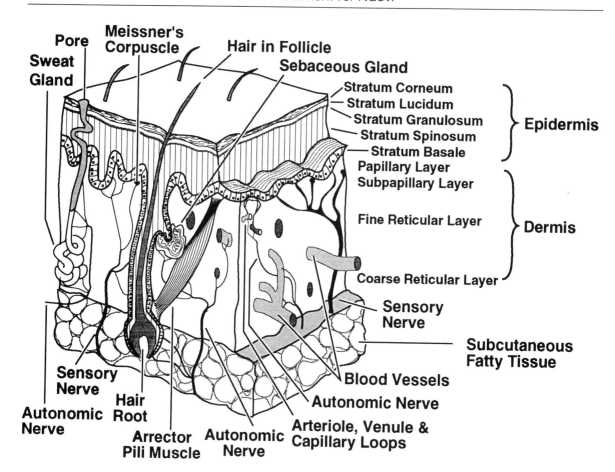

Fig 1.5: *Simplified schematic of the skin. Note the penetration of the living layers of the epidermis down into the hair follicle, important for considerations of epithelization in the intact skin condition and in any treatment involving epithelial peeling.*

the fingers, which are unique to each individual, and can be recorded as palm- and fingerprints.

Human skin consists of three distinct layers: the epidermis, the dermis (corium) and the subcutis.

1-2-1-(B) Epidermis

The epidermis is a nonvascular stratified epithelium of ectodermal origin, and consists of the surface epidermis, and the appendage epidermis, the latter subdivided into the pilosebaceous apocrine unit, the eccrine unit and the nails. The epidermis meets the dermis at the epidermo-dermal junction. Dermal papillae project up into the

epidermis, and a mirror-image of retia project down from the epidermis to surround the dermal papillae. Thus on cross section the dermo-epidermal junction appears in an irregular wave-shaped form. Binding the epidermis to the dermis at the dermo-epidermal junction is the basement membrane (or basilemma) which is closely connected to the basal layer of the epidermis, and is an amorphous extracellular layer with a complex mixture of muscle cells, Schwann cells and fat cells in a collagen matrix, to which type IV collagen is unique.

The epidermis is mainly made up of keratinocytes, with an admixture of melanocytes, Langerhans cells, dendritic cells and Merkel's cells. The upward mitosis of the keratinocytes is the basis of the keratinization process, by which the cells rise from the basal layer, adjacent to the basement membrane, and gradually move outwards to the horny layer of the skin where they cornify, and are gradually shed in minute flakes of keratin. The life cycle for the keratinocytes is a total of 40-56 days, of which 26-42 days are taken by the cells to go from the basal layer to the granular layer, and then a further 14 days to complete the final stage of the cycle.

The epidermis is composed of four layers. From the bottom, these layers are the basal layer, the prickle cell layer, the granular layer and the horny layer. Between the granular layer and the horny layer can be seen the clear layer (or stratum lucidum), but usually only in palmar and plantar skin (see Figure 1.5).

1-2-1-(B-1) The Basal Layer

The basal layer, or stratum basale, consists of a single layer of basal cells located in the depest portion of the epidermis, which are in contact with and receive nutrition from the basement membrane which connects the epidermis to the dermis. The cells are cylindrical in shape, with a vertical long axis. The cellular cytoplasm is basophilic, and the nucleus is ellipsoid and rich in chromatin. Melanocytes also exist in the basal layer, at a ratio of approximately 1:40 - 1:50 with the basal cells, and a vertical section ratio of 1:6 or 1:7. The function of the melanocyte is to manufacture the biologic pigment melanin, and the melanin is taken up by the upward moving skin cells by a process of phagocytosis from the melanocytes' dendritic processes. The melanin fragments into melanin granules, which collect at the upper pole of the skin cell, forming a protective nuclear cap over the cell's nucleus. This cap affords protection to both the epidermal cells and the dermis below them against harmful UV radiation (refer to Figure 1.3 above).

1-2-1-(B-2) The Prickle Cell Layer

The prickle cell layer, or stratum spinosum, exists between the basal layer and the granular layer, and is the largest epidermal layer, making up the majority of the epidermis. Skin cells are polyhedral at the bottom of the layer, with sharp angular processes which give the layer its name. As the cells proceed towards the skin surface, they gradually flatten. Cell layers vary in number from a very few to ten or more, forming a mosaic-like pattern. Compared to basal layers cells, prickle layer cells are larger and clearer, with a comparative lack of nuclear chromatin. The cells are called prickle cells, and seem to be connected to each other by their spiny angular processes which act as a cellular bridge, but these processes are identified as desmosomes under electron microscopy.

1-2-1-(B-3) The Granular Cell Layer

The granular cell layer, or stratum granulosum, exists between the prickle cell layer and the horny layer. It is composed of from one to three layers of flattened skin cells, which have shed their melanin granules, hence the name of the layer. The cytoplasm of the cells contains a large amount of basophilic keratohyaline granules.

1-2-1-(B-4) The Horny Layer

The horny layer, or stratum corneum, is the outermost layer of the epidermis, and is composed of multiple layers of flattened eosinophilic cells, which have given up their nuclei in the transition from granular layer to horny layer. The cells are very rich in keratin, and are finally constantly shed off from the outermost layer in minute keratinous flakes.

The clear layer, or stratum lucidum, is almost nonexistent anywhere else on the body except for the plantar and palmar skin. The clear layer, where it exists, lies between the granular and horny layers, and consists of a few rows of flattened clear cells containing eleiden (a refractile keratinous substance) in which the nuclei and cell boundaries are not distinguishable. The clear layer has strong transmission characteristics because of the incomplete keratinization of the cells.

1-2-1-(C) The Dermis

The dermis, also known as the corium or the cutis, is of mesodermal origin, and is formed of a connective richly vascularized living tissue layer under the epidermis, consisting of a random matrix of mainly collagen and a relatively small amount of elastin fibres. The dermis is several times thicker than the epidermis, and from the outside in is composed of three main layers: the papillary layer, the subpapillary layer and the reticular layer.

1-2-1-(C-1) The Papillary Layer

This layer gets its name from the dermal papillae, as mentioned above. These ultrafine prominent processes penetrate up into the epidermis, composed of ultrafine fibrous components. Each papilla contains a blood vascular capillary loop and a sensory nerve ending. The papillary layer is from 50 μm to 150 μm in depth.

1-2-1-(C-2) The Subpapillary Layer

The subpapillary layer exists under the papillary layer (150 μm - 250 μm/300 μm). This layer consists of a matrix of fine collagen and elastin fibres, and is rich in blood vessels and neural components.

1-2-1-(C-3) The Reticular Layer

the reticular layer (from the Latin *rete*, meaning a net) is the thickest of the three layers, and in fact comprises almost all of the dermis. The base of this layer is in contact with the subdermal layer of fatty tissue, very rich in coarse collagen fibres. Sometimes this bottom part of the layer is referred to as collagen fibre bundles. the reticular layer runs from 250 μm/300 μm to 1.5 mm-4 mm depending on the site. Of the fibrous components, approximately 90% is collagen, with the remainder made up of a mixture of elastin, reticulin and smooth muscle fibres. The fibrous matrix is constantly bathed in and lubricated by the ground substance, a rich amorphous material composed of proteoglycans, plasma constituents, water and ions: it is the transport medium for cellular components, such as fibroblasts, macrophages, histiocytes, mast cells, leukocytes and plasma cells released from the blood vascular system.

1-2-1-(D) Skin Appendages

In order to function as the multipurpose protective layer that it is, the skin needs the assistance of a number of specialized units which are located in the skin itself: these units are the skin appendages. They help the skin to remain waterproof and flexible, and assist in the complex body temperature regulation functions which are also part of the skin's function.

1-2-1-(D-1) The Eccrine Unit

The eccrine units (from the Greek *ekkrino*, to secrete), or sweat glands, are distributed all over the skin, with the exceptions of the mucocutaneous junctional regions, such as the red lips. They are especially plentiful in the palmar and plantar regions, and poor in the thighs. Their main purpose is, through sweating, to excrete H_2O, thus controlling the body temperature and keeping the horny layer of the skin moist. In the average human at rest, sweating is seen to start when the body temperature rises by as little as 0.1°C to 0.5°C, as the blood temperature is monitored by the brain centres. The sweat glands are under sympathetic nerve control. Thus if the skin is cut badly, severing sensory and sympathetic nerves, not only will there be loss of sensation in the distal part of the injury, but it will also lose the ability to sweat.

The sweat glands consist of two main parts, the coiled secretory gland and the excretory duct. The coiled part of the gland exists in the deepest portion of the dermis, very near the junction of the dermis with the subdermal fatty layer, and is tightly wound in a ball-like formation, consisting of one layer of clear cells and dark cells. This layer is surrounded by long columnar cells, and the outermost layer consists of the epidermal basal layer.

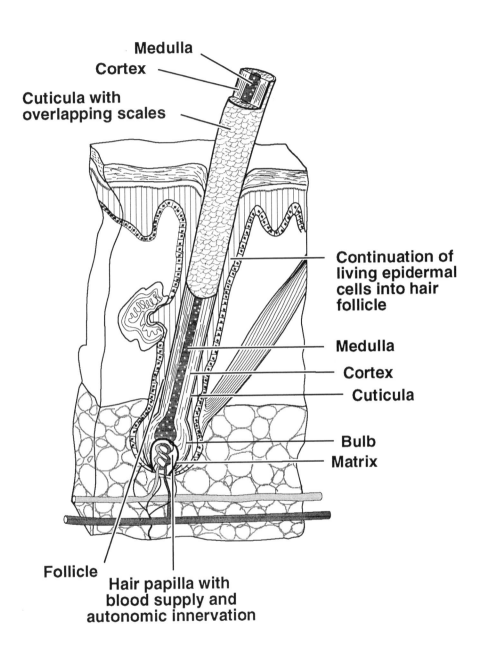

Fig 1.6: *Schematic showing detail of hair and hair follicle*

Sweat is produced in the coiled secretory gland, and is conveyed to the skin surface through the excretory duct. This duct is wound as it leaves the secretory gland, then proceeds directly through the straight duct in the dermis, and finally appears at the skin surface through the spiral duct (or acrosyringium) in the epidermis.

The straight duct consists of long columnar myoepithelial cells (which also line the spiral duct) surrounded by a contiguous extension of the epidermal basal layer.

1-2-1-(D-2) The Pilosebaceous Apocrine Unit.
The pilosebaceous apocrine unit consists of the hair follicle, in which grows the hair, the arrector pili muscle, the sebaceous gland, and in some specialized areas, an apocrine sweat gland. At the base of the hair follicle, the hair grows from the hair root, passing up through the follicle, and emerging into the outside world through the follicle foramen (Figure 1.6).

1-2-1-(D-2)-(a) The Hair Follicle and Sheath.
Hair follicles which are tube-like invaginations of the epidermis, containing the hairs, start in the subcutaneous fatty layer, and run obliquely up through the dermis and epidermis, opening out through the horny layer. They are lined with contiguous epidermal basal layer cells, and are surrounded by a fibrous sheath of dermal origin. The bottom of the follicle bulges to encompass the hair root bulb and papilla, and at a point above this bulge is inserted the arrector pili muscle, which has its origin in the upper dermis. The sebaceous gland opens out into the follicle between the point of insertion of the arrector pili and the foramen. If an apocrine unit is present, it in turn opens onto the follicle above the sebaceous gland.

The hair root sheath opens to the epidermis in an infundibulum shape. The hair originates at the hair root, connected to the hair shaft, and ends at the hair apex protruding from the skin surface. The root sheath is comparatively thick, composed of the inner and outer sheaths. The inner sheath consists of the sheath cuticula, Huxley's layer and Henle's layer (from the inner aspect). Cornification occurs at the opening of the sheath into the epidermis, contiguous with the horny layer. The inner root sheath connects with the outer root sheath, which is composed of an inner section of fibrous, ring-shaped connective collagen tissue surrounded by a layer of longitudinally-running fibres, and the arrector pili muscle is inserted into this tough outer root sheath.

1-2-1-(D-2)-(b) Hair

(Figures 1.5, 1.6) The hair root bulges at the base and is called the hair bulb, in which the hair papilla is contained. Each papilla has its own anastomosing blood supply, and this provides the nutrition for the healthy growth of the hair. The epithel of the hair follicle covers the hair papilla and is called the hair matrix, from which the hair root originates. Hair is composed of an inner medulla, which is surrounded by the cortex, the outer part of which is enclosed in the hair cuticula, a layer of overlapping, shingle-shaped cells that help to keep the hair shaft firmly embedded in its follicle by connection with the inner sheath cuticula cells. In human hair, medullae can be found only in the hair of the head and beard, and melanin exists in the medulla which gives the hair its colour.

Hair is distributed all over the surface of the skin, with the exception of the palmar and plantar areas, palmar and plantar aspects of the fingers and toes, respectively, the ungual portions of the dorsal aspect of the digits, the red lips, the glans of the penis and the inside surfaces of the labia major, labia minor and the clitoris. In the foetal stage, the skin is covered with fine, soft lanugo hair. After birth, the skin is almost all invested with soft, short, fine, fair, medulla-less vellus hair, some of in turn matures to form terminal hair. Terminal hair is rich in pigment, depending on the amount of melanin in the medulla, and is thick: terminal hair is found on the head, in the beard, the eyebrows, eyelashes, axillary and pubic hair, and so on.

1-2-1-(D-2)-(c) The Sebaceous Gland

Sebaceous glands are secretory glands consisting of single and multiple sebaceous lobules, located on the hair follicles between the arrector pili and the follicle foramen. The sebaceous gland opens onto the hair follicle through a short sebaceous duct. The outermost layer of the gland is composed of cylindrical, basophilic cells with no fatty component. In the central matrix of the gland there are many fatty cells with a large cytoplasm and central nucleus, in which the synthesized lipid is stored as droplets. As the cells mature and die, the excellulated lipid is transferred to the body of the sebaceous gland in the process known as pimelosis. This fatty secretion together with the substances from the collapsed cells, known as sebum, is secreted through the sebaceous duct and the infundibulum into the follicle, and combines with the moisture present from the eccrine glands to form a waterproof emulsification, which is called the skin surface film, thus at the same time maintaining horny layer flexibility and the water-proofing function of the skin. Free sebaceous glands, which open directly onto the skin or mucosal surfaces without being connected to hair follicles, exist on the red lips, the bucal mucosa, the mucosal surfaces of the vulval and perianal regions and on the nipples in the female. On the other hand there are no sebaceous glands found on the palmar and plantar areas, these aspects of the fingers and toes, respectively, or on the dorsal ungual phalanges of the fingers.

1-2-1-(D-2)-(d) The Arrector Pili Muscle

The arrector pili muscle has its origin in the upper dermis, and is inserted obliquely into the fibrous outer root sheath of the hair follicle at a point above the hair bulb, but below the sebaceous gland. The muscle is composed of smooth muscle fibre, and is therefore under autonomic system control. On contraction, the muscle function is to raise the hair, and in doing so creates the phenomenon in the skin known as 'goose pimples' or 'goose flesh'.

1-2-1-(D-2)-(e) The Apocrine Sweat Gland

The apocrine glands have the same origin as the eccrine sweat glands and hair, which is referred to as the 'hair germ'. The apocrine gland is a specialized sweat gland, and can be found in the axillary, alveolar, umbilicus, genital and anal regions. Like the eccrine sweat glands, apocrine glands consist of two parts, the coiled secretory portion and the excretory duct, which instead of opening directly onto the horny layer of the skin, opens onto the hair follicle, into the upper part of the sebaceous duct at the cornified follicular foramen. The excretory area of the apocrine duct is much larger than the eccrine duct, and on cross section, the apocrine duct diameter is several times larger. The wall of the secretory gland consists of one layer of secretory cells, surrounded by myoepithelial cells, and the basal membrane makes up the outermost tunic of the gland. The secretory cells are columnar, with the nucleus at the base of the cell, containing eosinophilic bodies. The wall of the apocrine duct consists of two cellular layers.

The function of the apocrine system usually begins at puberty, and the lipid excretion contains excretory materials from the cytoplasm. The excretion is extremely viscous compared to the eccrine gland. It is easily analyzed by bacteria with a characteristic unpleasant odour. Typical human body odour is basically formed by the apocrine unit excretion, and can be sexually stimulating to others.

1-2-1-(D-3) The Nails.

The human nail consists of the plate, the nail wall, the bed and the nail matrix. The nail plate is made up of differentiated horny layer keratin. Growth takes place at the nail matrix and from the nail bed, which can be seen as the white crescent-shaped lunule. Average nail growth is approximately 3 mm a month.

1-2-1-(E) The Blood Vascular System

With the exception of the epidermis, all parts of the skin are richly vascularized. Arteries perforate the dermis from the deep subdermal arterial plexus, and form the deep dermal arterial plexus in the deeper portion of the dermis. Arteries rise from there to the upper layer of the dermis to form the subpapillary arterial plexus. From the sub-papillary layer, smaller arteries rise to the papil-lae, branching to form even finer arterioles, which further subdivide to form the capillary loop pre-sent in each dermal papilla. From the papillae, venules descend and join to form veins, which make up in turn the subpapillary and deep dermal venous plexi, before draining down to the deep subdermal venous plexi. Dermal vascular plexi are particularly rich near skin appendages, espe-cially around the eccrine glands.

The exception to the arterial capillary loops can be found at the fingertips, toe tips and subun-gual areas, where there is direct arteriole/venule anastomosis. These anastomoses are interwoven with glomus cells and nerve fibres. This portion is called the glomus cutaneus.

1-2-1-(F) The Lymphatic System

The dermal intercellular and interfibrous liquid is drained into a series of lymphocapillaries, con-sisting of thin endothelial wall structure: the lym-phocapillaries convey the returning fluid and its contents to postcapillary lymphovessels in the dermis and subdermis, which form an infrastruc-ture of plexi surrounding the blood vessels and nerve fibres.

1-2-1-(G) The Nervous System

The skin is well-innervated with both sensory and autonomic nerves. The autonomic nerves are linked with the skin appendages. The sensory nerves have endings in the dermis, with occa-sional extensions into the epidermis.

1-2-1-(G-1) Sensory Nerves

Sensory nerves originate from and return to the posterior root of the spinal dorsal horn, where

they are connected to the spinal cord. They are myelinated fibres for most of their length, with a comparatively high rate of transmission. Tiny unmyelinated fibres branch off, and end in the dermal papillae, hair papillae and hair follicle sheath, and so on: they are sensitive to changes of temperature, to pain and to irritative stimuli such as itching. Sensations of touch and pressure are detected by Merkel's cells attached to the base of modified keratinocytes in the epidermis; Meis-sener's corpuscles in the dermal papillae, in par-ticular those of the fingers and toes; and Vater-Pacini corpuscles distributed in the upper dermis of the fingers. Other sensory apparati are Ruffini's corpuscle, the end bulb of Krause (sen-sitive to cold) and the genital corpuscles, and others, all of which exist as end corpuscles.

1-2-1-(G-2) The Autonomic Nerves

The autonomic nerves are distributed to and con-trol the apocrine glands, eccrine glands and seba-ceous glands. They also control the action of the arrector pili muscles, and are connected with the dermal microvascular system, enabling vasocon-striction or vasodilation of that very large compo-nent of the blood vascular system, for body tem-perature control, for example. The fibres are either of the adrenagic type, in which transmis-sion depends on the adrenal-like transmitter sub-stance norepinepherine (noradrenaline); and cholinergic fibres, which transmit impulses by the transmitter s ubstance acetylcholine.

1-2-1-(H) Subcutaneous Tissue.

The subcutaneous tissue consists mainly of groups of lipocytes or fat cells of varying sizes, bound together as blocks of adipose tissue and transected by thick collagen fibre bundles. the thickness and volume of this layer differs greatly according to the age, sex, dietary habits and physical condition of each individual

1-2-2 Physiology of the Skin

The main subdivisions of the physiology of the skin mostly relate to its function as the envelope organ of the body.

1-2-2-(A) Protection against External Stimuli

1-2-2-(A-1) Mechanical Protection

The flexibility of the skin (elastin fibres) and its integral strength (collagen fibres) can protect the body against external mechanical power.

1-2-2-(A-2) Water Protection

The oily emulsification excreted by the sebaceous glands can protect the body from external water. At the same time, there is also a waterproof band between the horny layer and the granular layer.

1-2-2-(A-3) Bacterial Protection

The natural acidosis of the skin (pH 5.5 ~ 7.0) helps protect the body from the invasion and growth of external bacteria and fungus.

1-2-2-(A-4) Photodamage Protection

The epidermis, especially the highly refractile and reflective horny layer, helps prevent photodamage from overexposure to solar and other light radiation. As a second fence of resistance to photodamage, the nuclear caps over the nucleus of each ascending skin cell in the prickle cell layer absorb harmful UV radiation. UV exposure stimulates the epidermal melanocytes to synthesize more melanin than usual, to increase the protective power.

1-2-2-(B) Body Temperature Control

The skin can keep heat in the body by acting as a nonconductive and nonradiant body for thermal control. In the same manner, the skin can help prevent excessive heat from the outside environment penetrating into the body. On the contrary, when required, the skin can lower internal body temperature, in case of high ambient air temperatures, or internal fever generated excessively by the body's own defence mechanisms. By dilation or contraction of the superficial dermal blood plexus, and perspiration control, the skin can maintain a constant body temperature.

1-2-2-(C) Sensory Function

The sensations of touch and pressure, pain, warmth and cold are relayed to the brain from the complex system of sensors located in the skin. The sensitivity of touch sensations together with those of pressure allows differentiation between hard and soft, tough and smooth, dry or wet. The sensation of itching is one of the pain sensations.

1-2-2-(D) Secretory and Excretory Functions

1-2-2-(D-1) Eccrine Perspiration

The eccrine gland has the control function over body electrolyte balance and body temperature. These glands also act as important accessories for waste product excretion. They give moisture to the skin to protect it from dryness.

1-2-2-(D-2) Sebaceous Units Function

The oily secretion of sebum from the sebaceous glands creates the skin surface film to provide an emulsified waterproofing to ensure the constant flexibility of the epidermis. This film also has an antibacterial function to prevent growth of bacteria and fungus.

1-2-2-(E) Synthesis Function

In addition to protection from photodamage, the skin synthesizes vitamins D_2 and D_3, ergocalciferol and cholecalciferol, and any of the other steroids in the vitamin D group, following the dermal absorption of short wavelength ultraviolet radiation. This vitamin group promotes the proper utilization of calcium and phosphorous, so ensuring proper development of bones and teeth. The skin also synthesizes cholesterol.

1-2-2-(F) Respiratory Function

Skin has a role in the metabolism of glucose, and can help to control percutaneous exchange of gases with the outside air.

1-2-2-(G) Absorption Function

Because of the existance of the oily skin surface film from the sebaceous glands in the horny layer and the waterproof band between the horny layer and the granular layer, percutaneous absorption of exogenous materials will result in only a small degree of absorption. Most of these materials are absorbed through the pilosebaceous apocrine units. In deliberate application of any steroid or anti-steroid anti-inflammatory ointment or cream this comparatively small degree of absorption must be taken into consideration in laser treatment for naevi.

The skin is thus one of the most important part of the human body, not only functioning as an inert envelope, but as a living, breathing, adaptable and protective organ. It is thick where it comes in for abrasive treatment; it is well-attached to the subdermal fascia where it is most liable to be tugged off; it is provided with friction ridges and a lack of excessive oily secretion on those areas where grip and anti-slippage are required. The skin is *"the finest fighting tissue"* in the words of the British anatomist Samuel E Whitnall (1876-1952), and: *".... even with our ingenious modern machinery we cannot create a tough but highly elastic fibre that will withstand heat and cold, wet and drought, acid and alkali, microbic invasion, and the wear and tear of three score years and ten, yet effect its own repairs throughout and even present a reasonable protection of pigment against the sun's rays. It is indeed the finest fighting tissue."*

CHAPTER 2:

THE LASER

2.1: THE LASER

This chapter will: give a brief outline of the historical background to the development of the laser; examine basic laser theory in some depth; recap the basics of the physical laws governing light in general and laser energy in particular; give an overview of the different types of laser and their characteristics; examine the optical elements and other components of laser systems; discuss laser output control and quantification; examine the basic laser/biologic tissue interaction; summarize the biomedical history of the laser; look at thermal and nonthermal effects; and will conclude with a brief discussion of side effects and their control.

2-1-1 LASER HISTORY

The first laser was developed just over 30 years ago: however the concept behind the laser is by no means quite so recent. The origins of the optical physics on which the concepts of laser generation are based can be traced back as far as Christiaan Huygens' *Treatise on Light*, published in 1690. In this, Huygens postulated that light traveled in wave forms, and was also able to deduce the laws of reflection and refraction. Huygens' contemporary, Sir Isaac Newton, rejected the wave theory, and instead held that light consisted of minute particles which emanated from luminescent bodies in a straight line. This was the so-called corpuscular theory. The wave versus the particle theories were debated fiercely until the early 18th century, when the work of Thomas Young on interference and Augustin Fresnell on diffraction and interference swung the balance in favour of the wave theory. James Clerk Maxwell, in the latter part of the 19th century, was able to explain almost all the laws of optical physics known at that time in terms of his theory of electromagnetic wave propagation. Heinrich Hertz demonstrated the existence of 'electrical waves', now known as radio waves, which were demonstrated to move at the same speed as visible light, and other members of the electromagnetic spectrum. Although this was certain proof that light traveled in waves, Hertz also demonstrated the photoelectric effect, by which certain metals emit electrons when illuminated by light of a certain wavelength, but which depended on its explanation for the recognition that light travelled in a stream of particles, referred to as photons.

This work led Max Plank to develop his theories about the little packets of light energy, which he called quanta, and the work on the quantum theory was well under way. These findings led physicists to the modern concept of light propagation, which allows for the dual nature of waveform travel in discrete energy particles. So, three hundred years later, both Huygens and Newton were in a way proved correct. Working on Plank's theories as his basis, Albert Einstein formed the basis of modern quantum mechanics, by postulating that light could in fact be imagined to consist of discrete bundles of radiation, the so-called quanta, or photons. In 1916, Einstein proposed the principles of spontaneous and stimulated emission of radiation, which form the groundwork for laser generation. Population inversion, the keystone of efficient sustained laser action, was examined by V A Fabrikant in 1940.

These principles were put into practice in the early and mid 1950's by a team including Nobel Laureates Arthur Schawlow and Charles Townes, who were working on a device that would intensify a beam of microwaves. Microwaves are not part of the visible spectrum, but have many practical uses. Radar is a good example of the practical use of microwave technology, as are microwave communications, and the ever-expanding microwave oven. Schawlow and Townes, and other workers in the field, such as Gordon, Zeiger, Basov and Prokhorov, made important contributions to the transition from microwave to the much shorter wave visible light amplification.

The device Schawlow and Townes were working on was called a MASER, an acronym for Microwave Amplification by Stimulated Emission of Radiation. In 1957, they began to explore the possibility of producing a similar device for the amplification of the much shorter visible light waves, in other words, an 'optical maser'. In 1958 they published their ideas in the journal *Physical Reviews*, under the title of "Infrared and Optical Masers". Shortly after that, synthetic ruby became a popular candidate for the first practical optical maser system, and the race to develop the first operative optical maser was well and truly on. Theodore Maiman was working on such an optical maser at the Hughes corporation. In July of 1960 he succeeded in firing the first practical optical maser. In Maiman's system, as light was being amplified instead of microwaves, it was termed Light Amplification by Stimulated Emission of Radiation, which gave the now-familiar acronym of LASER. In fact, the term "Laser" had been previously coined by another U.S. physicist, Gordon Gould, in notes he had made on a gas-discharge visible light laser in 1957, but because of adverse circumstances, Gould was unable to apply for a patent on his officially recorded proposals: eventually, in 1987, Gould was granted a broad-based patent, covering many different kinds of laser, which had important financial implications for all the companies producing lasers covered by that patent, which is still in force at the time of writing.

Maiman's laser used a synthetic pink ruby crystal, which emitted light in the deep red part of the visible spectrum. A popular demonstration of the power of this new light beam was to use the millisecond pulse of light to drill a tiny hole through a stack of razor blades. It was suggested then that the power of the laser should not be measured in watts, but in Gillettes. In 1961 a mixture of two gasses, helium (He) and neon (Ne), was used by Javan and his colleagues; the HeNe also emitted red light. In the same year Johnson developed a laser emitting in the invisible infrared using an yttrium aluminium garnet crystal doped with the rare earth, neodymium - the neodymium YAG or Nd:YAG laser. The argon laser, a gas laser giving a blue-green visible beam, was developed by Bennet in 1962. Two years later the work of Patel and his colleagues resulted in yet another gas laser, the carbon dioxide laser. Like the Nd:YAG laser, the CO_2 laser emits in the invisible infrared portion of the spectrum. It is interesting how close together these lasers appeared and up till the present remain among the principal lasers used in surgery and medicine for the past three decades, despite the fact that literally hundreds of thousands of other solids, gasses, liquids and vapours (including the fumes of good Scotch whisky), and semiconductor diodes have been found capable of producing laser energy.

2-1-2 BASIC LASER THEORY

Laser, as has been well stated, is an acronym for Light Amplification by Stimulated Emission of Radiation. In the literature of today, the word 'laser' is no longer used to describe the basic physical phenomenon behind the production of the energy unique to this energy source, but is also used to describe the systems producing this pure beam of energy, and to describe the energy, or laser light, itself. A laser beam is a beam of artificial light, which depends for its production on the highly specialized and individual characteristics of the laser system: the beam of light thus

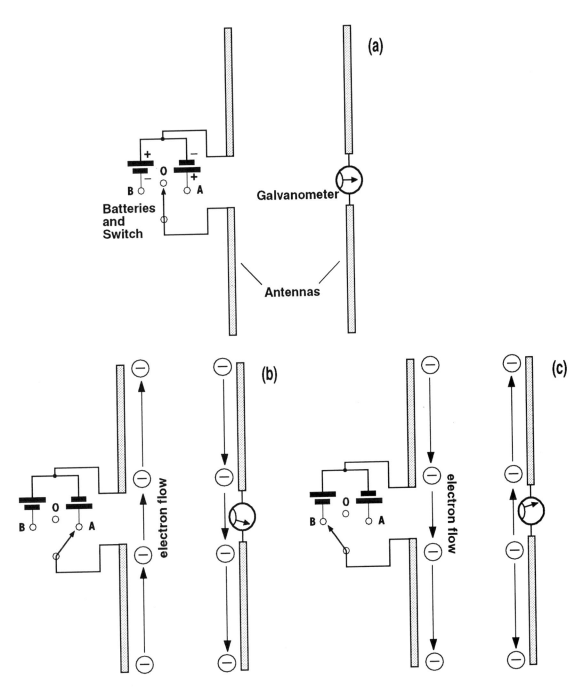

Fig 2.1 *Generation of EM wave:* **a:** *Basic apparatus, consisting of battery, connected through a switch to a dipole antenna (transmitter) and a second dipole antenna (receiver) connected to a galvanometer.* **b:** *Switch set to A, receiver indicates brief induced current flow in one direction.* **c:** *Switch set to B, receiver indicates brief induced current flow in opposite direction.*

has certain characteristics which are unique to it. In order to use this light in medicine and surgery effectively and safely, the laser surgeon or therapist must therefore fully understand these unique beam characteristics, and having understood them, will then be able to use the laser in treatment or therapy with the safety of the operator, ancillary staff and the patient assured. In this section, then, the essential and basic physical properties of laser generation and laser propagation will be examined, to provide a solid basis for the correct understanding of the beam, which is necessary in then applying the beam in practical clinical use.

2-1-2-(A) Absorption and Emission of Photons

Light is a member of an energy family called the electromagnetic (EM) spectrum. The EM spectrum is vast, and the section of light used for medical and surgical laser applications occupies only a small portion of this spectrum, but all members of the EM spectrum have one thing in common: they are all forms of radiation which are capable of travelling through space. How can we generate or demonstrate EM wave radiation? Consider the apparatus shown in Figure 2.1a. This consists of two batteries connected by a switch to a dipole antenna. By rotating the switch to the appropriate contact, the circuit is off, or live, with either of the batteries selected depending on the position of the switch at B, O or A. As can be seen from the diagram, the polarity of the two batteries as connected to the circuit is opposite. The second part of the apparatus consists of a second dipole antenna, separated from the first and connected to a galvanometer, capable of detecting and showing current flow in either direction.

When the switch is set to select battery A, (Figure 2.1b) a very brief flow of negatively-charged electrons is induced, as is shown by the arrows. Even though the antennas are set apart, the galvanometer in the other circuit will then indicate a current flow, showing that electromagnetic energy is somehow being transmitted between the two antennas in what is referred to as a wave form. Imagine a stone dropped into a still pool of water. After the stone enters the water, a series of concentric waves will spread out from the spot of impact. In the same manner, electromagnetic energy is transmitted from the first antenna to the second one in a series of invisible waves. Reversing the flow by selecting battery B produces the situation as seen schematically in Figure 2.1c.

From this schematic, it can be seen that an accelerated electron flow through the left-hand circuit causes a brief emission of electromagnetic waves, which is received and absorbed by the other right-hand antenna, causing acceleration of the electrons. The speed at which the waves travel is the speed of light, approximately 3×10^{10} cm/s.

2-1-2-(A-1) Wavelength and Frequency

If the switch is moved in one complete cycle from O to A to O to B to O over one second, in other words a *frequency* of one cycle per second, we arrive at a waveform as seen in Figure 2.2a, with a distance of propagation of one complete wave cycle from X to Y of 300,000 kilometres, with a transmission time from X to Y of 1 second. Frequency is usually expressed in *hertz* (**Hz**), where 1 Hz = 1 cycle/s). The *wavelength* is measured from the beginning of the cycle to the end of the cycle, and the wavelength in this instance is thus 300,000 km. If the rate of switching between battery A and B is increased to a frequency of 4 Hz, the waveform will also change as shown in Figure 2.2b to show 4 complete cycles from X to Y. As wavelength is measured from one complete cycle, the wavelength of the beam generated with a switching frequency of four is 75,000 km: in other words, the higher the frequency, the shorter the wavelength, altering in exact inverse proportion. A frequency of 8 Hz would thus produce a wavelength of 32,500 km, and so on. From this we can derive the formula:

$$\frac{\text{Speed of Light}}{\text{Frequency}} = \text{Wavelength}$$

As the frequencies increase, we arrive at waveforms known to wireless listeners as long wave (LW), medium-wave (MW), short wave (SW),

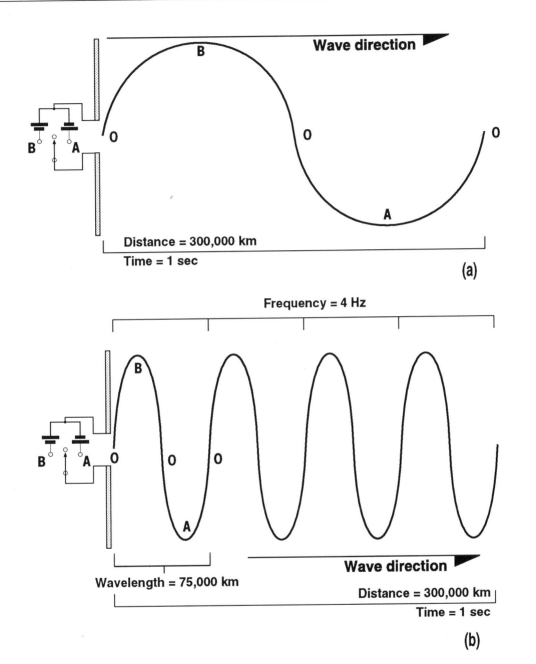

Fig 2.2: Schematic demonstrating concepts of wavelength (**a**) and frequency (**b**). Frequency value is seen to increase in direct proportion to decrease in wavelength value. In other words, the shorter the wavelength, the higher the frequency.

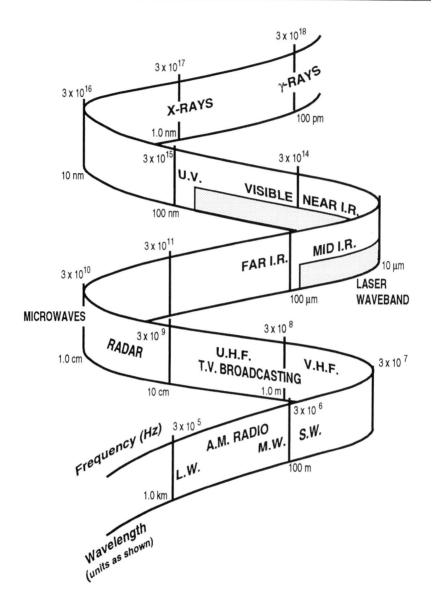

Fig 2.3:   *Schematic demonstrating extent of electromagnetic (em) spectrum, with examples of devices using em spectrum components.*

very high frequency (VHF) and ultra-high frequency (UHF). Television broadcasts use the latter wavebands. In theory, therefore, if we could move that switch fast enough between batteries A and B, we could actually produce "light". To do that, however, we would need to move the switch at a frequency of 4×10^{14}

Hz (400,000,000,000,000 times per second), and substituting values in the above formula, that would produce a wavelength of:

$$\frac{3 \times 10^{10}}{4 \times 10^{14}} = 0.75 \times 10^{-4} \, cm = 750 \, nm$$

giving a beam of barely visible near infrared light (visible light waveband = 400 nm - 700 nm).

Figure 2.3 shows the electromagnetic spectrum, and some associated devices, ranging from long-wave radio to ultrashort-wave cosmic radiation.

2-1-2-(A-2) Particle Theory of EM Propagation
Following the above discussion, an electromagnetic (EM) wave is induced by forced movement of electrons in the transmitting antenna and electron movement occurs by energy absorption of the EM wave in the receiving antenna. We would now like to examine the emission and absorption of EM waves at the atomic level. An atom consists of a positively charged nucleus orbited by one or more negatively charged electrons. These orbits are governed by the energy state of the electron. The orbit of an electron is not in a continuously determined state, such as that of a satellite orbiting the earth. At the atomic level, the range of wave characteristics of an electron is very wide and the actual site of the electron is always changing, like a cloud. Each electron has its own wavelength to be considered, and a stable electron state can only be attained in the case of a stationary wave. Thus an electron's stable state orbit is governed intermittently, just as the resonant frequency of an open guitar string is restricted and governed by a number of physical parameters. The actual orbit which an electron can attain is determined by its energy.

There are two kinds of energy associated with electrons: potential energy and momentum energy. Electrons in an outer orbit have a lower momental energy, with an increase in the potential energy: the opposite is true for the inner orbit electrons. The sum of the two energy types, i.e. the total energy of an electron, varies directly with the size of the electron's orbit. Stimulation of an electron to move into a larger orbit can occur when the electron absorbs energy from an external source, such as from absorption of a photon. The difference between these total energies equals the photon energy. In the case of absorption of energy by the electron, the absorbed energy (light or otherwise) moves the electron to a higher energy level, at which it remains for only a brief period, before returning, or decaying, back to the ground energy level or to an intermediate energy level. In decaying, a photon is released into space. The energy of that photon is equal to the difference in energy between the electron's energy levels.

In Figure 2.4, an electron is shown in the resting state, or at ground energy level E_0. Incident energy, (light, electrical, RF or chemical, for example), strikes the electron and is absorbed, sending the electron up to a higher excited level E_α: the value of α will depend on the degree of

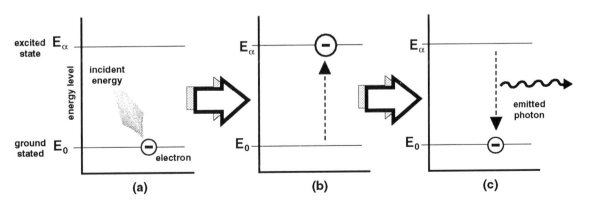

Fig 2.4: *Principle of electron energy absorption and spontaneous emission.* **a:** *An electron at ground state E_0 absorbs incident energy.* **b:** *After absorption, electron is raised to excited energy level E_α, where it stays for only a brief period.* **c:** *Electron spontaneously decays back to ground energy level, releasing stored energy in the form of a photon: this is spontaneous emission of radiation.*

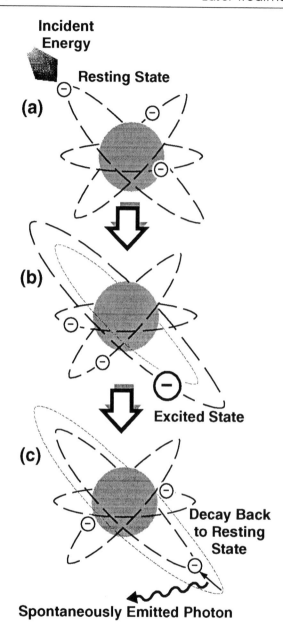

Incident Energy

Resting State

(a)

(b)

Excited State

(c)

Decay Back to Resting State

Spontaneously Emitted Photon

Fig 2.5: *Schematic of atomic model for absorption* **(a & b)** *and spontaneous emission* **(c).**

energy imparted to the electron. The electron can remain at state E_α only for a brief period, and then must decay back to E_0, ground energy level, but in doing so, the electron must release its stored energy, *no matter which form of energy was first*

absorbed, in the form of a photon, our small unit of light energy. Figure 2.5 is an atomic model representation of the same phenomenon, showing that the higher excited energy level of the electron is associated with a larger orbital path, and on decaying back to ground energy level, the original orbit is resumed.

It has been experimentally shown that, when one photon is emitted by one electron, the energy of the photon is expressed as

$$E = hc/\lambda$$

where h is Planck's constant and c and λ are, respectively, the velocity and the wavelength of light. From this consideration the concept of the photon, specifically for light energy, as a single particle of light energy can be understood. From the above, it is also clear that the shorter the wavelength, the higher the photon energy. This has importance in deciding the basic energy/target reaction, as will be dealt with later in the appropriate section.

2-1-2-(A-3) Spontaneous Emission

A model for absorption and emission of energy has already been covered above. The electron at the excited level quickly and spontaneously decays to a lower energy level, in such case spontaneously emitting the stored energy as a photon. Consider Figure 2.6. A ball is very carefully balanced on a stair tread, representing the excited energy level of an electron. Because of its size relative to the tread, the ball may remain in balance only for a short while, (an electron may only remain in its excited state for $1 \times 10^9 \sim 1 \times 10^7$ s) but eventually the ball will spontaneously fall to the ground (return to ground energy level), and in doing so will make a specific sound: this represents spontaneous emission of energy, as happens with the excited state electron, which in a laser medium emits not sound but light energy in the form of a photon.

2-1-2-(A-4) Stimulated Emission

This decay from excited level to ground energy level can also be induced, however, in other

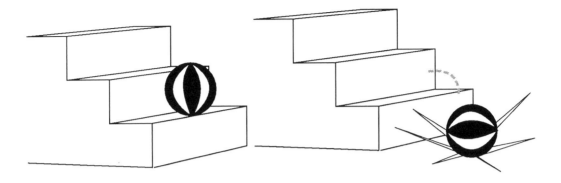

Fig 2.6: *Ball in 'raised energy' state on a stair, spontaneously falls to the ground creating a sound (spontaneous emission analogy).*

words, stimulated. In Figure 2.7, the ball is once again balanced on the stair tread as before, but behind the stair riser is a powerful loudspeaker. Before the ball can fall spontaneously to the ground, the loudspeaker emits a sound of specific volume and frequency. The resultant sound wave strikes the riser, and stimulates the ball to fall back to the ground. This is a simplified model for stimulated emission of energy.

In the case of the electron in its excited state, a photon of a particular wavelength and direction, released previously by spontaneous emission, collides with the electron in its upper energy level, and stimulates it to return to ground energy level, but in doing so it must emit its stored energy in the form of a photon similar in all characteristics to the photon which collided with the electron. So now, where there was only one photon, travelling in a particular direction, there are now two photons exactly alike, travelling together in the same direction. This is known as amplification, and thus the phenomenon of light amplification by stimulated emission of radiation (LASER) occurs. Figure 2.8 is a composite atomic model for the whole process of absorption, spontaneous emission, and stimulated emission. Before amplification by stimulated emission can occur, however, other criteria have to be met: one of these is the state known as population inversion of electrons.

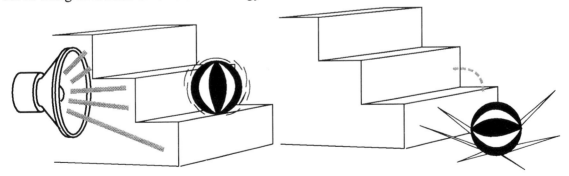

Fig 2.7: *Same ball on same staircase: a loudspeaker behind the staircase is activated, the sound waves from which stimulate the ball to fall from the stair to the ground, creating a sound on striking the ground. Analogy for stimulated emission.*

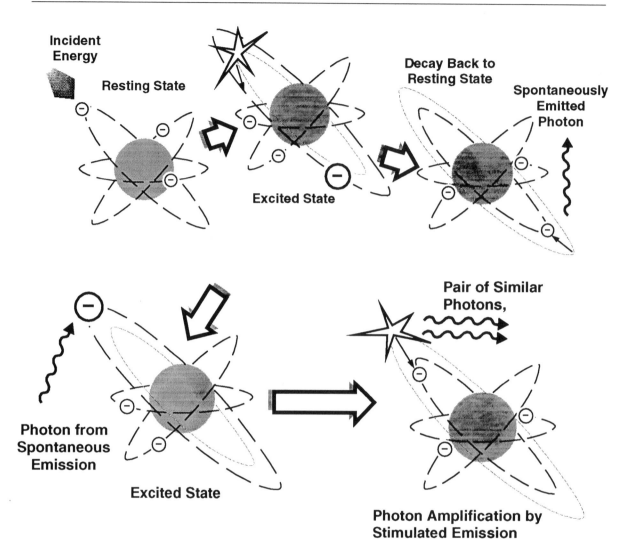

Fig 2.8: *Atomic model showing absorption, spontaneous emission of photon radiation, and stimulated emission caused by spontaneously emitted photon striking electron already in an excited state, stimulating it to emit a photon similar to the one striking the electron. This is the basis of light amplification by stimulated emission of radiation (LASER)*

2-1-2-(A-5) Population Inversion

The greater the increase in the temperature of matter, the more light energy is emitted. This means that as the number of electrons at ground or a low energy level decreases, the number of electrons at higher energy levels increases and spontaneous emission of photons increases, as seen in Figure 2.9a and b. When matter is in a state

of thermal equilibrium, Boltzmann's distribution of electrons exists. In such a distribution, no matter how much the temperature rises, the higher the energy level the lower the population of electrons.

It has already been discussed that an electron in a lower energy level will go up to a higher level on absorption of light energy, and will then spontaneously decay, or will be stimulated to decay to

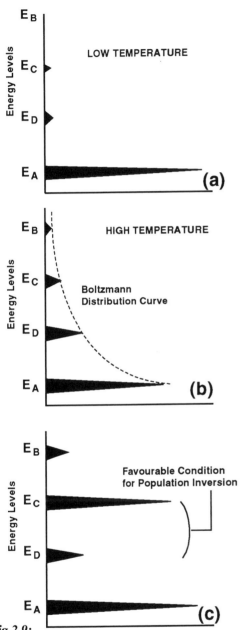

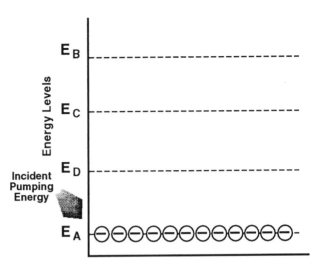

Fig 2.10:
Pumping of electrons from ground energy level up to higher energy levels to obtain population inversion. Electrons are all in ground energy level E_A, when they are forced to absorb incident pumping energy.

a lower level, emitting light energy in the process. When light travels through such matter, a lot of absorption will occur because there are many electrons in the energy lower level. On the other hand, when the electrons in matter are in the energy state as shown in Figure 2.9c, there will be a greater rate of stimulated emission of an appropriate wavelength than absorption. In this case the incident light energy will be amplified, provided it is of an appropriate wavelength.

2-1-2-(A-6) Pumping

In order to reach the state of population inversion, it is necessary to scoop the electrons in the lower energy level up into the higher energy level. Such an operation is called 'pumping'. In lasers, the pumping source may be light, as in a flash lamp, electrical energy, radio frequency energy, or chemical energy, but the sole object of the pumping is to produce population inversion. Pumping will now be examined in more detail with an example. Figure 2.10 shows a number of electrons at ground energy level E_A. The upper energy

Fig 2.9:
*Demonstration of population inversion. **a:** photons in a material at low temperature. Vast majority are at ground energy level, or resting state. **b:** Increasing temperature of material increases slightly electrons at higher energy levels, giving a typical Boltzman distribution. No population inversion yet exists because majority of electrons are still in resting state. **c:** Large amount of photons have been raised or pumped up to a higher energy level: this is a favourable condition for population inversion between levels E_C and E_D.*

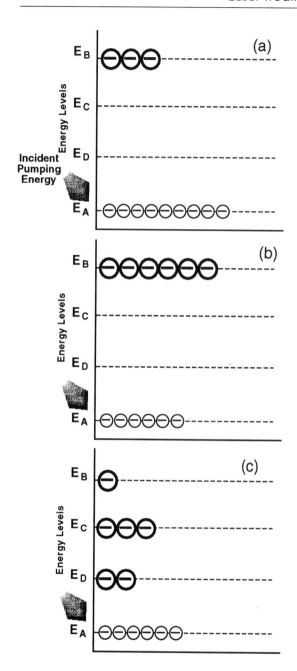

Fig 2.11:
a: *Some electrons are forced up to level E_B by pumping, and in* **b:** *are joined by more. Population inversion can now occur between E_C and E_B.* **c:** *Electrons at E_B soon drop to longer-lived state E_C. As E_D becomes vacant, population inversion with spontaneous and stimulated emission will occur between E_C and E_D.*

levels of E_B, E_C and E_D are also shown. When the energy of the pumping photons is E_B-E_A, incident pumping energy takes the electrons of energy level E_A up to energy level E_B, and we have the situation in Figure 2.11a and b.

In this example, the lifetime of energy state E_c is much longer than E_B or E_D. The electrons at E_B will soon drop down to level E_C, and the population of E_C will increase. Those levels which have reached level E_D from the upper levels will soon drop down to ground level E_A, thus giving population inversion between E_C and E_D (Figure 2.11c).

Unexpectedly, population inversion can never take place between E_B and E_A, even with a very powerful pumping light. This is because the pumping light will also induce stimulated emission, and the electrons in level E_B are forced back to ground level E_A.

From the foregoing it can be seen that the pumping light must have a large inherent energy, i.e. composed to a certain extent of shorter wavelengths.

2-1-2-(B) Laser Resonator

In the infinite space of the cosmos, it is not necessary to use any kind of resonator to amplify electromagnetic waves, because of the availability of the vast limitless area of space: this naturally-occurring phenomenon has been observed and reported on. In the small space of a laboratory or clinic, however, an resonator is necessary to produce a laser beam of a practical intensity.

The main object of using a resonator in a laser device is to increase the length of the light path in the laser medium. Even in the case where a short medium produces only a small rate of light amplification, by increasing the length of the passage of light through the medium, a laser beam of practical power can be generated. As the physical size of the medium is restricted by the constraints of environment, at least on Earth, an effective method is to force the light to make multiple passes through the same medium.

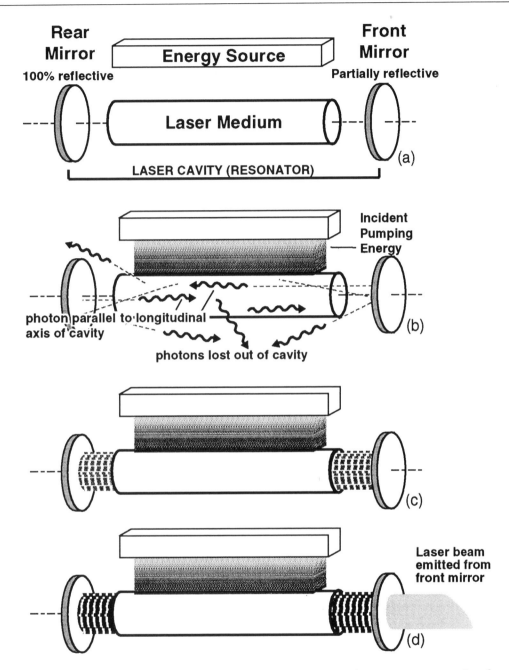

Rear Mirror
100% reflective

Energy Source

Front Mirror
Partially reflective

Laser Medium

(a)

LASER CAVITY (RESONATOR)

Incident
Pumping
Energy

photon parallel to longitudinal
axis of cavity

photons lost out of cavity

(b)

(c)

Laser beam
emitted from
front mirror

(d)

Fig 2.12: **a:** *Typical laser resonator consisting of medium bounded by mirrors (the cavity or resonator) and an external energy source for pumping the medium.* **b:** *Energy (light, electrical or chemical) is forced into the medium from the energy source, and random spontaneous emission begins to occur. Note some of the photons will be exactly parallel to the longitudinal axis of the cavity, and stimulated emission will also occur in the same plane.* **c:** *These photons are dynamically reflected back and forth through the medium, building up strong resonance.* **d:** *A certain proportion of the light inside the cavity at any time passes through the partially reflective front mirror in the form of a laser beam.*

The basic concept behind an optical resonator is almost the same as the electrical resonator found in electric circuits, or acoustic resonators such as guitar strings or the column of air in the tubular body of a flute: they are all storage devices or accumulators of vibrational energy.

2-1-2-(B-1) Structure of Resonator

An example of one type of laser resonator is shown in Figure 2.12a. There are many styles of optical resonator, but in most popular cases they are bounded at both ends of their horizontal axis by two parallel mirrors. The mirrors must be extremely accurately positioned in order to maximize the quality of the resonator. If the mirrors are not positioned precisely parallel to each other, light cannot make multiple passes back and forth between the mirrors because of light loss, and the quality of the resonator is reduced. Mirrors are thus installed on micro-adjustors so that their inclination and collimation can be precisely set.

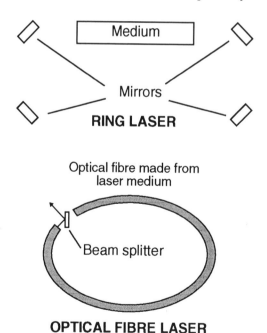

Fig 2.13: Examples of other laser cavity types: the ring laser and the optical fibre laser.

The mirrors and the medium form what is termed the *resonant cavity* of the oscillator. The board, or optical table, on which the mirrors and the medium are installed, must be extremely rigid to resist flexion.

The basic function of this type of resonator is to amplify the original generated beam by forcing the beam to pass many times back and forth through the medium by the mirrors at each end (Figure 2.12b and c). The kind of mirrors used can include both flat surface mirrors and concave mirrors. In the case of high-powered laser systems, convex mirrors are also used, since in such high densities of light the light-gathering characteristics of the medium itself can be seen.

The generated laser beam can be got out of the cavity in a number of ways, using a beam splitter, for example, to divert a portion of the intracavity beam. More common is the application of a semireflective mirror as one of the pair of mirrors used in the optical cavity, leaving the other mirror 100% reflective, and a portion if the intracavity beam escapes through the partially reflective mirror (Figure 2.12d).

There are many other resonator types. For example, the ring laser is constructed using three or more mirrors, forcing the light to travel in a circular path; the optical fibre laser uses a fibre constructed from a medium material (Figure 2.13), and so on.

2-1-2-(B-2) Condition of Resonant Oscillation

In order to produce efficient laser oscillation in the resonator, the light amplification rate must be greater than the loss rate. For example, if 90% of the beam is allowed to pass through the semireflective mirror and other light losses are negligible, then the remaining intracavity 10% must be amplified more than ten times in one single passage back and forth through the medium to maintain the intracavity beam to ensure oscillation. The trigger photons for the oscillation can be obtained by spontaneous emission, but only a portion of the spontaneously emitted photons is used as the trigger, since only those photons travelling exactly parallel to the longitudinal axis of the cavity will oscillate back and forth through the medium on exactly the same path. Usually below 10^{-10} of spontaneously emitted photons fall into this category of the useful trigger beam, even in a well-adjusted resonator. In many laser cavities, spontaneous emission by the medium occurs at the rate of more than 10^{20} per second: thus the oscillation trigger using spontaneously emitted photon beams is possible.

2-1-3 CHARACTERISTICS OF LASER

2-1-3-(A)   Characteristics of Light

A laser beam is basically a beam of electromagnetic energy, similar to 'light'. The 'L' in LASER after all stands for 'light'. Laser beams can therefore be reflected, refracted, transmitted, diffracted, scattered and absorbed, depending of the specific interaction between the laser beam and the target material, and the special characteristics of laser light itself.

A thorough understanding of the physical properties of light must also be important factors in understanding the physical phenomenon of laser/tissue interaction. The main phenomena which influence the effect of a laser beam incident on tissue are reflection, transmission, scatter, absorption: these phenomena will vary greatly and be much influenced by the wavelength of the light. A deep understanding of these properties will stand the laser clinician in excellent stead when looking at a desired clinical effect, and how best to achieve it with the laser. This chapter, although possible 'old hat' to many laser clinicians is none-the-less extremely important, and the author recommends that everyone, expert and novice alike, give this chapter a good deal of attention and real study.

2-1-3-(A-1) Reflection and Transmission

Electromagnetic energy, of which laser energy is a member, travels like waves, and interacts with charged particles by the energy units known as photons: a beam of energy in the wavebands which lasers occupy may be invisible (UV, <400 nm; and IR, >700 nm), or visible light with a wavelength from between 400 nm (violet) to 700 nm (deep red), or a mixture of any or all of the above. When light energy encounters a target substance, the interaction with the incident stream of photons will depend on the wavelength of the light and the make-up of the substance.

The energy may be *reflected* (Figure 2.14) from the target substance: visible light striking a polished bright metal surface, for example, will be mostly reflected from that surface: if the metal is large enough in area and flat, and the light strikes at an angle, the angle of incidence ($\theta°$ in Figure 2.14), the beam of energy will be reflected back at the same angle, the angle of reflection. Most of the photons in the beam of light seem to be neither absorbed by the structure of the metal target, nor can they pass through, and they simply seem to bounce off. The reader must always remember the saying: "Electrons move by collision with photons." In this case, the same concept holds true.

Most of the photons in the beam of incident light will be absorbed once by the electrons of the metal target, but because of the nonexistence of an upper orbit of the electrons, spontaneous emission will occur almost simultaneously. The

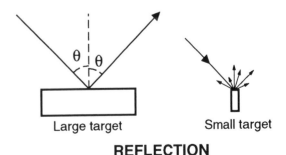

REFLECTION

Fig 2.14: Reflection illustrated schematically, from large and small surfaces (relative to the size of the beam).

newly-born photon is thus different from the absorbed incident photon. It could be imagined that the photons would be emitted (or 'reflected') in all directions, but because of the phenomenon known as the 'diffraction index' the direction of emission is not random. However, the author would not like to explain that in detail at this point. In the case of incident light of shorter wavelengths, the probability of interaction between the photon and the electron may differ. If the wavelength of the incident beam is equal to or shorter than X-rays, however, at that wavelength the metal reflectance is lower, and a certain proportion of the radiation energy would be allowed pass on into and through the target, depending on its thickness, the kind of matter, the wavelength of the incident beam, and so on.

When a beam of visible light strikes a sheet of clear, optically isotropic SiO_2 glass, perpendicular to the surface plane of the glass, a portion will be reflected while the remainder will be allowed to pass on through the glass, emerging on the opposite side unaltered in its path. This is *transmission*. In this case the photon is duly absorbed and emitted by the electrons in the target material. The difference between a transmissive material and metal is that the free electron density is very small. There is a relatively long period from absorption to emission by free electrons, but the period is much shorter in an insulator or dielectric body. If the incident beam were not composed of visible light, but of photons with a wavelength of 10,600 nm in the mid infrared, (the wavelength of the CO_2 laser), the glass ceases to transparent at that wavelength, and the CO_2 beam will not pass through. In this case, the energy of the photon is changed to molecular vibration (i.e. thermal energy).

For materials such as air and glass, the reflectance at the boundary of two transparent materials can be calculated by Fresnell's formulae, in which the reflectance is determined by the refractive indices of the two materials and the incident angle of light (see dictionaries of optics).

2-1-3-(A-2) Refraction and Scattering

Refraction is the process by which the speed of light is changed as it enters a medium of different electromagnetic properties, for example, the dielectric constant or magnetic permeability, than the one in which it has been travelling. The basic law of refraction, which was first proposed in 1621 by the Dutch scientist Willebrord Snell, relates the magnitude of refraction to the velocity of light in the two media and expresses it in the index of refraction, or refractive index, of the media. Consider a horizontal piece of glass: the line drawn perpendicular to the surface is called the normal. A beam of light entering the glass from air is bent toward the normal; on exiting the glass, the beam is bent away from the normal. In this example, because the surfaces of the glass are parallel the beam that emerges will be parallel to its incident beam but laterally displaced (Figure 2.15)

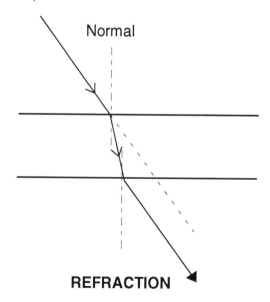

Fig 2.15:
Refraction illustrated diagramatically. A beam entering a substance of greater refractive index is bent towards the normal, and bent away from the normal when entering a substance of a lower index of refraction.

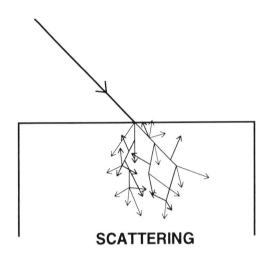

SCATTERING

Fig 2.16:
Scattering shown schematically. As both forward and back scattering can occur at the same time, there may be areas of greater photon density within a target material than at the surface.

If the glass is not clear, but homogeneously translucent, such as milky-white glass, then the ordered progress of the light stream is interrupted: while it is still allowed to pass into the glass, most of the light is turned aside or deflected by the random arrangement of small particles of different refractive indices from the clear body of the glass: this form of modified transmission is known as *scattering*.

Scattering tends to turn a narrow beam into a wider beam. There are three main types of scattering which can affect the transmission of light through matter. *Rayleigh scattering* is the scattering which occurs when light is scattered by much smaller particles than the wavelength of the light passing through them. The wavelength shift caused by Rayleigh scattering is very small. *Mie scattering* is caused by light interaction with larger particles, similar in size to the wavelength, such as found in smoke or fog. In Raman scattering, wavelength shifts occur in a beam of light passing through a clear medium, depending on the composition of the medium, resulting in the

incident wavelength bands being surrounded by satellite bands of greater or lesser wavelength.

Depending on the density of the target, multiple scattering may occur within the target, so that when the remainder of the light emerges from the opposite side of the target it is less in density, and travelling in different directions than before it entered the target. Because of multiple forward- and back-scattering, the actual photon density may be greater under the surface than at it. Generally, in theory, the shorter the wavelength, the greater the degree of scattering, but in biological tissue this phenomenon is of particular importance in the deeper-penetrating wavelengths in the near infrared, and for the practical applications of LLLT. Scattering is shown schematically in Figure 2.16.

2-1-3-(A-3) Absorption and Wavelength

While reflection, refraction, transmission and scatter are very important in understanding or predicting a laser/tissue reaction for a given laser wavelength and tissue, the following concepts are even more important when considering the final effect and treatment or therapeutic result. Absorption of the incident light in biological tissue, or any target substance, will determine the reaction: the first law of photobiology states that there must be absorption before any reaction occurs. The wavelength of the incident energy will determine the mechanism of the absorption through the *chromophores*, the wavelength-specific absorbing agents. Wavelength is coupled with the frequency of the incident energy, and the frequency determines the unit energy inherent in the wavelength, more or less independent of the incident power. The wavelength/tissue reaction, more than anything else, will determine the penetration depth of the incident beam, without taking incident power levels into consideration.

Absorption: If the incident light energy passes into the target, and the energy is taken up by the target, this is called *absorption* (Figure 2.17). Absorption is the final event in the complex chain of events which can involve reflection, transmis-

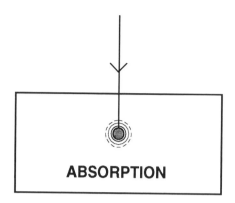

ABSORPTION

Fig 2.17: *Absorption of energy within the target material.*

sion and scatter, and is a very important concept for the laser clinician. In taking up or absorbing the incident energy, the recipient target material must change in some way, as the energy from the incident beam must go somewhere, and do something.

Light is an electromagnetic wave, for which the first stage of absorption is by electrically-charged particles such as electrons. The change of energy level of an electron involved in this process has already been discussed. The changes in a material caused by light absorption depend on the movements of these charged particles. When the velocity of an electron is high enough, it is capable of moving from its usual position to another position. If that electron is the member of a chemical bond, then the properties of the bond may change resulting in a chemical reaction. This is known as a photochemical reaction. On the other hand, considering electron motion, interaction may occur with adjacent particles, which force the moving electron off its set path, which in turn causes the electron to emit a long wavelength photon, resulting in heat. Heat is caused by the vibration of particles in the material such as atoms or molecules.

The resonant frequency of a chemical bond is determined by the structure of each particular bond. The energy from this frequency may be stored after absorption, and it may take a long

time for the energy to exit the resonator. The stored vibrational energy will however continue to cause vibration in adjacent atoms to a certain extent, and the stored energy will finally be transformed to heat. There is a particular group of chemical bonds which are highly frequency-specific in their absorption characteristics, leading to quick absorption of their specific frequency. These are referred to as chromophores, as they are specific for a particular colour frequency or wavelength.

Wavelength: Laser energy is grouped along with other energy forms in a band called the electromagnetic spectrum (EM spectrum), as already discussed above. The wavelength of the beam is, as has already been said, the distance the beam takes to make one complete cycle. In clinical applications of laser, the accepted unit of measure of wavelength is the nanometre (nm) [1 nm = 1 x 10^9 m]. Occasionally, for longer wavelengths such as the CO_2 laser (10,600 nm), the micrometre or micron is used (1 μm= 1 x 10^6 m).

2-1-3-(A-4) Frequency

The frequency of the beam is determined by the number of complete cycles the beam makes in 1 second, as already demonstrated. From that discussion, the reader is reminded that wavelength and frequency vary directly as the inverse of each other: the longer the wavelength, the lower the frequency: the shorter the wavelength, the higher the frequency. Frequency is important when considering the chemical or physical effect of a photon's absorption by its target. The higher the frequency, the greater the individual photon energy level measured in electron volts (eV).

eV is defined as the motion energy when an electron is accelerated by V volts. The voltage may be calculated by the following formula:

$$V = \frac{h\nu}{e}$$

When the wavelength is 500 nm, the acceleration voltage of one photon can be calculated by substituting the following values:

$$h = 6.6 \times 10^{-34} \text{ J s}$$

$$\nu = \frac{\text{Velocity of Light}}{\text{Wavelength}} \text{ Hz}$$

$$= \frac{3 \times 10^8}{500 \times 10^{-9}} \text{ Hz}$$

$$= 6 \times 10^{14} \text{ Hz}$$

$$e = 1.6 \times 10^{-19} \text{ C (coulumb)}$$

The value V = 2.475 volts is thus obtained.

For light in the visible waveband, the electron voltage is measured in units of volts, within the same range of voltage as batteries used daily in many examples of common electronic equipment such as cameras, cassette tape players, and so on. Batteries are devices which generate electricity from a chemical reaction, and so the reader may therefore quickly understand that photochemical reactions easily occur from absorption of visible light. Table 2.1 shows the relation between wavelength and voltage as calculated by the formula already given above.

That one single photon can transfer to an electron in excess of one million volts acceleration in the γ-waveband is a sobering thought. This will cause the electron to shoot off at an extremely

high velocity and capable of travelling very far, thereby possible destroying molecular structures. The incident energy is thus converted to heat or chemical energy.

In contrast, when an electron absorbs a photon in the visible waveband, the electron stays very close to the area of its original atom, and the degree of chemical reactivity is thus comparatively low, compared with γ-radiation. For absorption of photons in the infrared or microwave bands, the electron cannot leave the area of its atom at all, and instead transfers the absorbed energy in a vibrational change, resulting in heat.

Multiple Photon Absorption: The voltage rise which occurs in an electron by absorption of a broadcast waveband photon is less than 1 μV. However, when the output of a transmitter is measured at an antenna very near the transmitter, voltages well in excess of 1 mV can be recorded. This phenomenon is due to the rapid absorption of many photons by a single electron, leading to high energy levels in the electron, and is referred to as multiple photon absorption.

This phenomenon may not occur with low photon densities, therefore it is very rarely seen

Table 2.1:   *Relationship between wavelength and electron voltage*

Wavelength	Voltage	Class of Energy
0.5 pm	2.475 MV	γ-rays
50 pm	24.75 KV	X-rays
5 nm	247.5 V	X-rays
500 nm	2.475 V	visible light
50 μm	24.75 mV	Infrared
5 mm	247.5 μV	EHF band
500 mm	2.475 μV	UHF band
50 m	24.75 nV	HF band
5 km	247.5 pv	LF band

EHF = extra high frequence; UHF = ultra high frequency; HF = high frequency;
LF = low frequency (all radio waves)

with conventional visible light sources, but may well occur when a laser is used which has the capability of generating high photon densities with very small focused spots, or in very high-powered laser systems. In this case, an electron with extremely high energy levels will be the result, and even with visible or infrared lasers, a photochemical reaction may easily occur.

2-1-3-(B) Specific Characteristics of Laser

In addition to sharing the above physical characteristics with all forms of light, laser energy has certain aspects unique to it, directly caused by the method of generation and the properties of the resonating cavity.

2-1-3-(B-1) Monochromaticity

Sunlight is composed of many colours, easily demonstrated by passing a beam of sunlight through a prism, and breaking it up into the component colours of the rainbow. However, even the beam of 'red' light seen in that experiment can be

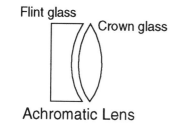

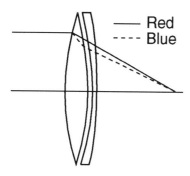

Fig 2:18: *Principle of the achromatic lens. Different wavelengths can be brought to the same focal point.*

further divided by a diffraction grating into other different components. Monochromatic light is defined as light having a single narrow waveband. A light emitting diode (LED) can emit light of a fairly narrow waveband. Many laser systems emit light of a much narrower waveband than an LED.

Monochromacy has the merit of being able to be focused to a very small spot. A light beam consisting of a mixture of wavelengths is subject to chromatic aberration, in other words, the exact point of focus of each component of the light differs depending on the wavelength, and must be corrected by a combination of lens types (Figure 2.18). Pure monochromatic light, especially from a point source such as a laser, could in theory be focused to a spot equal in diameter to a single unit of the wavelength of the light, thus enabling extremely high photon densities at the point of focus.

2-1-3-(B-2) Directivity

Directivity of a beam is the ability to produce a beam with very little divergence. A searchlight is capable of collimating noncoherent light, so that it can travel further with minimum divergence: a lighthouse uses the same principle, enabling the beam to be seen by far-off vessels. These devices can attain divergences in the region of 100 milliradian. Because of the nature of the laser resonator, a typical laser beam can emerge from the cavity in a practically parallel fashion. The larger the generated laser beam is in diameter, the smaller the divergence can be, because of the properties of light. Among commercially-available laser systems, it is possible to find many laser products obtaining divergences of less than 1 milliradian.

A beam of one milliradian divergence will expand in diameter by only 1 mm in 1 m, or 10 cm in 100 m. This means that the entire beam is easily gathered and focused to a very fine spot, enabling high photon densities at the focal point.

2-1-3-(B-3) Coherence

Coherence can be expressed as the ability of a light beam to demonstrate interferometric characteristics. Interference is the phenomenon by

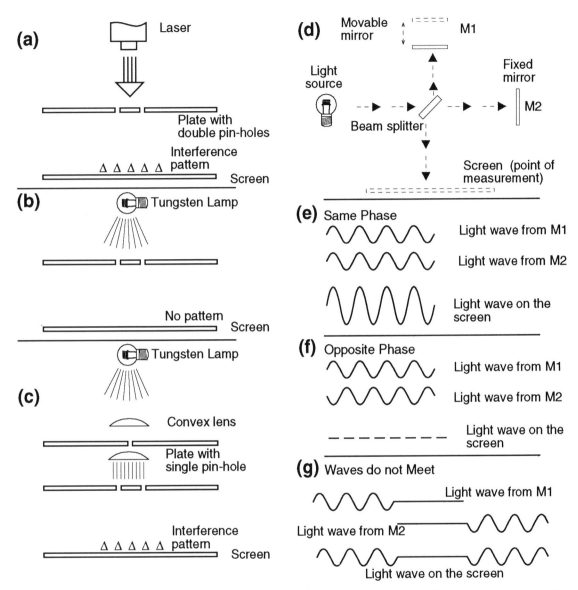

Fig 2.19: *In* **(a)** *and* **(b)** *the principle of light interferometry for measuring and demonstrating spatial coherence is shown.* **c:** *Apparatus for creating spatial coherence from a tungsten light source.* **d: - g:** *Michelson's interferometer: an apparatus used to measure temporal coherence.*

which the light amplitude equals the sum of the respective elements of the light wave when more than two light waves converge on one point. Figure 2.19 demonstrates various methods for assessing coherence using interferometry. In Figure 2.19a the classic interferometry experi-

ment using a light source, a barrier with two pin holes and a screen is shown. If the light source is a laser, an interference pattern will be projected on the screen. If, as in 2.19b, a tungsten lamp is used as the light source, no interference pattern can be seen.

However, if the beam from a tungsten lamp is collimated, or made parallell using the apparatus in Figure 2.19c, then the interference pattern can be seen. A form of coherence has thus been imposed on the tungsten lamp beam when it is collimated: this is called spatial coherence. Another form of coherence exists, known an temporal coherence, which is assessed using Michelson's interferometer, as seen in 2.19d. The incident light source is divided by the beam splitter into two sources, one of which is sent to M1, the other to M2. The beams recombine at the beam splitter and are either reflected or transferred so that they meet at the screen.

If the two beams have the same phase, then they will produce an image as in 2.19e. If the phases are opposite (i.e. inverse phase), then the pattern will be as seen in Figure 2.19f. If the beams are totally out of phase, then the pattern as in 2.19g will be the result.

In other words, light beams with the same phase produce double amplitude, and with inverse phase they cancel each other out. As the difference of the optical path of the beams increases, the two waves cannot meet on the screen, and so interference cannot occur. With a normal light source, temporal coherence may be obtained up to light paths of 1 metre, but for lasers the distance may well be in excess of 100 m.

2-1-4 LASER DEVICES

In theory, it is possible to get laser output from several hundred thousand different substances, but in the surgical and medical field, the practicality of laser generation and delivery of the generated beam limits the types that have been traditionally used. The main types of laser used in surgery and medicine will now be looked at in detail, classifying the system by the type of laser medium.

2-1-4-(A) Gas Lasers

If the medium of a laser is composed of a gas or a mixture of gases, then it is classed as a gas laser. In metal vapour lasers, the medium is a solid at normal temperature, but it takes the form of a superheated vapour in actual operation, and so the author would like to include these under the category of gas lasers. Figure 2.20 shows the diagrammatic structure of a typical gas laser. There are two main types of gas laser: the internal mirror and external mirror types, depending on the position of the mirror relative to the gas discharge tube. Usually in either type, excitation occurs through electrical discharge through the gas contained in the tube. There are two classes of discharge: the longitudinal axis (Figure 2.20) and transverse axis types (Figure 2.21). Table 2.2

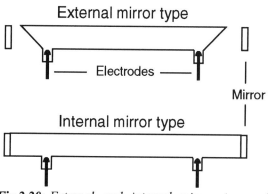

Fig 2.20: *External and internal mirror types of longitudinal axis discharge gas laser tube.*

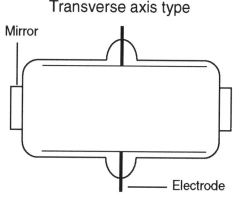

Fig 2.21 *Transverse axis discharge gas laser tube.*

Table 2.2: *Main gas lasers used in medicine & surgery and their characteristics*

LASER TYPE & WAVELENGTH	OUTPUT POWER	SPECIFICS	APPLICATION
Helium Neon (HeNe) 632.8 nm (main wavelength) Also available (in nm): 543, 596, 612, 633, 730, 1015, 1523, and 3392	typically C/W, Less than 100 mW	Visible red beam Small and compact, air cooled, easy to transport and handle	As guide beam for invisible CO_2 or Nd:YAG lasers: In laser Doppler systems Measuring or range-finding equipment
Argon (Ar) 488 - 514.5 nm	C/W, typically under 10 W	Visible blue/blue-green beam Sizes vary, not generally portable: usually water cooled, but some air-cooled models exist	Coagulation of small blood vessels. Tissue coagulation Used in dermatology, ophthalmology or in endoscopic procedures.
Krypton (Kr) 476, 531, 647 nm	C/W, less than 5 mW	Visible red beam	mainly ophthalmologic applications
Carbon dioxide (CO_2) 10,600 nm	C/W or superpulsed mW up to 100 W	Invisible infrared beam, with high energy conversion efficiency. Some portable systems, but more usually mobile systems used in operating and treatment rooms	Used across many specialities for "laser scalpel" incisional and vaporizational applications.
Carbon monoxide (CO) 53 μm	C/W up to 100 W	Invisible infrared beam with high energy conversion efficiency	Used as laser scalpel, but not so common.
Nitrogen (N_2) 337 nm	Pulsed beam (10 ns) approx. 30 MW	Invisible near ultraviolet beam.	Mainly dermatological applications, especially in treatment for skin cancers.

shows the main types of gas lasers used currently in the medical field, their characteristics and their application.

The Column: Gas is contained in a closed tube, and two electrodes are inserted to provide two poles. An electrical potential difference (PD), or electric power, is then applied to the electrodes. However, a low PD cannot induce current flow in the tube. By increasing the PD, at a certain point current will flow through the gas in the tube. When the gas contains relatively fewer ions, cur-

rent flow through the tube is very difficult to achieve. By triggering an initial extra strong pulse of electrical energy through the gas, ions of the gas in the tube are accelerated, which in turn attack the gas molecules, causing ionization of the gas molecules as one of the electrons is cut free by the incident ion. These freed ions again accelerate, and in turn cause further ionization. Such a serially-occurring phenomenon produces a cascade of ions, increasing the flow of current through the gas in the tube. During this phenomenon, the distance between the molecules of gas can be expected to increase to some extent. However, the acceleration of the ions must be enough to cause serial ionization of other molecules, otherwise the necessary ion cascade will not occur. A good everyday example of this is the common fluorescent tube. In the inert or resting state, before switching on the power to the light, the distance between the molecules of gas in the tube must be large enough to allow the build-up of acceleration of the ions, when they are produced. However, a large initial trigger PD must be applied to get the ion cascade under way, and this is brought about by the familiar starter, or choke, which builds up a large PD and suddenly lets it free: the basic principle is similar to the camera flashlamp, where a small dry battery of a few volts is capable, through a trigger circuit, of producing a PD of several thousand volts for a fraction of a second. In the fluorescent tube, (and the laser tube), after the initial burst of high power has instigated the ion cascade, the PD across the poles is then reduced to a normal level, and the ion cascade is maintained, thus also maintaining the current flow through the tube between the electrodes. Ultraviolet light is produced in the course of the reaction between the ions and the electrons, and visible light is produced as the UV light reacts with the phosphor envelope, but there are no mirrors. In the case of a laser gas tube, the mirrors at either end will then build up the familiar photon resonance, good population inversion and a high amplification rate of light will occur because of the energy generated from high current density in a tube of comparatively small cross-section, giving laser oscillation.

Metal vapour lasers currently used are mainly the copper and gold vapour systems. However, warm-up time is long, and at the time of writing there are problems maintaining a stable output and useful output power over extended periods. However future development may well make them a valuable addition to the range of visible light lasers, especially from the point of view of their multiwavelength capability for selective haemocoagulation applications. Figure 2.22 shows a schematic of a typical metal vapour laser.

Another member of the gas laser family is the excimer laser. *Excimer* stands for '*EXCI*ted di*MER*'. Excited dimers are unstable molecules which can exist only in an excited state. In the excimer laser, laser emission is caused by molecular disassociation. The main lasers used in the medical field are the xenon chloride (XeCl), krypton fluoride (KrFl) and the argon fluoride (ArFl). They all operate in the ultraviolet waveband, and deliver ultrashort pulses. They are mainly used in the ophthalmologic field for corneal sculpting in the procedure known as refractive keratoplasty. However, some applications in angioplasty for clearing plaque-blocked vessels are now appearing.

2-1-4-(B)   Solid State Lasers

If the laser medium consists of a solid material, then the system is classed as a solid state laser. A typical example is the neodymium yttrium-aluminium-garnet laser, commonly referred to as the Nd:YAG laser. The medium consists of a synthetic ion-doped crystal in the form of a rod. If the rod ends are polished and coated, then no external mirrors are needed, but the rod can be used with external multicoated mirrors, with antireflective

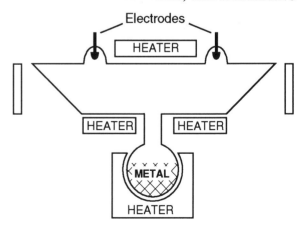

Fig 2.22: *Schema of a typical metal vapour laser.*

Table 2.3:   *Main solid state lasers in current clinical use and their characteristics*

LASER TYPE & WAVE-LENGTH	OUTPUT & POWER	SPECIFICS	APPLICATION
Ruby (Ru) 694.3 nm	Pulsed/Q-Switched Up to 200 J/pulse 100 MW (Q-switched pulse)	Visible red beam. Water-cooled, high-powered system	Dermatological applications for blood vessel anomaly group and some melanin anomaly group. Q-switched pulsed systems good for tattoo removal
Nd:Glass 1060	Pulsed Extremely high power	Near infrared beam. Glass is not a crystal, so can get very large medium, capable of generating very high powers.	Dermatological applications. Possible applications in laser-mediated fusion experiments.
Nd:YAG 1064	C/W: pulsed; Q-switched Up to 100 W in C/W, up to 10 J/pulse.	Near infrared beam. Wide scattering effect in tissue, good for deep coagulation. High power conversion efficiency	Wide variety of applications. Fibreoptic delivery enhances surgical flexibility. Used with sapphire tips in contact excisional surgery. Q-switched beam used in ophthalmology as photodisruptor.
Er:YAG 2.94 mm	C/W, pulsed or Q-switched. Up to around 2 W	Infrared beam, but well-absorbed in water	
Ho:YAG 2.1 mm	C/W, pulsed or Q-switched. Up to around 0.8 W	Infrared beam	Ophthalmologic applications as photodisruptor. Possible applications as low-powered laser scalpel
Alexandrite Tunable, 700-820 nm	C/W or pulsed, 10J: Q-switched, 1J Up to 10 W	Visible/ Near infrared beam. problems with stability.	Has the strong points of both ruby and Nd:YAG lasers: high repetition rate, with high energy per single pulse High efficiency Dermatologic applications. Ophthalmologic applications for retinal photocoagulation

coating on the rod ends. An optical source of pump energy, usually an arc lamp or flashlamp (krypton or xenon), is placed near the rod, surrounded by carefully designed reflectors, and the whole of the unit is usually encased in a water cooled jacket. Figure 2.23 shows a typical Nd:YAG laser design. When a different crystal is substituted for the Nd:YAG rod, then naturally the coated mirrors must also be changed, as the coating is wavelength-specific for each medium used.

These systems can be used as Q-switched systems, with the addition of a Pockels cell or another electro-optical or acousto-optic element. The mirrors can be either slightly concave, or plane surfaced, and a HeNe laser is often used through the same optical system as the guide beam for the invisible infrared Nd:YAG beam

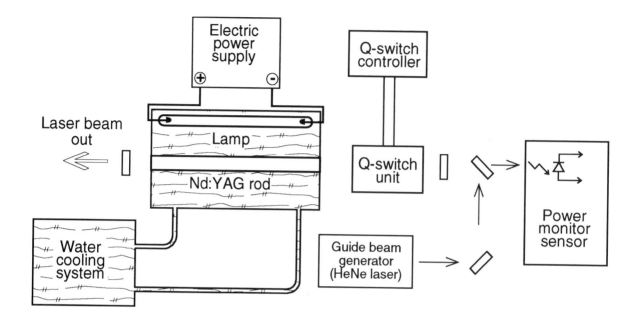

Fig 2.23 *Schema of typical Q-switched Nd:YAG laser system components.*

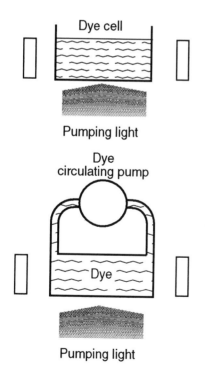

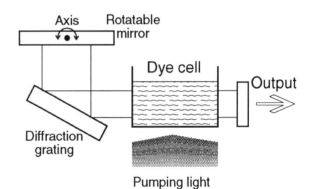

Fig 2.25: *Variable wavelength control from a dye laser employing an intracavity diffraction grating and a rotatable back mirror.*

(see Figure 2.23 above), although some systems use a non-laser light source. In both cases, the aiming beam shares the same axis as the treatment beam. Table 2.3 (previous page) summarizes the main members of the solid state laser group currently used in clinical applications.

Fig 2.24: *Two types of dye laser.*

Table 2.4:   *Dyes, characteristics and wavelengths*

Compound	Wavelength (nm)
p-Origophenylene group	
B M-terphenyl	308-360
p-terphenyl	322-365
Oxazole,ozadiazole derivatives: *inadequate - long rise oscillation time needed*	
PBD	352-388
POPOP	390-445
Stilbene derivatives: *low efficiency*	
stilbene 1	390-450
stilbene 2	403-493
Coumarin derivatives: *dye deteriorates quickly*	
4 MU	385-574
DAMC	440-505
coumarin 120	420-575
Xanthene group of dyes: *most popular, high efficiency*	
rhodamine 110	530-580
rhodamine 6G	560-650
rhodamine 101	610-690
Oxazine group of dyes: *high efficiency*	
cresyl violet	620-700
oxazine 1	695-800
Cyanine group of dyes: *important group in IR waveband*	
DOTCI	720-870
HITCI	780-930
DNXTPC	1107-1285

2-1-4-(C) Liquid Lasers

The liquid media can be subdivided into organic dyes, inorganic dyes, and organic chelate compounds (where a central metallic ion is attached to an organic molecule in two or more places) such as cobalt or chromium. Only organic dye lasers are in practical clinical use. The dye is contained in what is referred to as a dye cell, from which it can be fairly easily replaced when exhausted, or replaced with another dye to give a different wavelength. The cell is then pumped with either a powerful flashlamp or another laser to produce lasing action in the dye, and is easily cooled. Figure 2.24 shows a typical schematic of a dye laser set-up. In general, dye lasers can emit multiple wavelengths. By using a prism or an intracavity diffraction grating to select the desired resonant wavelength, selection of laser wavelengths is possible within a certain limit (Figure 2.25). Table 2.4 lists the dyes currently used and their characteristics.

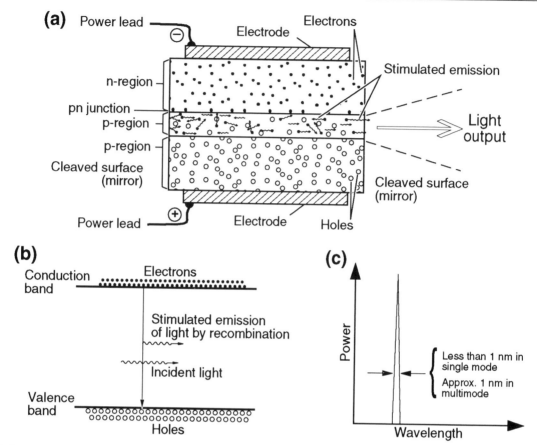

Fig 2.26: **a:** *Diagram of typical semiconductor (diode) laser. Recombination of electrons and holes in the active area of a p-n semiconductor generates photon emission when an electric current is applied to the electrodes.* **b:** *recombination illustrated schematically between electrons from the conduction band and holes from the valence band.* **c:** *typical waveband of diode laser, of less than 1 nm in single mode and approximately 1 nm in multimode application.*

2-1-4-(D)   Diode (Semiconductor) lasers

There are several hundred types of semiconductor lasers, but in practical applications the P-N junction type is usually used, as illustrated in Figure 2.26. In this type of laser, the P-N junction is the oscillation field. When a moderate electric current is passed through the semiconductor, radiative recombination of electrons and holes occurs in a forward bias operation (Figure 2.27). The recombination of electrons and holes generates photon emission, giving laser generation in appropriately-designed semiconductors (Figure

2.28). The simplest semiconductors tend to emit from the top and edges of the chip, but by cleaving two opposite surfaces they form the semireflective front and rear surfaces, with the adjacent surfaces being roughly etched to limit lateral modes. Note the highly divergent elliptical beam of generated laser emission from the front and rear surfaces of the example shown in Figure 2.28.

With an increase in applied power, the temperature of the diode will increase also, lowering the efficiency, so an effective cooling system,

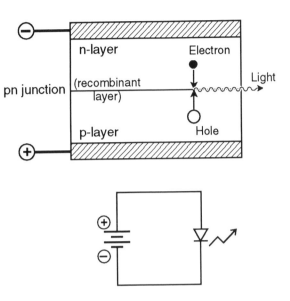

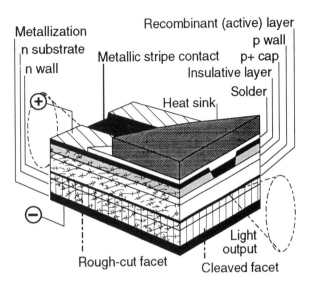

Fig 2.27:
Recombination in a schema of a diode laser (above) and a typical representative circuit (below) showing the symbols for a battery on the left and the light-emitting diode on the right of the circuit.

Fig 2.28:
Layer construction of a typical injection-stripe geometry epitaxial-layered double heterostructure (DH) GaAlAs edge transmission laser diode with directed emission. The heat sink is connected to the metallic stripe injector by a layer of solder to give efficient conduction of heat away from the stripe injector layer. The stripe geometry limits current distribution in the positively-charged p-cap and p-wall, thereby limiting the area of emission. The front and back walls of the diode are cleaved to give a semireflective facet, while the side walls are rough-sawn to eliminate lateral modes by allowing free passage of laterally-travelling photons out of the cavity. Note the highly divergent elliptical beam typical of this type of laser diode, emitted simultaneously from the front and rear facets.

usually involving bonded heatsinks, is necessary for efficient continuous operation. 1 to 3 volts is usually used as the constant operating level in this type of laser. The diode laser is an efficient energy converter, but because of its dielectric construction is very susceptible to damage from environmental static electricity. Diode lasers are very simple to use, and are reliable laser generators in the mW region, although some visible light diodes have been announced capable of generating an output of a few watts, up to 20 W being available at the time of writing. the most-used systems vary from the mW - 10 W range. Diodes are available which can give wavelengths from 630 nm to 3,000 nm, depending on the material of the chip. Applications are found in experimental equipment, low reactive-level laser therapy (LLLT), and in ophthalmology.

2-1-4-(E)   Other Laser Types

In the developmental stage at the time of writing are the chemical and free electron lasers, and are mentioned in this chapter simply because they are there. However, they are too complex, too large and above all too expensive for practical clinical application, but in the future they may well have practical applications. Figure 2.29 shows in schematic form a chemical laser: these lasers are analogous in operation to a flame thrower. The

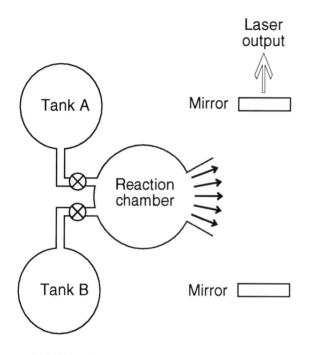

Fig 2.29: *"Flame-thrower" basis of a chemical laser.*

"flame thrower" forces a flame into the oscillator where a byproduct from a chemical reaction exists, and stimulated emission is induced.

The free electron laser uses a beam of electrons travelling at nearly the speed of light to produce a high-powered beam of laser radiation. The electrons are forced to travel through a system of transverse magnetic fields, which force a waveform on the electrons: this part of the system is called the wiggler (Figure 2.30). The energy source depends on the wave motion of the electrons which emits synchrotron radiation. A resonator can be formed by placing mirrors at both ends of this system, and laser oscillation can occur. By adjusting the magnetic field and the energy of the electrons, the laser wavelength can be tuned over a wide range. Peak powers are in the area of 10 MW and pulse width are in the picosecond range, with typical average powers of around 10 W.

In its preliminary development, the free electron laser could only oscillate within the infrared region. However recent reports have claimed oscillation in the UV band at 240 nm, although this was only in an experimental laboratory setting.

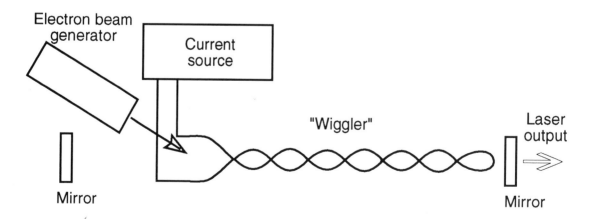

Fig 2.30: *Much simplified schematic of a free electron laser.*

2-1-5 OPTICAL ELEMENTS AND PARTS

It is very important to know and understand not only the theoretical aspect of lasers, but also to be familiar with the actual components found in a laser system. Occasionally, modification of a system already on the market will be required; sometimes system repair will be required; simply because there are many medical applications of the laser, and one configuration will not satisfy all clinical specialities' requirements.

When we consider any of the members of the electromagnetic spectrum, we have to visualize a plane of polarization in the electric component of the wave as it travels through space, as seen diagramatically in Figure 2.31. When this polarization plane is stable in any given time frame, it is referred to as linear polarization. Light emitted from a standard incandescent lamp has multiple planes of random polarization: in other words, nonpolarized light. If this light is then passed through a polarizer, we can get a linearly polarized beam from the lamp. Figure 2.32a shows the plane of polarization in a light beam and the polarizer, in this case a simple wire frame. In such a case, the electric component of the wave strikes the wire frame and is obstructed by it: it cannot pass through. But in 2.32b, the plane of polarization is rotated through 90°: the electric component of the beam can now pass unhindered through the wire frame polarizer. In a typical laser system, such a polarizer is often found in the so-called 'Brewster's Window', often found at either end of an argon laser and other gas laser tubes.

2-1-5-(A) Mirrors

the mirror has already been discussed as an essential part of the laser system. However, the laser mirror is not as simple as the mirror found in the home, or in a lady's handbag.

2-1-5-(A-1) Normal Coating

The standard household mirror is usually coated on the reverse side of the glass, into which we

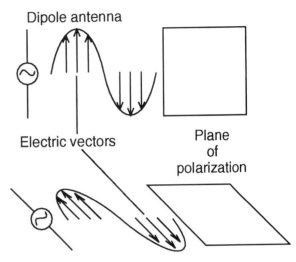

Fig 2.31:
The plane of polarization of a beam of em radiation is determined by the direction of the electric vectors of the beam, rather than the magnetic vectors.

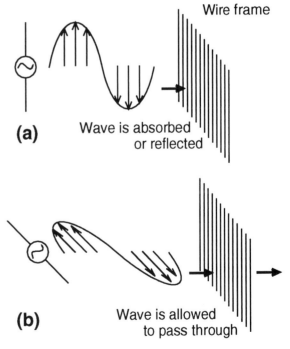

Fig 2.32:
Simple wire-frame polarizer will allow horizontal electric vectors to pass through but will prevent vertical vectors from passing by absorption or reflection.

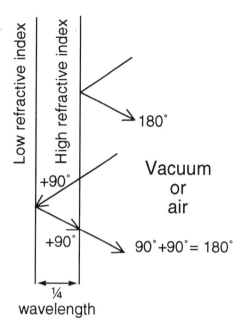

Fig 2.33:
Dielectric coating: a high refractive index coating on a glass substrate equal in thickness to one-quarter of the incident wavelength. Phase difference between beams reflected from the surface of the coating and the surface of the glass substrate is zero degrees, giving increased reflection rates by interference.

look to see our reflection. If such a reverse-face coating is used in a laser system, there will be a large amount of the incident energy reflected off the glass before it has a chance to be reflected correctly from the coating. Even if the optimum metallic coating is used as a reverse coating, it is impossible to achieve anywhere near 99% reflection in the visible light range, because of the problems of the absorption rate. in a high-powered laser system, the mirror would quickly heat up to the point where some form of distortion or even destruction would occur. The advantage of this type of mirror is the ease of manufacture, and even though it is not applicable in any application requiring extreme high quality at high power ranges, it will always find applications in everyday use.

2-1-5-(A-2) Dielectric Coating

If incident light is perpendicular to the boundary surface between two materials of different dielectric properties. the amplitude of the reflected light is expressed as follows:

$$R = \frac{n1 - n2}{n1 + n2}$$

where n1 and n2 represent the refraction indices of the materials. In the course of reflection from the boundary, the phase of the incident light will be altered. When light is transmitted from a low refractive index material to one with a high refractive index, the phase of the reflected light will be altered by 180° (π radian). In the opposite case, i.e. transmission from high to low refractive indices, the alteration will be 0°.

Let us consider the case where the surface of a plate of glass is coated with a material of a higher refractive index whose optical thickness is one-quarter of the incident wavelength [see subsection 2-1-5-(A-4) below]. In this case, the phase shift of the reflected light incident on the coated surface will be 180° from the first surface (the coating material) and 0° from the second surface (boundary between coating and glass). However, the reflected beam from that second surface must then re-enter the coating with a resultant phase shift of 180° (Figure 2.33). Thus the phase difference between the two beams is actually 0°, and they strengthen each other. When multilayered coatings of materials of alternating low and high refractive indices are employed, the reflection rate can be as high as 99.9%.

In the above principle the reflection rate depends on the relationship between the coating thickness and the specific wavelength to be reflected. If only one particular wavelength is required as the output from a laser, then this kind of mirror is very useful. This type of mirror can be constructed with a high damage threshold because it has a lower absorption rate compared with metal mirrors, and can thus be used in many high-powered laser systems.

2-1-5-(A-2)-(a) Wave and Particle Characteristics of Light

The phenomenon of the mutual strengthening of reflected light beams caused by the phase difference in optical thin films is recognized even in beams of noncoherent or weak light. This concept becomes very difficult to understand if we look at light as consisting of particles (the corpuscular theory already mentioned above). Accordingly, in modern physics we must adopt the concept that: "everything in this world occurs in waves," after which the above phenomenon can be more easily understood. For those readers not familiar with quantum dynamics, this concept may seem strange. We can thus further modify the above concept as follows: "the reason that light particles seem to exist is that energy transmission occurs as a discrete unit only where the waves interact, as if actual particles existed."

For example, light energy exists as a wave, and has the appearance of a particle only when the energy interacts with other particles such as electrons, protons, positrons and so on. The light we 'see' is not light which exists at the moment of seeing it, but is former light energy which has been extinguished in the act of absorption by the retina. There may well be some differences between the 'real' (or wave) world, and the world we actually see.

2-1-5-(A-2)-(b) Optical Thickness

The velocity of light in a vacuum (approximately 300,000 km/s) is different from the velocity of light through any other medium. Light velocity in a material (vM) is calculated as follows:

$$v\,\mathrm{M} = \frac{v\,\mathrm{V}}{ri\,\mathrm{M}}$$

where vV is the velocity in a vacuum and riM is the refractive index of the material.

For example, the velocity of light in a material with a refraction index of 2.0 would be 150,000 km/s. From the above equation it is obvious that the velocity of light in any material other than a vacuum will be less than 300,000 km/s: however, although the velocity is changed, the frequency remains constant. Thus if the wavelength of light in a given material is halved, and if the thickness of the thin film is 1 μm, the phase shift of incident light would be greater than the shift from a 1 μm thin film in a vacuum. In order to equalize the phase shift of the light in the material with that of a 1 μm thick film in a vacuum, given an index of refraction for the material of 2, the thickness of the material must be 0.5 μm. In other words, when a thin film has an index of refraction of 2 and a thickness of 0.5 μm, its optical thickness is equal to 1 μm.

2-1-5-(A-3) Beam Splitter

If a laser beam is to be divided into two (or more) components, then the easiest method is to employ a beam splitter. If only a few percent of the beam is required to be split off from the main beam, then the simplest beam splitter is a plane glass plate, arranged at the angle as seen in Figure 2.34. By applying the dielectric membrane coating as discussed above, it is thus possible by varying the thickness or the material of the coating to split off the desired percentage of the incident beam, and also control the rate of throughput.

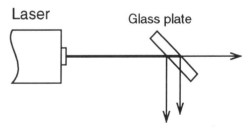

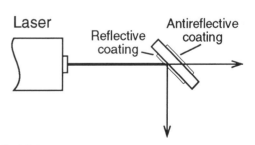

Fig 2.34:
Performance of a beam splitter, with and without reflective and antireflective dielectric coatings.

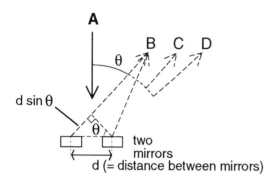

Fig 2.35:
Demonstration of the reflection principle of a mirrored diffraction grating.

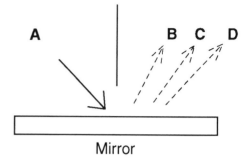

Fig 2.36:
Reflection from single mirrored surface must include total surface reflection. In actual practice, the reflected electric vectors at points C and D will be negligible, with the strongest light at point B.

2-1-5-(A-4) Diffraction Grating

There are many kinds of diffraction grating including, for example, the plane, concave, transmission and reflective types. In this section, I will explain the plane and reflection type. This type of grating is made of a refractive material, for example many metals, and has a flat surface etched with a series of many parallel linear groves, with a density of from 600 to 1200 lines per millimetre. As the angle of reflection depends on the wavelength, this type of grating is used in spectroscopes. The resolution of this device is much greater than a prism, because of which such a diffraction grating can be used in a wavelength-tunable laser resonator as the wavelength selection device.

Ex-1) Light Reflection and the Diffraction Grating

In a normal mirror, the angle of incidence is equal to the angle of reflection, but this rule does not hold true for a diffraction grating. The light waves can be reflected in many directions. In the case of a diffraction grating, mirrors of almost one wavelength in size are arrayed as in Figure 2.35. thus the light coming from point A will be reflected off separate mirrors. To simplify the illustration, only two mirrors are shown.

Consider the following situation. The incident light is perpendicular to the diffraction grating and the distance between the mirrors (d in figure 2.35) is comparatively short. In this example the optical distance from the left hand mirror to point B is different from the right-hand mirror to the same point. The difference is expressed as almost d sin θ (θ = angle of reflection). If this difference is equal to one wavelength, then the light is strengthened. If the difference is equal to one-half a wavelength, then the light is weakened, or is nearly zero. From the following, different wavelengths will thus reach point C or point D, respectively.

For continuous reflective surfaces such as mirrors, when calculating the reflection path it is necessary to take into account the total reflected light from the entire surface of the mirror. Consider Figure 2.36. Even when the incident light beam seems very small in diameter, light emitted from point A will reach almost the entire surface of the mirror. and will be reflected in many directions. Considering the sum of the electric vectors of the reflected light beams, however, the strongest light will be found at point B, with the value at points C and D equal to almost zero. This apparatus is used to prove the statement that the angle of incidence is equal to the angle of reflection.

2-1-5-(B)   Other Elements and Effects

2-1-5-(B-1) Beam Delivery Systems

When we want complete and accurate control of a laser beam during its use, then some method of flexible beam delivery must be used to carry the beam from the laser cavity to the desired target field. These fall into two main types: the flexible fibreoptic, and the multimirrored articulated arm. To achieve further sophistication in flexible fibre-optic-based systems, a beam splitter system can be used to allow the operation of multiple treatment rooms from the one laser source, increasing the cost-efficiency of the laser system to the institution.

2-1-5-(B-1)-(a) Laser Fibre

The first basic optical fibre was the homogeneous type as seen in Figure 2.37a. The incident light is propagated on through the fibre due to repeated internal reflection of the light at the boundary between the material of the fibre and the air. This type of fibre is very simple in construction, but if any other material is allowed to come in contact with the fibre, the condition of total internal reflection is destroyed, and light may leak out of the fibre.

An improvement to this design of fibre was the step type of fibre, comprising a central core of a high refractive index surrounded by a cladding material with a lower index. The step type fibre has a homogeneous refractive index in the core, and resembles a 'step', hence the name. Light is propagated on through the fibre by total internal reflection at the junction between the core and the cladding (Figure 2.37b).

The third type of fibre, the graded type, is also a step-type of fibre, but has a gradient of refraction in the core. The light is propagated along the fibre, gradually changing direction to the centre of the core which has a high refractive index (Figure 2.37c).

Quartz fibres cannot transmit all wavelengths, however. The transmission range is from 200 nm in the ultraviolet to 3,000 nm in the

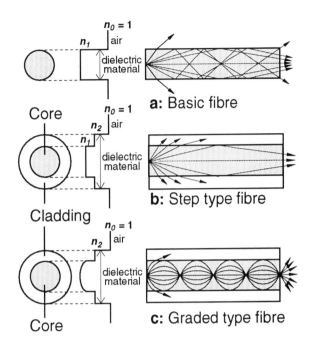

Fig 2.37:
Schematic showing differences between a basic optical fibre, and two types of stepped optical fibres.

infrared, with the optimum around 1,500 nm. In order efficiently to transmit wavelengths greater than 3,000 nm, such as the CO_2 laser wavelength of 10,600 nm, a different fibre is required, or another means of beam transmission. Many compounds have been tried for the CO_2 fibre, but they were potentially poisonous or had other problems, and so had not found widespread practical application. Recently the AgCl/AgBr fibre has been developed, and is used mainly in the fibrescope. The most practical method of CO_2 beam transmission in dermatological applications remains the multimirrored articulated arm.

2-1-5-(B-1)-(b) Multimirrored Articulated Arm

For those wavelengths where a fibre is not yet a practical means of transmission, or where output power is unusually high, the mechanical articulated arm has to serve as the light guide, fitted at the joints with mirrors specially coated to reflect

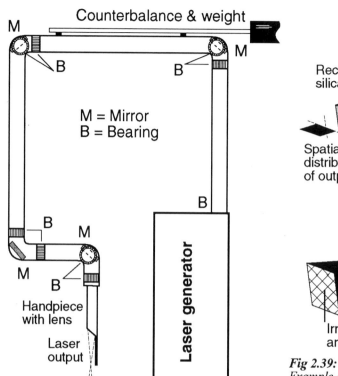

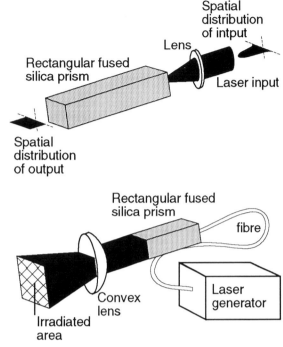

Fig 2.38:
Schematic of a multi-mirrored articulated arm, most commonly used for transmission of CO_2 laser energy from the laser generator to the target surface.

Fig 2.39:
Example of a kaleidoscope system designed to give a homogeneous beam output from a nonhomogeneous input (for example, Gaussian distribution). (Upper) Principle of the system. (Lower) Schema of practical system component arrangement.

the wavelength being transmitted. Figure 2.38 shows a schematic of such an arm, with the mirrors in the joints fitted at an angle of 45°. Such an arm will usually allow flexibility with the ability to move the handpiece at the end of the arm through three degrees of freedom. The disadvantages of such an articulated arm are: limitation in length, thus keeping the laser system very close to the sterile operative field; problems with the alignment of the mirrors; and a problem with inertia, causing the arm to continue to move, even after the handpiece has been held still.

2-1-5-(B-1)-(c) Kaleidoscope System

In the usual single mode Gaussian beam distribution, the power density is greater in the centre of the beam, and decreases towards the periphery. When this type of beam is used in the treatment

of naevi, the treatment results will thus not be equal at the centre and at the periphery of the treatment beam, which may well result in unequal colour removal in the area after treatment.

Many methods have been considered to try to equalize the power distribution in a Gaussian beam, to give an equal power density at any point the beam. Using a fibreoptic-based delivery device, for example, alters the mode-locking of the beam, and gives a more homogeneous multimode beam, depending on the quality of the optics in the system. The kaleidoscope system is however considered the most efficient delivery device for giving good homogeneity of the treatment beam. The construction is shown in Figure 2.39. The rectangular or square rod is made from a transparent material, and the light is transmitted by re-

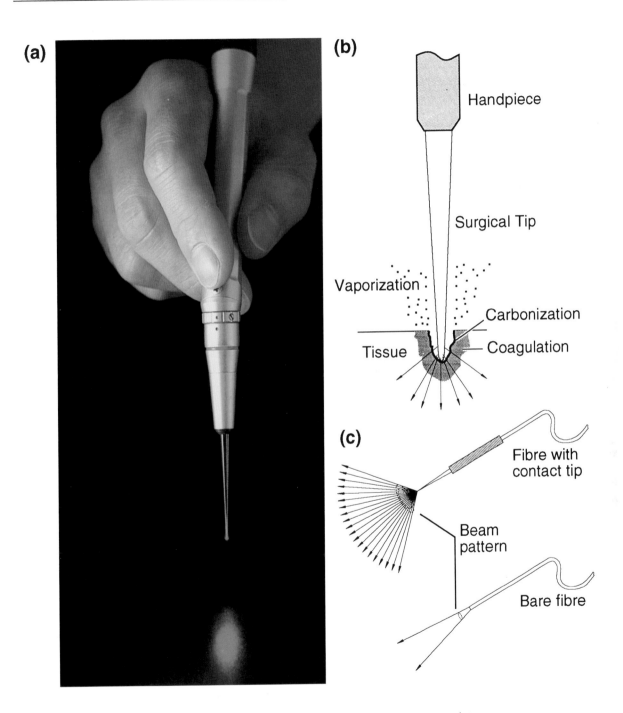

Fig 2.40: *Example of and principles behind sculpted contact surgical tips.*

flecting many times from the boundary surface of the rod.

By moving forward a certain distance, the light distribution at the tip of the rod can be very even. A convex lens is placed near the rod tip which projects an image of the tip on the treatment area. The light distribution in this image is excellent, and is capable of giving a high-quality beam for use in laser treatment of naevi.

2-1-5-(B-1)-(d) Sculpted Surgical Contact Tips

The main difference between a conventional scalpel and the laser 'light knife' is the lack of tactile response when cutting target tissue. Surgeons are trained to use this tactile response to judge depth of cut, tissue being incised, etcetera. In order to return tactile feedback to the surgical laser, the contact laser scalpel or 'light rod' was developed. Examples are seen in Figure 2.40.

The Nd:YAG laser has been mainly used for this application. Laser energy enters the contact tip at its connection with the fibre optic delivery

cable, and is conveyed to the cutting tip or edge of the tip by multiple internal reflection. the power density at the tip is very high, high enough to cut tissue, but the surgeon can still retain some degree of tactile feedback between the delivery device and the tissue. In addition to incising, the contact tips offer a high degree of haemostasis. Some laser systems, notably the KTP/532 system from Laserscope (CA, USA), have delivery devices designed to use the bare fibre in incision, vaporization and coagulation, without the need for an ancillary tip.

2-1-5-(B-2) Luminescent Elements

The following are devices which are used to give some form of light output for pumping.

2-1-5-(B-2)-(a) Arc Lamp

An arc lamp is shown schematically in Figure 2.41. The basic structure consists of a transparent quartz or glass envelope, filled with an appropriate gas, in which are situated bipolar electrodes. A powerful electric current is passed between the

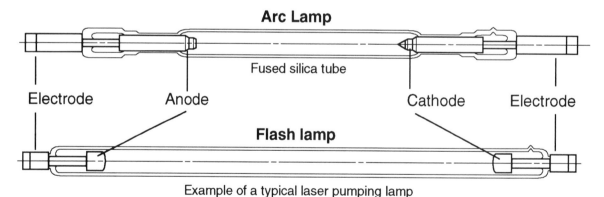

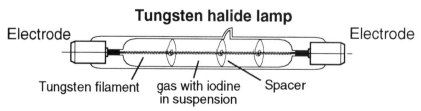

Fig 2.41: *Typical cross-sections of an arc lamp, a flash lamp and a quartz tungsten-halide lamp. Note the different designs of the electrodes in the arc and flash lamps to minimize wear and maximize lamp life.*

elements and forms a discharge. A popular example of a form of arc lamp is the common fluorescent tube. Xenon and krypton arc lamps are usually used as the energy pump source in laser systems, but in order to strike the arc, an extremely high trigger voltage is needed, so this adds to the complexity of the electronics circuitry.

2-1-5-(B-2)-(b) Flash Lamp

The flash lamp (Figure 2.41) is very similar in structure to the arc lamp, but it is constructed to provide a brief powerful flash of light from the application of a pulsed strong current. The difference from the arc lamp, designed to produce continuous output with a smaller current, is found in larger electrodes of a slightly spherical shape. A high uniformity of discharge is obtained on the electrode surface in order to prevent the destruction of the electrodes by the very strong trigger current.

2-1-5-(B-2)-(c) Tungsten Lamp

The tungsten filament lamp is one of the most popular domestic light sources, and is also used for automotive light bulbs, etcetera. The bulb consists of a glass envelope, which may be filled with an inert gas, in which the fine tungsten filament is suspended from supporting posts, which also carry the current to the filament. As electric current passes through the filament, because the resistance of tungsten is comparatively high, it generates a lot of heat, and the filament becomes incandescent, providing both light and heat. It is not efficient enough to be used as a pump source.

A more efficient form of filament-based light is the quartz-halide or halogen lamp. These lamps are filled with a suspension of a halide in gas, usually iodine, and the iodine reacts with the incandescent tungsten filament to help effect repair of any damage. This gives these lights a much longer life and makes them brighter than conventional tungsten filament lamps. They have many applications including projector and microscope lamps. They still cannot emit as much light as a flash lamp or arc lamp and the time rise is longer,

so their application in laser systems is limited to continuous pumping.

Arc lamps are in many ways superior to halogen lamps, but the halogen lamp has the advantage of a low operation voltage and no need for triggering, so the driver circuits can be very simple.

2-1-5-(B-2)-(d) Light Emitting Diode and Laser Diode

The basic principle of radiative recombination at the P-N junction of the diode chip has been covered already. Light emitting diodes or LED's, (also called luminescent diodes) are used as indicator lamps, as they draw a minimum current, yet provide a comparatively bright light. Figure 2.42a (left) shows a typical light emitting, or luminescent, diode, with the chip set in a reflector to catch and reflect the light emitted from the lateral edges of the chip. They emit very narrow-band light,

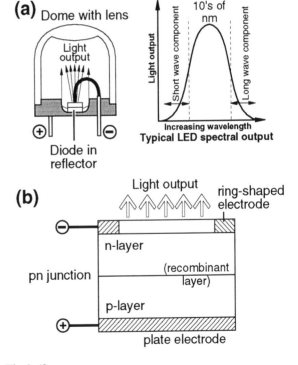

Fig 2.42:
Schematics of light-emitting diodes (LEDs). **a:** *(Left) Multi-surface emission chip mounted in a reflector and incorporating a lens in the covering dome. (Right) typical LED narrow waveband spectral output.* **b:** *Directed-emission ring electrode LED.*

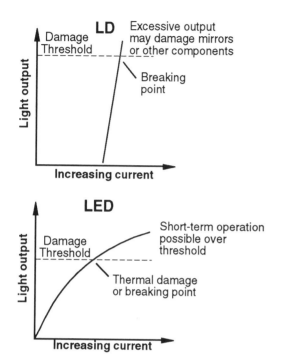

Fig 2.43:
Comparison of the input/output characteristics and damage thresholds of a typical LED and a laser diode.

almost monochromatic, but noncoherent (Figure 2.42(a), left), and demonstrate good linearity between the degree of current passed through the chip and the light output. Figure 2.42(b) shows a schematic of the ring-electrode type of LED with directed output.

Laser diodes give a 'brighter' light, because they emit partially coherent light at a quite narrow waveband. Laser diodes are now being used as pump sources for Nd:YAG and other solid state lasers, because their energy conversion efficiency is extremely high, and they are now capable of delivering over 25 W in continuous wave.

Semiconductor lasers, however, have a very narrow current range within which they operate at maximum efficiency with no damage (Figure 2.43). A small change in current can dramatically shorten the life time of the diode chip.

2-1-5-(B-3) *Electro-optic effects*

Application and elements of electro-optic and acousto-optic effects: An electro-optic effect (EOE) is defined as the alteration of the physical properties of a material, such as its index of refraction, by applying an electric potential across the material. There are two classes of effect: Pockels effect, and kerr effect, which in turn give their names to the electro-optic unit as a Pockels cell or a kerr cell. The Pockels effect is a primary EOE, while the kerr effect is a secondary EOE (Figure 2.44(a)): a primary EOE is defined as an effect where the volume of the effect is relative to the applied potential difference, and a secondary effect where the effect volume is relative to the square of the PD. Pockels cells are usually constructed from such materials as ADP, KDP and $LiNbO_3$. Kerr cells are constructed of nitrobenzene or CS_2. Such cells are usually used as an electronic shutter, combined with a polarizer. Figure 2.44(b) (upper) shows a schematic of a typical Pockels cell. Electrodes are attached to a crystal demonstrating a Pockels effect, thus enabling its use as an electronic shutter. When the voltage across the cell terminals is zero, then the cell allows the transmission of light through it. When a certain voltage is applied across the terminals, it causes a difference in the refraction index between the horizontal and vertical directions. When polarized light has a 45° inclination, the light can be analyzed into an x- and a y-component (Figure 2.44(b), lower).

As has already been discussed, the velocity of light in a material is determined by the material's index of refraction. In the case of the Pockels cell, on applying voltage across the terminals the vertical refractive index will differ from the horizontal. The frequency is not changed, but the wavelength will change. When a voltage equivalent to one-half of the incident wavelength is applied, a phase difference of 180° will be seen as the beam passes through the crystal. Figure 2.44b shows a schematic representation of these two components. Note that the direction of polarization is rotated through exactly 90°. In such an example, the polarizer on the opposite side of the cell must be rotated, or light will not pass through.

Exp-1: Acousto-optic Effect

The acousto-optic effect (AOE) phenomenon acts very much in the same way as the EOE described above, except that the distortion is caused by acoustic wave distortion of the cell material, rather than an electrically-generated dealignment. The ultrasonic wave causes a periodic change in the concentration of the cell material. This change is subdivided in to two classes: Bragg diffraction and Raman-Nas diffraction. Suitable materials for this kind of cell are GaAs, $LiNbO_3$, SiO_2, Al_2O_3 and TeO_2. Both EOE and AOE switches can be used as the spoiler in Q-switching systems, dealt with in detail below.

2-1-5-(B-4) Application and Elements of Non-linear Optical Effects

When listening to a radio or Hi-Fi system at an appropriate volume, the sound is clear and true across the entire frequency range for which the systems speakers were constructed. In other words, the sound waves are coming out in a pure waveform. If the volume is turned up so that the output exceeds the wattage for which the speakers were designed, the sound becomes distorted because of the inability of the speaker cone to handle the loading imposed on it. In other words, the waveforms have been distorted from the pure waveforms being generated before, creating extra 'sounds' not in the original signal. This distortion of waveforms can also be found in light waves when passed through certain materials, for example certain crystals, as shown schematically in Figure 2.45. When the light beam is of low amplitude, the incident and emergent waves are the same. When the amplitude is increased, depending on the crystal lattice structure, the emergent

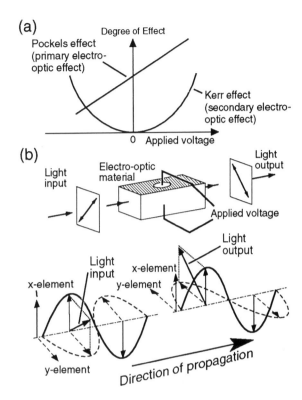

Fig 2.44:
a: *Difference demonstrated between primary and secondary electrooptical effects.* **b:** *(Upper) Typical Pockels cell in operation as a light shutter. (Lower) Analysis of x- and y- components of 45° polarized light.*

waveforms are distorted, changing the frequency of the wave, and thus altering the wavelength. Such nonlinear effects are used in frequency-doubling crystals, which are capable, for example, of giving an emergent visible green 532 nm beam from an incident 1064 nm Nd:YAG beam. Representative materials are KTP ($KTiOPO_4$), KDP, ADP, BBO and LN ($LiNbO_3$).

2-1-5-(B-5) Photoreceptor Devices

These devices detect and absorb photons, transforming them into an electronic signal. Photocells, CdS cells and solar cells are all included in this category of device. Specific types of photoreceptor devices will now be examined.

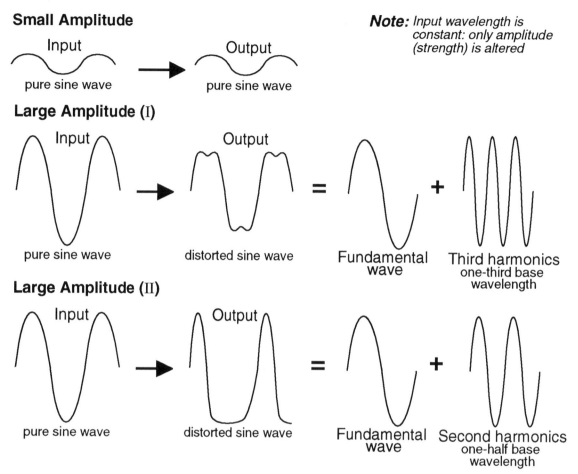

Fig 2.45: *Distortion of light waveforms resulting in production of third and second harmonics.*

2-1-5-(B-5)-(a) PIN Photodiode

The PIN photodiode has the P and N structure, and an intrinsic semiconductor zone. (Figure 2.46) The reaction speed of these materials is extremely fast, better than 1 ns, and sub nanosecond devices are now available. The linearity between the input signal and output signal is excellent (Figure 2.47), so PIN photodiodes are often used in laser output monitors. Many laser diodes now include a PIN photodiode already built into the chip mounting as standard, to allow constant and accurate detection of the laser output. Re-

verse bias voltage is usually applied to this type, and forward current is not usually used.

2-1-5-(B-5)-(b) Avalanche Photodiode

The avalanche photodiode (Figure 2.48) is very similar in structure to the PIN photodiode. Although the reaction time of this photodetector is much shorter than the PIN photodiode, the linearity between input and output signals is not so good because of the avalanche breakdown phenomenon. This type of photodiode is used in the measurement of picosecond laser pulses or for high speed digital communication.

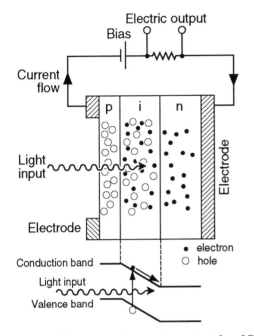

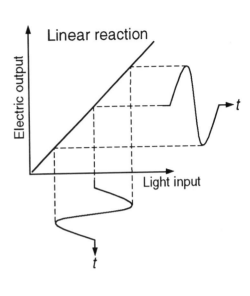

Fig 2.46: *Schematic of operation principle of PIN photodiode.*

Fig 2.47: *Demonstration of input/output linearity of PIN photodiode.*

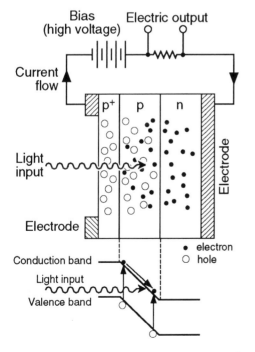

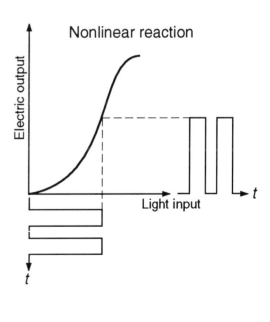

Fig 2.48: *(Left) Construction and operation of an avalanche photodiode and (right) nonlinear input/output.*

2-1-6 LASER CONTROL TECHNOLOGY

There are many methods of controlling the laser beam once it has been generated in the cavity, including alteration of the cavity itself, and some form of modulation applied to the beam once it has exited the cavity, or a combination of both of those.

2-1-6-(A) Generation of Pulsed Laser Beam

When considering a strong pulse of light, a good example is the photographic flash. In the standard flashgun, a capacitor circuit builds up a very strong electric charge, which is released on demand as an extremely high voltage trigger pulse, which causes a very short pulse of brilliant light as this electrical discharge is applied to the flash tube. Pulse widths are usually less than one millisecond. Immediately after discharge, the level of electric charge is zero, until the capacitor is once again fully charged and ready to fire. The same principle is applied to flashlamp-pumped laser systems, where the powerful arc lamp pumps the medium in the cavity with an intense beam of powerful light energy: the medium responds by generating a single intense millisecond or submillisecond pulse of high power laser energy, thus giving us the simplest form of short-pulse pulsed laser. To stabilize the output, a simmer mode is added, whereby the trigger voltage is applied, and then a low current is continually applied from the simmer current source, and so the electrical discharge continues. The simmer mode is particularly useful in generating stable Q-switched pulses of laser energy.

2-1-6-(B) Q-Switched Laser

In the case of a ruby laser, the active medium is a synthetic ruby crystal. When pumped with an ultrashort beam of intense light, the ruby crystal responds with a comparatively long pulse, as the active elements in the crystal have a long excited life: the typical ruby pulse is seen as a large peak power, followed by a series of random smaller peaks as the crystal gradually returns from the

excited to the normal state. It is possible to change the 'quality' of the cavity, so that all of the power is released in one single, ultrashort, very high powered pulse, and the switch that can do this is called the quality-switch, or Q-switch for short. In a Q-switched system, the quality of the cavity is controlled by a switch placed between one of the mirrors and the medium, usually the rear mirror, and when activated, it denies access to that mirror: thus although many of the photons in the cavity are lost, population inversion continues to increase, placing more electrons in the excited state and generating very high levels of spontaneous and stimulated emission. The switch is then activated, releasing all the pent-up energy in the cavity in a single, powerful, ultrashort pulse. This is shown diagramatically in Figure 2.49. With

1: Initial pumping

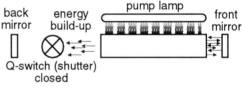

2: Energy build-up and storage

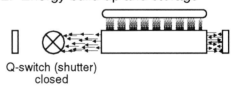

3: Energy release and oscillation

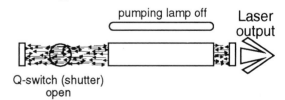

Fig 2.49:
Principle of the three stages in high-powered ultrashort pulse generation by Q-switching in a flash-lamp-pumped pulsed laser.

such high-powered pulses, optical components with a high damage threshold must be used.

The quality (Q) of the resonator can be expressed as follows:

$$Q = 2\pi \times \frac{\text{Total Energy Stored in Cavity}}{\text{Energy Lost in Single Cycle}}$$

Thus if the energy lost in a single cycle increases, the quality decreases, and conversely if the value of energy lost decreases, the quality increases. There are many types of Q-switch (Figure 2.50).

2-1-6-(B-1) Mechanical Q-Switch

This type of switch depends on a rotating or vibrating mirror. When the mirror is rotated or vibrates, the usual oscillation does not occur, but there is a constant build-up of energy within the medium. Restoring the mirror to its normal state allows this built-up energy to be swiftly released. depending on the speed of rotation or vibration of the mirror, microsecond or nanosecond levels of pulses can be obtained, and repeated to provide a train of ultrashort pulses separated with a comparatively long interpulse interval: this is the basis for the quasi-continuous wave laser.

2-1-6-(B-2) Ultrasonic Wave Q-Switch

This type of switch depends on the acousto-optic effect for its action. With this method, pulse widths of 100 ns are obtainable, which can also be repeated in a train of quasi-continuous wave pulses.

2-1-6-(B-3) Electro-optic Effect Q-Switch

The EOE has already been discussed above. Practically-speaking, the Pockels Cell Q-switch is very popular, especially in pulsed flashlamp-pumped laser systems, giving nanosecond levels of pulsing, or shorter. Q-switching proceeds as follows.

During flash-lamp activation, a one-quarter wavelength voltage is placed across the Pockels cell so that the light from the cavity passes through the polarizer and the Pockels cell, and returns back through the cell, but is therefore out of phase by a total of one half of its wavelength, having now passed through the cell twice. This

gives a 90° difference in linear polarization of that light, so that it cannot pass through the polarizer into the medium, and so the quality of the cavity is spoiled, and oscillation cannot occur, although the energy levels in the medium are constantly rising. At the end of the pump flashlamp pulse, the voltage to the Pockels cell is rapidly decreased, the energy being lost to the oscillation process is restored, the quality of the resonator increases suddenly and dramatically, and a single ultrashort giant pulse is generated from megawatts to hundreds of megawatts in output power, provided the system has remained undamaged.

2-1-6-(B-4) Dye Saturation Q-Switch

In some types of dye, absorption of light will continue until the saturation point of the dye is reached, at which point the dye becomes transparent. The dye saturation Q-switch is constructed by inserting such a type of dye cell in the resonator. When the dye becomes transparent, strong

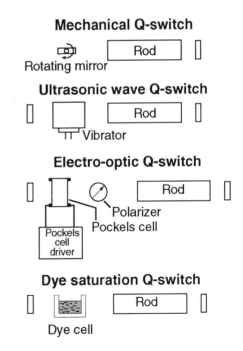

Fig 2.50: *Different methods of Q-switching*

oscillation will occur. This kind of Q-switch is easy to construct, but the life of the dye is short, so maintenance is a problem.

2-1-6-(C) Stabilization of Laser Output

It is more difficult to stabilize the output of medical laser systems than many other medical instruments. However, some extent of stability must be reached, or consistency and repeatability of the treatment method may be lowered, and there may also be some danger to operator or patient.

Causes of change in output include change of temperature, humidity, fluctuations in the voltage of the power supply or current, maladjustment of a mirror by external vibration, air-borne dust, deterioration of an optical element, contamination of the cooling water, and so on. The following steps are followed to counter any influence from the above factors:

1)

Sta-1) Stabilization of the electric voltage or power supply

Sta-2) Current stabilization of the pumping lamp or laser tube

Sta-3) Purification of the cooling water

Sta-4) Stabilization of working temperature and humidity

Sta-5) Incorporation into the equipment of some form of shock absorbing mechanism

Sta-6) Filtration to remove air-borne contaminants, such as dust.

Many medical laser systems already incorporate these steps: in some systems from areas of low temperature and humidity, however, some of these precautions may be lacking, which will necessitate partial modification before such systems can be used with confidence.

Other techniques of output stabilization include negative feed-back control, where there is a power monitor connected to a current controller, so that the current to the laser tube or lamp is automatically changed depending on the monitoring of the output by the control circuit. When the output falls below the correct level, power to the cavity will be increased, and vice-versa. This type of control technology can therefore maintain laser system output within a certain region.

2-1-7 BASIC LASER QUANTIFICATION

In the clinical and experimental applications of laser, it is extremely important to decide all irradiation conditions and parameters in order to achieve the desired results and effect in the target tissue. Of particular importance are the power and energy densities, and the individual components which go to make up these values. Even more important that deciding on these parameters, is the correct reporting of them so that other researchers or clinicians can faithfully duplicate the experimental or clinical protocol, in order to corroborate the results, or to achieve the same clinical effect as originally reported. Correct, complete and accurate reporting of parameters is thus essential when reporting experimental or clinical protocols in the literature, and the following list is the minimum description necessary. Please provide:

Pa-1) Laser Details
The Laser type, model number or name and the name of the manufacturer

Pa-2) Wavelength
The wavelength of the system

Pa-3) Power at Tissue
The output power, incident to the tissue (watts [W] or milliwatts [mW]). If it is a pulsed laser, then provide the pulse width, the interpulse interval, the peak power, but above all the *average power*.

Pa-4) Spot Size
The spot size (irradiation area) per exposure, expressed either as the diameter or as the area (cm^2)

Pa-5) Power density
From the incident power and the spot size, the power density can be obtained, in W/cm^2

Pa-6) Energy and Energy Density

The exposure time per shot (in seconds), per session, and the total number of sessions. By multiplying the incident power by the exposure time, the incident energy in J can be calculated. By multiplying the power density by the exposure time, the energy density can be obtained, in J/cm².

Only if the researcher and clinician provides all of these parameters will others be able to repeat their work: repetition of work for corroboration of results is the backbone of scientific research, and underpins the ability to achieve consistent surgical effects in the actual treatment of patients.

2-1-7-(A) Measurement of Power and Energy

Commercially-available power meters can be used for this purpose, which will usually consist of the detector portion and a display console of some kind. There are many kinds of detectors.

Exp-1) Surface Absorption Type

The surface absorption type consists of a thermodetector coupled to a coating of a material of high optical density, which is capable of measurement of comparatively low peak pow-

ers, i.e. below 500 kW/cm². The response time is relatively short.

Exp-2) Multireflection Type

The multireflection type is another type of surface absorption detector, but it is capable of measuring comparatively high peak powers of over 100J, but the response time is slower than the normal surface absorption type.

Exp-3) Body Absorption Type

The body absorption type detector consists of a thermodetector coupled to a thick absorbing medium with a relatively low optical density. Because of the low rate of thermal conduction, the time needed to complete a measurement with this type is relatively long, for example from 10 s to 100 s. It is however much more able to resist damage from high peak powers in excess of 10 GW.

Exp-4) Nonthermal Detectors

Solar cells and PIN photodiodes are employed in the nonthermal type of power detector. Because of the nature of the detector elements, there is not a flat sensitivity distribution over a wide waveband, so some kind of internal calibration control circuit is required for measurements over a wide waveband.

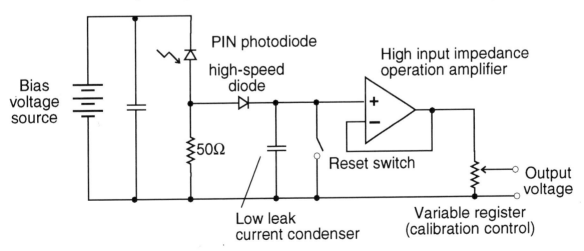

Fig 2.51: *Circuitry for construction of a typical peak power meter.*

2-1-7-(A-1) Measurement of Pulse Peak Power
There are several methods for measuring the peak power of a laser pulse. After measuring the energy of a single pulse, the pulse width should then be obtained (see below) and the peak power is calculated by the following equation:

$$\text{Peak Power} \approx \frac{\text{Energy (J)}}{\text{PulseWidth (s)}}$$

Otherwise, a peak power meter can be used. This can be constructed by using a PIN photodiode connected with a peak-hold circuit (Figure 2.51).

2-1-7-(A-2) Measurement of Pulse Width and Waveform
Solar cells can be used for the measurement of pulse widths down to and around 30 - 40 ms. For measurement of shorter pulse widths than that, systems based on PIN photodiodes or avalanche photodiodes are used. Pulses of 200 ps or more can be measured using high-speed PIN photodiodes. Avalanche photodiodes are capable of measuring shorter pulse widths, but distortion may occur in the measured waveform, and some form of corrective circuit may be necessary.

The detectors convert incident light signals into electric signals, which are sent to storage or sampling oscilloscopes, where the electric signal is converted to a visible signal on the oscilloscope cathode ray tube (CRT). naturally, an oscilloscope with a suitably high response speed is necessary for the measurement of ultrashort pulses.

There are many definitions of pulse width, which is usually calculated as the period of duration of above half the peak power.

2-1-7-(B) Measurement of Spot Size
The easiest way to measure the spot size of a laser is to irradiate a piece of 'footprint' paper (a black coating on a contrasting backing), and then to measure the diameter of the resulting spot with a rule.

For measurement of CO_2 laser spot size, provided the output power is sufficient, the flat surface of a styrofoam or formed plastics block can be irradiated, and the diameter of the entry hole measured with a rule.

With homogeneous high-power beams, these methods are quite satisfactory. An inhomogeneous or low-powered beam cannot be accurately measured by the above methods, and a graphic display of the power distribution must be produced.

A pin hole is made in an opaque plate, and the plate is attached to some method of easily determining the position of the plate, such as a micromanipulator. The output power is then measured with the plate in several positions, while the laser delivery device remains fixed. The relationship between the power and the positions is then plotted on a sheet of paper, by connecting the spots of equal power. This will give a series of contour lines representing the spatial distribution of the power in the beam. If the result is circular, the spot size can be measured. A practical spot size is usually regarded as the diameter of the area with over $1/e$ of the maximum power distribution. If required, however, the following items may be included in the report, especially if it is a report directed to a government agency to determine the safety and efficiency of a laser device.

i)   The diameter of the area over 90% of the maximum power distribution.

ii) The diameter of the area over 10% of the maximum power distribution.

In the event of the pinhole method not producing a rough circle, then the shape and its area should be described and calculated, together with the graphic representation of the power distribution.

2-2 LASER AND BIOLOGIC REACTION

When we look at the origin of the word *laser*, we must never forget that the 'L' in laser stands for 'light'. We tend to take light so much for granted, when in fact it is a most essential factor in our life. The sun is our most important light source, and has been shining constantly for around 6 billion years. With its brief, thirty-plus years of existence, the laser is a mere light-child. Having dis-

cussed above the physical properties and basics of the laser, in this section some of the clinical history of medical applications of light will be explored, and the reader will be introduced to how light, and laser energy, interact with tissue. The role of the laser in laser medicine and laser surgery will also be examined.

2-2-1 HISTORY OF THE MEDICAL APPLICATION OF PHOTOTHERAPY

Before examining the medical implications and applications of the light-tool we call the laser, we will look at the influence of light on our very living, and at the early applications of light in medicine; the origins and development of phototherapy, of which medical and surgical laser applications form a part.

2-2-1-(A) Light and Life

For the vast majority of living things, plant or animal, light is essential to life. There are very few exceptions: some kinds of lichen can live in caverns which have never seen the light of day. A very few species of marine life live in the depths of the ocean, in complete darkness, too deep for the penetration of even a feeble glimmer of the sun's rays. For the rest of us, on or near the surface of the continents and oceans, light can be equated with life. Even at night there is a trace of light, from the moon, or stars.

Light enables plants to carry on their endless task of photosynthesis, and plants will actively seek light when deprived of it, growing towards the feeblest of light sources. In fact, the food cycle could be said to depend on light: photosynthesis stores energy in plants, and filters carbon dioxide from the atmosphere, replacing it with oxygen during the daylight hours. The energy-rich plants provide fodder for herbivorous animals, and in doing so release a small fraction of the stored energy into the bodies of the animals which eat the plants. The animals are in turn eaten by other carnivorous creatures, passing an even-smaller

quantity of that original light-mediated energy on to the consumer. The death of these creatures transfers that tiny portion of energy, through decay, to the earth, and back once again to the plants, so the cycle begins all over again.

Animals have their lives governed by light, the circadian cycle, even those animals which are nocturnal by evolution. Interfering with the natural light-dark cycle can cause biological abnormalities: night-shift workers, for example, and those whose style of work forces them to turn night into day, and sleep during the daylight hours, will often demonstrate a lowered autoimmune system: in the case of females, menstrual irregularities can and do occur. Battery hens are stimulated to lay eggs at a greater rate by keeping them in an artificial environment with an accelerated light-dark cycle.

It has been suggested that cells transcribe and store information in their genetic materials, from the light which first activated them. Re-exposure to light, carrying the same information, can thus bring about reactivation of the cell, or activation to a different state than normal. This could explain that some processes which do not require light, or which at least usually take place in darkness, can be activated by light, such as repair and replication of UV-damaged DNA.

All living beings are based on some form of cellular structure, from the monocellular protozoic amoebae to the complex multicytotype structure of the mammal, including the human being. We depend on the cell for our life, and the cell in turn depends on other influences for its life, including, of course, light. Light has played an enormously important role in the building of what we recognize as 'life'. The formation and the production of the first primitive cell, a simple non-nucleated DNA-containing envelope: light-mediated changes in the primordial 'soup' in which the cell developed to form a membrane-enclosed cytoplasm surrounding a clearly bordered nucleus: the addition of motion with the development of a single flagellum: the first grouping of cells to make a primitive multicellular life form: in all of these processes, light has probably played some role. The three simple cells forms, the non-nucleated prokaryote, the nucleated eukaryote and the mobile flagellate can all find family members in the human cell structure. Viruses and bacteria are prokaryotes: normal mammalian cells, including fibroblasts, mast cells, lymphocytes and other leukocytes, are eukaryotic; and spermatozoa are flagellates. Cells respond to exogenous stimuli, as do we as human beings: they need to eat, to breathe, and to replicate. Most of all, they respond to light.

The first living cells are reckoned to have appeared 3.5 billion years ago, and for even 2.5 billion years before that, the sun was the most important source of light, and life, to this earth, and continues to be so. We tend to take it for granted, however, especially as we have "tamed" the force of electricity to enable us to flood the night with light at the flick of a switch. With the flick of a different switch, we can turn on a man-made light source which can, point for point, outshine the sun in brilliance. It is natural that, having used the curative powers of the sun for centuries, we should want to explore the therapeutic properties and medical potentials of our powerful light-child, the laser.

2-2-1-(B) History of Phototherapy

The history of the use of the laser in medicine and surgery is comparatively recent, just over 30 years, in fact. A laser is simply a specialized form of light-producing tool, and the use of light in medicine has a much longer pedigree. Before going on to examine the clinical applications of the laser, it is important to look first at the earlier medical applications of light, or phototherapy. The first phototherapeutic source was, of course, the sun. Before looking at the development of heliotherapy, the specific application of sunlight in medicine, let us look briefly at the mystery of the sun and sunlight.

The Ancient Egyptians of 4 000 years ago were sun worshippers, and they were certainly not alone in instinctively or empirically recognizing the sun as our source of light and life on earth. A single, supreme sun-god Amen-Ra, or Ra, emerged as the chief of the Egyptian deities, and in the fourteenth century BC, the Pharaohs began to identify themselves with the sun, and attached Ra to their names. They even began to consider themselves the Sun-God incarnate. Figure 2.52 shows a portion of a frieze from the second millennium BC, depicting the rays from the sun ending in helping 'hands', which are patting humans and plants alike. Note also the *ankh*, Egyptian symbol of life, at the end of the one of the rays just in front of the Pharaoh and the lady in the frieze, showing that even over 3,000 years ago, the Ancients recognized the importance of the life-giving properties of the sun.

Many other ancient people, both civilized and primitive, held the sun in awe and majesty, and worshipped it in varying degrees of intensity. Some, like the Aztecs and, later, the Maya of central America, propitiated their Gods with human sacrifices, in which the heart of the victim was pulled, still beating, from the living body, and offered to whichever of the Gods was being approached for their favours. Special prearranged battles, known as the "Flowery Wars" were waged between two tribes, in order to provide the requisite number of victims to ensure the Gods' pleasure, when victims were otherwise in short supply. In Japan, as in ancient Egypt, the mystery of the sun is elevated to a theistic plane. The Sun Goddess, Amaterasu, is considered in the Shinto religion to be a founding ancestor of the imperial family. It is said that she sent her son Niniji to pacify the Japanese islands, and her great-grandson, Jimmu Tenno, became the first Emperor of Japan. The chrysanthemum, symbol of the royal family, very closely resembles a sun surrounded by rays: the Japanese national flag, the *Hino Maru*, is a bold red sun on a white background, while the national symbol is a rayed rising red sun on a white background.

For the most part, sun worship and the myths that surround the sun were an emotional response to natural phenomena now scientifically explained in physical laws; however, documentation exists showing that the Ancient Egyptians of 4,000 years ago were using a form of dermatological phototherapy, in the treatment of a number of skin conditions. The treatment of vitiligo, depigmented patches on the skin, involved photosensitization of the affected area by rubbing it with the crushed leaves of a plant very similar to parsley, followed by exposure of the treated area to sunlight. The psoralen compound, affiliated to furocoumarin, in crushed parsley leaves photosensitizes the skin cells in the treated area to light in the near ultraviolet-A (UV-A, 320 nm - 400 nm) and short-wavelength visible blue light (400 nm - 480 nm). 24 to 48 hours after exposure, the photosensitized areas developed a severe erythema, or sunburn, which was followed by a deeper and more persistent postinflammatory hyperpigmentation, or suntan. This was caused by the body's natural defence mechanism to light induced skin damage, as we now know in some detail from the work of Smith, Parrish, Magnus and others.

While the knowledge and techniques of heliotherapy died out with the end of the Ancient Indian, Chinese and Egyptian civilizations, the sun of course remained, especially as the central element in primitive religions. The occasion of a solar eclipse, for example, was a time of great fear, as the Sun God had taken His light from His worshippers. Not until the middle of the 19th

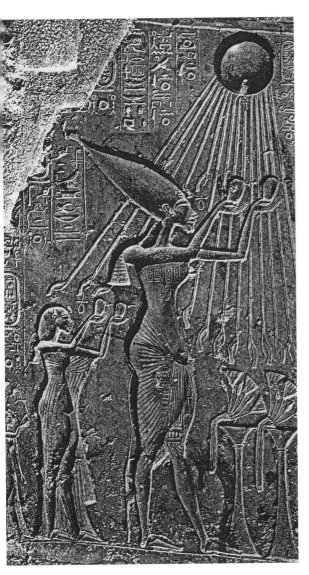

Fig 2.52:
Portion of 1,375 BC Frieze showing Pharaoh Amenhotep IV and even his flowers benefiting from the healthy 'hands' from the sun: note the 'ankh' life symbol on the ends of the rays directly in front of the faces of the Pharaoh and his lady-friend.

century did any sort of systematically reported clinical application of sunlight begin to re-emerge. "Sun bathing" was offered as a general tonic for depression. As the skies over Europe, particularly Great Britain, began to be filled with the smoke pouring from the factories and engines of the industrial revolution, the amount of UV-A radiation reaching the earth from the sun was diminished, and a number of calcium deficiency-related conditions became the scourge of the rapidly industrializing areas: foremost among these was rickets, or rachites, the disease in infants and young children resulting in stunted and deformed bone development, remaining with the affected person through life. UV-A is absorbed in the skin, and forms a precursor of vitamin D. In the small intestine, this precursor is transformed into the free form of calcium ion, and is carried to the bones via the blood stream. Interruption of the UV-A results in a vitamin D deficiency, and hence imperfect bone formation. Exposure to 'pure' unfiltered sunlight in the 'clean' air of the sea or mountainside was found to halt or even reverse the course of rickets. Consumption and tuberculosis were also rife, due to poor air and even poorer working conditions. The seaside or mountain sanatorium became a common sight along the coasts and mountainsides of Europe, for both treatment and convalescence for those who could afford it.

The sun, however, is a fickle agent, especially in northern Europe, and it was not until the late nineteenth century that a man-made and controlled source of therapeutic broad band UV and infrared (IR) light was developed by the Danish scientist and clinician, Dr Niels R. Finsen, the father of modern phototherapy. At this time it was recognized that particular bands of radiation or light were more effective than others in curing particular diseases and conditions. 'Red-light therapy' was extremely effective for treatment of melancholia, in which the patient was placed in a red-windowed room. With his near IR and long-wave visible red lamp, Finsen treated the fever

and eruptive stages of measles (*rubella*), chicken pox (*varicella*) and smallpox (*variola*). Other early photobiological research (Fubini, 1879) demonstrated the effects of red light on altering the respiratory rate of cells and cultures *in vitro*.

Finsen found UV-A and short wave visible blue light to be particularly useful in the treatment of tuberculosis of the skin (*lupus vulgaris*), and went on to win the Nobel Prize in Medicine in 1903 for his advances in this research. His institute can still be visited in Copenhagen, and the Finsen Medal is one of the most coveted international awards in modern photobiological research. Finsen's arc-based lamp employed a complex and clumsy series of filters and condensers to deliver the required waveband, but clumsy as it was, this was a major step forward: an artificial light source was finally available, which could be used at any time of the day or night, or in any weather, in any season, for phototherapy.

This interest in phototherapy lasted into the first two decades of the present century, but once again, with the development of specialized drugs and topical medications, broad-band phototherapy fell into disuse some 40 years before the first laser appeared. Since then, however, several more dependable therapeutic light sources have been developed, including incandescent, high- and low-pressure gas and fluorescent lamps, but in 1960, Doctor Theodore Maiman, working out of the Hughes Research Laboratory in Malibu, California, was the first to succeed in the race to produce a man-made powerful pulse of intense, pure red light, point for point more powerful than the most powerful light source known then: even more powerful than the sun. Science fiction had become science fact - the laser was born.

2-2-1-(C) History of the Laser in Surgery & Medicine

2-2-1-(C-1) History of Laser Surgery (HLLT)

The effectiveness of the laser as a surgical tool was tentatively explored in the early sixties very soon after its initial development by Maiman, and with its unique properties, laser light was quickly recognized as having real potential, especially in ophthalmology for retinal laser photocoagulation for retinal tears and detachments, and diabetic retinopathy; and in dermatology for transdermal coagulation of vascular and other pigmented lesions. This precise photothermal destruction of targeted tissue underpinned the early development of laser surgery, and many applications now exist. The main applications and specialties can be summarized as below, but the reader must realize that this is not intended to be by any means an exhaustive list, merely an attempt to give a broad overview of the multiplicity of laser photothermally-based surgical procedures.

In dermatology and related specialties, laser effects pigment-specific, tissue-selective, sell-selective bloodless excision, vaporization and coagulation for removal of pigmented and non-pigmented cutaneous lesions

In ophthalmology, laser is used for welding of detached or torn retinal tissue to the sclera; obliteration of neovascularization of the retina in diabetic retinopathy; and sealing of bleeding vessels causing cloudiness in the vitreous

In oncology, neurosurgery, urology and general surgery, laser allows selective vaporization of benign and malignant growths, with the added advantage in the latter indication of instant sealing of the blood and lymphatic vessels so as to help prevent viable tumor cell seeding. The laser can be applied through rigid and flexible endoscopes to internal structures, giving minimally-invasive surgery. General surgery and urology also utilize laser lithotripsy, the photothermal, or photoosmotic destruction of urinary calculi, stones in the bladder.

In otolaryngology, head and neck surgery, laser precision is ideal for delicate procedures in the bones of the middle ear such as laser stapedotomy and stapedectomy, to return hearing lost through calcified fixation of the bones; laser turbinectomies; laser tonsillectomies, especially in the adult for whom tonsillectomy is a potentially life-threatening procedure; and in the removal of benign growths on the vocal cords

In gynaecology laser is capable of selective removal of carcinoma of the cervix by vaporization or conization; excision and vaporization of condyloma acumminata, so-called vaginal warts; control of dysmenorrhoea; and in minimally-invasive laser laparoscopy for endometrial implant removal, or adhesiolysis

In orthopaedic surgery laser is used in minimally-invasive arthroscopic procedures for trimming and repair of damaged articular tissues

Laser is indicated in vascular surgery, for the welding-assisted repair of blood vessels; and for endovascular recanalization of blocked blood vessels by the vaporization of artheriosclerotic plaque, either in open endarterectomy or endoscopically through catheters threaded up to the affected vessels.

2-2-1-(C-2) History of Laser Medicine (LLLT)

In addition to its well-known photothermal tissue-destructive applications, the laser is also being investigated and used in several nonthermal surgical applications. These include the photodynamic activation of a photosensitizing chemical which, having selectively infiltrated precancerous or cancerous cells, destroys them without damaging uninvolved normal cells. A special type of pulsed laser, depending for its action on selective thermal photodisruption, is used in ophthalmology in the treatment of glaucoma, for the cutting of opaque elements in the vitreous, and the removal of the opaque membranes which can form on the lens capsule left after cataract or lens implant surgery. Also in ophthalmology, new 'cold' photodisruptive excimer (excited dimer) lasers are being used in corneal sculpting, or refractive keratoplasty, as an alternative to the conventional or laser scalpel-based radial keratotomy, for the correction of bad sight. The laser has seen great advances especially in the past decade in photobiological activation and low reactive-level laser therapy (LLLT), including wound healing, pain attenuation, laser acupuncture, bone fusion, anti-inflammatory action, collagen normalization, and so on. These have been dealt with in detail in two earlier volumes, also published by Wiley: *"LLLT: A Practical Introduction"* (1988), and *"LLLT: Practical Applications"* (1991), in addition to *"Progress in Laser Therapy"* (1991), the proceedings of the first congress of the International Laser Therapy Association.

Although the application of lasers in surgery and medicine is only just over thirty years of age,

it has applications even now in virtually all the medical specialties. As new and different lasers emerge, and as more physicians understand and apply them to a widening variety of clinical problems, laser photosurgery and phototherapy will become progressively more and more an essential tool for the surgeon.

2-2-2 Laser/Tissue Interaction

The reaction between incident laser energy and target tissue is classified into photothermal reactions, where the reaction is entirely due to heat created in the tissue as a result of absorption of the light energy by the target tissue, and nonphotothermal reactions, where there is direct absorption of light energy at a tissue, cellular or subcellular level, with no immediate rise in temperature: instead, the transfer of light energy to the target tissue causes one of a number of nonthermal reactions.

2-2-2-(A) Photothermal Reactions

Photothermal reactions following absorption in tissue of a laser beam are naturally restricted to laser surgery, rather than laser therapy, following Ohshiro's definition of low reactive-level laser therapy. Photothermal reactions can in turn be subdivided into the radiant heat effect, the conducted heat effect and so on.

When a material is irradiated by an electromagnetic wave the absorbed energy is transformed in some degree into heat. The heat which originates directly from the absorption of electromagnetic energy is referred to as **radiant heat**. Thus any effect occurring in tissue as a result of this reaction can be clinically termed a radiant heat effect. Radiant heat effects are restricted to the areas in which they are produced. When the heat spreads from these areas to surrounding tissue, a different effect occurs, which is clinically referred to as the **conducted heat effect**. Consider a laser beam incident on a single human tissue cell, which has a diameter of approximately

20 µm. The absorption of the incident beam is restricted to that cell only. As the temperature of the cell rapidly rises due to the radiant heat effect, some heat is transferred to the surrounding tissue cells by conducted heat, and their temperature also starts to rise. After 1 millisecond of heating, the rate in the rise of the temperature of the irradiated cell (the radiant heat effect) slows down clearly compared to the beginning of the reaction (Figure 2.53).

The reduction in the rate of temperature rise in the target cell is due to the increase in the heat

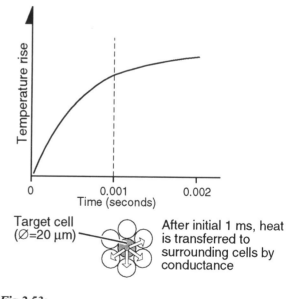

Fig 2.53:
Computer-program generated data of heating effect within and after 1 ms in a laser-irradiated cell of 20 µm in diameter and its surrounding unirradiated cells.

conduction from the target cell to the surrounding tissue. If the incident beam continues to target the material at the same incident power for longer than the 1 ms period most of the incident energy is spent raising the temperature of the surrounding cells, and is thus not used further to raise the temperature of the original cell by the radiant heat effect. From this consideration, at least at cellular-size levels, when a beam of laser energy is incident on a cell for less than 1 ms, the radiant heat effect is very high: at exposure times of longer than 1 ms, the conducted heat effect becomes stronger. When higher laser output powers are coupled with shorter exposure times the creation of radiant heat is limited to the target cell, which undergoes a sudden sharp rise in temperature leading to cell necrosis. Because of the short exposure time, the heat effect in the surrounding cells is much smaller than in the target cell, and the surrounding cells will be damaged less. Appropriate control of incident doses of laser light can thus limit damage to the tissue with the target cells, sparing the surrounding cells. This is referred to as cell-selective treatment, in which the radiant heat effect is restricted to the target cell, and the conducted heat effect can be ignored. Such kind of cell-selective treatment can in theory be used on abnormal coloured cells such as naevi cells to cause cell-selective necrosis of the targeted cells without damaging the surrounding normal cells.

The above model used to explain the concept behind cell-selective treatment is very much simplified: in practical clinical applications, the phenomena involved are much more complex, so that even with a sub-ms pulse of high laser power and energy, it is difficult to minimize the conducted heat effect in many cases. The following conditions must all be met for this purpose:

Con-1)   An appropriately short pulse must be used.

For example, a pulsed Q-switched ruby laser giving pulse widths in the order of several tens of nanoseconds (ns) is much more efficient for the selective removal of pigment than a normal pulsed ruby laser with pulse widths of several ms.

Con-2)   The target cells or material which is to absorb the laser energy must be limited.

If the target cells in a tissue block account for 1% of the total cells in the block, then it is practical and possible to limit damage selectively to these target cells without damaging most of the surrounding normal tissue, as mentioned above. If the ratio of target cells to normal cells rises above 1:100, then limiting damage to the target cells becomes progressively more difficult, since the greater the number of cells in tissue exhibiting the radiant heat effect, the more heat will be available for transfer to surrounding tissue by conducted heat, and thus the temperature of the surrounding cells may well rise to above the threshold of cell death. The control of the output power in conditions where there is a high ratio of target cells to normal cells therefore becomes more critical, and ultrashort pulsed laser systems must be used. When a laser system is capable of delivering a very high incident power density of some tens of MW/cm^2 at an ultrashort pulse width of some tens of ns, then selective vaporization of the target cells with very low conducted heat effect is possible, because the vaporization is accomplished in a very short time and the heat conduction period will also be very short.

Con-3)   The spot size must be sufficiently small.

If an incident laser beam has a spot size of 2 cm in diameter, then it can take nearly 1 min for the irradiated tissue to return to normal temperature following laser irradiation. In the central portion of the irradiated area, the temperature remains high for a longer period and thus conducted heat damage to the surrounding normal cells is more likely. In the case of an appropriately small spot size, the temperature of the irradiated cells will quickly return to normal thus lowering damage to the surrounding cells.

Con-4) The output power must be appropriately controlled.

Even in the case of a laser giving a high output power in a comparatively short pulse, if the delivered energy is over the dose required to kill the target cells the excess energy is transferred to conducted heat which can damage the surrounding normal cells.

Con-5) The temperature of the tissue must be kept as low as possible before irradiation.

When the preirradiation temperature is high, normal surrounding cells are easily damaged even in the case of a comparatively small rise in temperature. In this situation, achieving cell selective treatment becomes very difficult. If the opposite is achieved, in other words a low preirradiation temperature in the tissue, then the cell selectivity is very high, even where critical control of the laser output power is not possible. Neglecting preirradiation temperature control of the target area as a whole, even in the case of pulsed laser treatment, will result in poor cell selective treatment. For example,

if the laser beam is targeted on an area adjacent to a just-treated area, the rise in temperature of the second area will be greater than in the first-treated area (Figure 2.54), because there must be some temperature rise in the second area as a result of the first shot. Palpation of treated areas to test the temperature must be used to prevent this from happening. If a rise in temperature is detected, then the surgeon must wait until the temperature in the treated area has dropped back to normal before the next irradiation of contiguous zones: this can be accelerated by some form of cooling such as electric fans or blowers, cold water, ice packs and so on.

It goes without saying that the wavelength of the laser must be selected to achieve a good cell- or material-selectivity. For this purpose, the absorption rate of the target tissue for the selected wavelength should be high, and that of the normal surrounding tissue low.

2-2-1-(A-1) Application of Radiant heat Effect

Tattoo materials are vaporized at temperatures below 6,000°C. When they return to a solid state, they will be in the form of small particles. If the

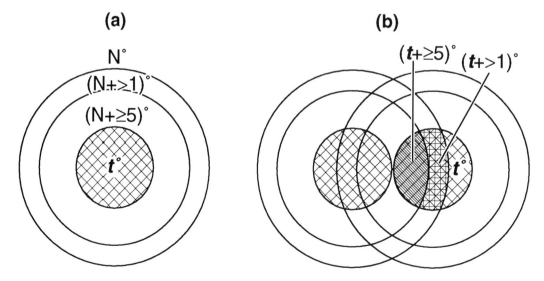

Fig 2.54: *Synergistic heating effect of periphery of previously-irradiated area* **(a)** *on centre and periphery of subsequently irradiated area* **(b)** *leading to higher tissue temperatures.*

particles are small enough, they will be phagocytosed by the macrophage cells, and carried off from the skin. As a result, removal of tattoos from the skin is possible.

Using ultra-short acting pulsed laser irradiation, if the concentration of target materials is low, there may be only a small rise in temperature in the adjacent normal tissue, giving the possibility a much smaller scar formation and better configuration than with conventional therapy.

Treatment of deep-sited lesions is more effective with the combination of high power densities and short pulse widths. Usually it is necessary to use a very large dose to assure enough of the incident light will reach the deep-sited target tissue. However, with a high enough peak power, a relatively low amount of total energy can destroy the target cells or materials. With a high power level and a short-acting pulse (i.e. below 1 μs), the low total energy can still achieve a high rise in temperature and rapid vaporization or plasma formation, in other words, an explosive effect in the small subcellular organelles in the target cell. The cell itself is eventually induced to explode, and is thus destroyed. There are some differences compared with thermal cell damage: this can be referred to as explosive therapy, and by this effect a deep-sited target can be effectively destroyed with a relatively small temperature rise in surrounding normal cells.

For treatment of excessive pigment in the melanin anomaly group, the use of the above laser types or the ultrashort-acting pulsed dye laser is recommended.

2-2-2-(A-2) Application of Conducted Heat Effect
Considering laser treatment for haemangioma simplex (HS), the ideal result is to achieve selective damage in the blood vessel walls of the haemangioma lesion. In practice, however, such a selective absorptive wavelength specific to the blood vessel wall does not exist. The primary laser target in HS treatment must instead be the erythrocytes within the vessel walls, rather than the walls themselves. Following irradiation, the heat generated in the target erythrocytes by radiant heat will be conducted to the blood vessel walls in several milliseconds. In other words, the temperature of the cells in the vessel walls will rise, and they will be damaged secondarily to the irradiation of the erythrocytes by the conducted heat effect. By careful control of the laser output power, pulse width and other conditions it is thus possible selectively to damage the cells in the blood vessel walls without large amounts of damage to the normal tissue surrounding the walls. The recovery time of the irradiated area is then kept short and scar formation is minimized. Even in the case of the conducted heat effect, with proper control of the irradiation conditions, it is possible to achieve a tissue- or cell-selective treatment.

When treating cases which do not require cell- or tissue-selectivity, there are many applications of the conducted heat effect. For example, irradiation of the Nd:YAG beam onto white or fairly transparent tissue does not produce a large amount of absorption or enough of a rise in temperature to destroy tissue because of the beam characteristics of the 1064 nm Nd:YAG laser. Painting the surface of the target to enhance laser absorption will produce radiant heat in the absorptive material of the paint, which will in turn with appropriate irradiation conditions be transferred to the underlying target cells. Thus indirect heating is possible, and many superficially-limited tumours can be treated by this method.

Other heat transfer systems exist in the body, such as convection and the blood and lympho-circulation; yet other systems may exist. However, clinical applications involving these types of heat transfer are rare, so they are omitted in this book for the purpose of practical applications in laser treatment for naevi.

2-2-2-(B) Nonthermal Effects
In addition to the photothermal effect of laser/tissue interaction, there are a variety of nonphotothermal effects, some particularly associated with high power surgical lasers, and some with

low incident power density systems such as laser therapy systems, and many shared by both.

When a pulsed laser strikes tissue, it does so with an almost percussive force. For example, when the carbon dioxide laser is employed in the so-called "superpulsed" mode (quasi-C/W), where the beam is composed of a train of high peak power, short pulse width pulses, the sound of the laser beam hitting the target tissue becomes perceptibly louder and higher pitched. This photoacoustic effect is concomitant with rapid thermally-mediated swelling; vaporization; or discharge on the occasion of the high electric field of a high-powered laser; and so on, and photoosmotic effects can be recorded. However, if the osmotic effect is too high, it can also cause physical damage to cellular structures of affected cells or tissue, or cause hearing loss.

A laser beam, surgical or therapeutic, is part of the electromagnetic spectrum, and by definition is composed of both electric and magnetic components. They have their own particular effects on tissue, and so there are associated photoelectric and photomagnetic effects in the target tissue.

At the periphery of a surgical laser beam, as the power densities in the target tissue drop dramatically, another range of nonphotothermal effects is seen, as the light energy is absorbed directly into the cell membrane or subcellular organelles, depending on the wavelength, without immediately raising the temperature or changing the architecture of the involved structures. However, a series of nonthermal reactions then occurs, including immediate photochemical or photophysical responses. They in turn trigger off a complex cascade of events, which have as their result a secondary range of effects, which include photochemical, photodynamic, photoenzymatic and photoimmunological consequences: some of these will be examined in detail under the heading of low reactive-level laser therapy (LLLT).

In laser surgery, we have been exploring mostly the photothermal effects of the laser/tissue interaction. Early reports from pioneers of laser surgery documented unexpected beneficial side effects, when comparing laser surgery with other forms of thermally-based surgery, such as electrocoagulation, or even the conventional cold knife: less postoperative pain following laser surgery, and better early-stage wound healing were two such effects. It was obvious that there was a nonphotothermal effect connected specifically with the laser, compared with the purely thermal effects of electrocoagulation, and excision or excision with the nonthermal conventional scalpel.

Well-documented experiments have shown that the immediate heat rise in the target tissue following extended LLLT irradiation in the rat model (60 mW, 830 nm, 0.3 cm^2 irradiated area, for 30 minutes) is negligible (1.1 °C after 4 min., no change thereafter). In addition to its applications in the total treatment concept in laser treatment for naevi, laser therapy has been successfully used for pain attenuation in all types of nerve, soft tissue and musculo-skeletal pain; for control of postanaesthetic numbness; to increase the patency of grafts and flaps; to restore circulation in circulatory disturbance-related diseases; to induce wound healing in slow-to-heal or nonhealing defects; to enhance bone fusion in delayed union fractures with better remodelling; and for laser acupuncture in both humans and animals. Other interesting and developing applications include activation of inactive or malfunctioning metabolic systems, such as in the therapy for hyper- and hypopigmentation, or hypertrophy and depressive scarring; normalization of the circulatory control system for treatment of hyper- and hypotension; to ensure speedy, neat and strong repair of injured tendons, with minimal remodelling and excellent tensile strength; to restore normal function to damaged or deteriorating nerve systems; for control of the immune system, such as in therapy for allergy-related complaints, such as atopic dermatitis, and autoimmune diseases. LLLT presents an ideal treatment method, since it is completely pain-free, easy to apply, noninvasive and is well-tolerated by all ages of patient, even the youngest children. To date at least, LLLT has exhibited no severe side effects, and has in fact been used in the control of side effects following laser surgery or other forms of surgical treatment, although the exact pathways and mechanisms by which LLLT and photobioactivation work are not yet completely clear.

Another nonphotothermal laser application is photodynamic therapy (PDT). PDT is a low invasive technique for the selective treatment of precancerous and superficial cancerous regions. A photosensitizing compound such as haematoporphyrin derivative (HpD) is injected into the patient. 48 to 72 hours later, this compound has been cleared from normal cells, and has aggregated in the cancerous or precancerous cells. Irradiating the suspected areas with low incident powers of visible red or yellow laser light causes the HpD to fluoresce. The borders of the involved tissue are thus clearly diagnosed. Subsequent irradiation with higher incident laser powers causes a cytotoxic reaction within the cell, connected with the production of singlet oxygen, a potent cellular cytotoxin, plus other superoxides, and the HpD impregnated cells are killed. Thus only the abnormally mitotic cells are destroyed, with low thermal effect to spread to surrounding normal tissue. The drawbacks to this therapy are firstly the effective depth to which the laser energy can penetrate in tissue, and secondly the systemic photosensitization of the patient to normal visible light. The depth problem is being addressed by inserting fibreoptic lightguides with diffusing tips into the body of the tumour through needles, and multiple treatment sessions. For the photosensitization side effects, prevention from exposure using gloves, wide-brimmed hats, avoiding sunlight, etcetera is the only answer at present. Reports have also appeared on the possible application of HpD in the treatment of psoriasis vulgaris, since it has been discovered that the compound will also be selectively taken up in the comparatively more mitotic cells in psoriatic lesions. The higher degree of photosensitization of surrounding normal tissue is a major obstacle to the practical applications of this, coupled with the difficulty of 'bathing' large areas of the body with laser energy.

Quasi-nonphotothermal effects can be found in the current advances in photodestructive effects. In photodisruption, the absorption of very high-energy ultrashort pulses of laser energy (pulsed Nd:YAG laser in ophthalmic procedures, for example) causes disruption of the molecules, causing them to fly apart. At the same time, a brief plasma spark is created, which in its turn is self-limiting to further penetration of the laser beam. These photodisruptive effects can therefore be extremely precisely administered, with very low radiant heat and conducted heat effects.

Another example of true nonphotothermal laser application well into its pioneering clinical stages at the moment is UV-wavelength excimer (excited dimer) laser treatment. The excimer laser is mostly applied in ophthalmology, for 'cold' ablative corneal sculpting procedures, known as refractive keratoplasty, amongst other applications. However, experimental work in other biologic tissue is proceeding, including endovascular applications in arterial plaque ablation. Laser beam delivery through fibreoptics small enough to fit in available catheters, the lack of thermal effect removing the problem of postirradiation thermal damage repair and possible restenosis, and the precise layer-by-layer application would seem to be ideal in plaque removal for recanalization of arteriosclerotic vessels. Other dermal applications of the excimer, possibly for naevi treatment, may well be seen in the not too distant future.

2-2-3 Photobiodestruction and Photobioactivation: HLLT and LLLT

What the clinician should primarily know is the surgical treatment or medical therapeutic effect of tissue absorption of a laser beam, as well as the actual laser system which is producing the beam. Accordingly, it is very important to look carefully at the terminology used when describing or discussing surgical laser treatment, and more particularly, medical laser therapy, and also to talk about clinical research projects in both areas of clinical laser application.

In the previous section, photothermal and nonphotothermal effects were discussed: strong photothermal effects destroy, or irreversibly alter the architecture in the irradiated tissue: this is what the author would like to call **photobiodestruction**. The target tissue is instantly heated to above its survival threshold: the level of tissue reaction is therefore highly destructive. The author thus classifies all photodestructive surgical laser treatments under the term High reactive Level Laser Treatment, or HLLT.

In medical laser therapy, on the other hand, there is very little or no thermal effect, and no visible change to the irradiated tissue architecture. The immediate effect is rather at the cellular and subcellular level, and consists of direct absorption of the low incident levels of light energy in the cell, either in the membrane or in the intracellular organelles, depending on the wavelength. This results in an increase in the energy level of the affected components which then reach a more active state. This in turn affects the whole metabolism of the cell, which gradually affects the surrounding cells and tissues, and eventually a systemic whole-body effect can be noted. There is no irreversible destruction, only reversible activation. The reader is asked to remember that activation of a system does not always result in acceleration. *Activation* of the braking system in a car, for example, will cause deceleration. *Activation* of the accelerator has the opposite effect, and stimulates greater speed by feeding more fuel to the engine. Activation has thus the double

meaning of stimulation, and control. The author has therefore proposed the term *photobioactivation* to describe the basic biological effects which can appear below the cellular survival threshold after laser irradiation of a biological system. The entire term becomes Low reactive Level Laser Therapy, or LLLT. These terms have been internationally accepted as a good catch-all to describe the clinical applications of laser. It is often mistakenly said that the laser is low-level, a low level laser was used, but the incorrect term can be seen sometimes in scientific papers. It is not the *laser instrument* that is "low level", but the reactive level of the laser/tissue *therapeutic effect* that is low! Correct terminology is very important to correct reporting of parameters or methods and results, and the author therefore hopes to use correctly the terms LLLT and photobioactivation, rather than the large number of hardware-based terms such as low-power laser and low-energy laser, or marketing-driven terms such as soft, cool, cold laser and so on.

2-2-3-(A) Arndt-Schultz Law

In the late 19th century, a law of stimulation therapy or physiology was proposed by Rudolph Arndt and Hugo Schultz of Germany. This is the Arndt-Schultz law which states that weak stimuli will activate an organism, moderately strong stimuli will favour its action, strong stimuli will retard its action. With the acceptance of Endre Mester's work, and the continuing work of his sons Adam in Hungary and Andrew in the USA, that law, which had fallen a little into disuse, has been revived. The author in 1987 proposed Ohshiro's hypothetical curve seen in its latest form in Figure 2.55. The strength of the stimulus is shown on the horizontal axis, increasing to the right, and the strength of reaction is shown on the vertical axis. From stimulus strength A to B_1 the curve shows a level area with little or no reaction. From stimulus strength B_2 to C there is a sharp rise, which slows down to reach its peak at strength D. Thereafter there is a sharp decline in the level of stimulation back to normal level, and to complete arrest at E_2. E_1 shows the normal level.

Figure 2.56 shows a graph of the results of an experiment reported in *Laser Therapy* by Kudoh *et al* in 1988. The experiment involved the *in vivo* irradiation of rat saphenous nerve using a GaAlAs diode laser (60 mW, 830 nm, 15 s - 120 s exposure). The graph shows different levels of sodium-potassium adenosine triphosphatase (Na-K-ATPase) activity on the vertical axis plotted against levels of laser dosage on the horizontal axis. The curve echoes very nearly Ohshiro's hypothetical curve as seen in Figure 2.55. Since that experiment, a number of others conducted independently on different subjects, both *in vitro* and *in vivo*, have demonstrated the same dose-de-

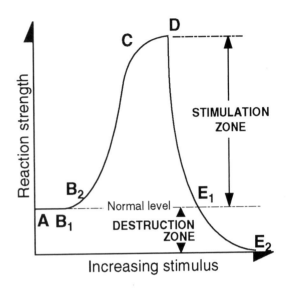

Fig 2.55: Ohshiro's hypothetical Arnd-Schultz curve.

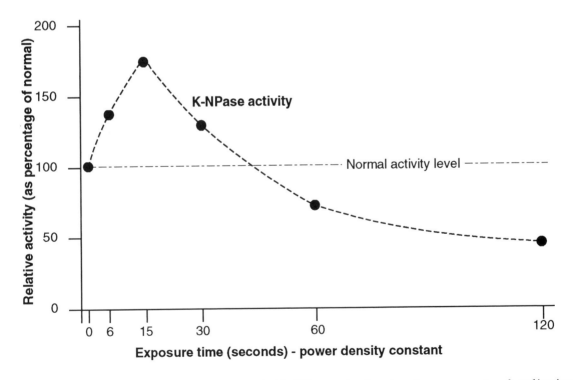

Fig 2.56: *Arndt-Schultz law seen in operation on Na-K-ATPase action in rat saphenous nerve irradiated* in vivo *by GaAlAs diode laser. The similarity to Ohshiro's hypothetical curve is clear. (Adapted from Kudoh et al (1989): Effects of gallium aluminium arsenide diode laser irradiation on rat saphenous nerve Na-K-ATPase activity. 'Laser Therapy', 1:2, 63-68, used with permission).*

GOOD FACE

Whole-Body Toning

Photosynthesis

Vision

Warmth and Light

Vitamin D Synthesis

Photoresponse

Heliotherapy

Killing Pathogens

BAD FACE

Biocidal action

Carcinogenesis

Skin Damage

Sunburn

Mutation

Sunstroke

Phototoxic Smog

Photoallergies

Photosensitization

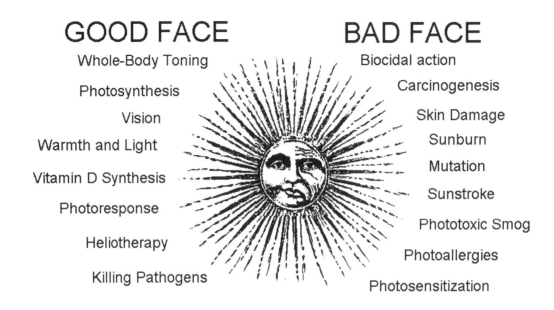

Fig 2.57: *"Bad" and "Good" faces of sunlight.*

pendent pattern, more or less looking exactly the same as Ohshiro's curve.

Looking again at Ohshiro's curve, the most effective LLLT dosage should be maintained from level B to E_1. HLLT would take effect in the E_1 - E_2 range with photodestruction.

2-2-3-(B) The Sun: Janus of Photoeffects

It would be impossible to leave this section on photoeffects without looking briefly at one of the longest lasting, if somewhat fickle sources, of light: the Sun. Harsh, strong light of the sun can create dry, arid, lifeless deserts. However, gentle sunlight can give leaves their green, and can bring colour to ripening fruit. The sun is without a doubt something of a Janus, a two-faced deity. On the

one hand, too much sun is harmful for man and nature, but on the other hand, sunlight sustains life, including that of mankind. Figure 2.57 shows in pictorial form the dichotomy of the effects on man caused by light from the Sun. On the one hand, there are the many beneficial effects, but they are balanced by the harmful effects, especially the ones due to overexposure. Exposure to sunlight is a photostimulus, and as such, follows the Arndt-Schultz law discussed above. The beneficial effects all fall within the biophotoactivative dosage levels, so LLLT could be thought of as being a family member of the gentle face of the sun, but like sunlight, must not be abused.

2-2-4 Biological Chain Photoreactions

Absorption of light energy by a cell instigates a well-recognized cascade of reactions, leading from the actual absorption, or photoreception, to the intermediate stages where the incoming signal is transferred from organelle to organelle within

the cell, gradually being amplified as it does so, to the final reaction of the cell, the photoresponse, This chain reaction of photoreception-signal transduction and amplification-photoresponse is made up of a series of intermediate chain reac-

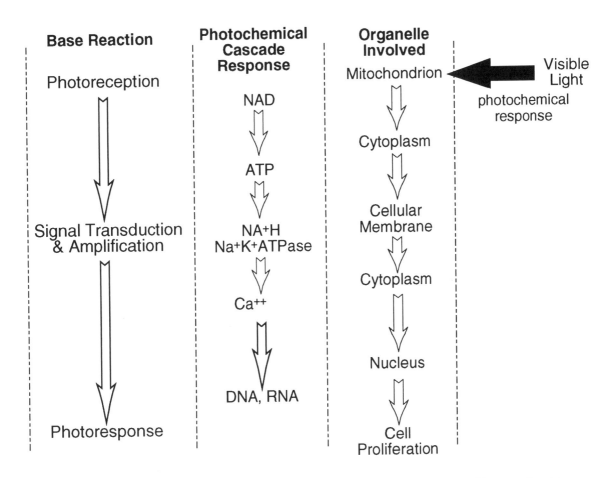

Fig 2.58: *Karu's model for photochemical action of visible light on the redox chain of the mitochondrion, initiating a cascade of photoresponses leading (amongst other things) to cellular proliferation.*

tions. However, the reaction is different for visible light compared with infrared radiation: the most popular LLLT systems are HeNe lasers, at 632.8 nm, visible diode lasers at around the same wavelength, or near infrared lasers, diode or Nd:YAG. There is a basic conundrum posed by this, as visible light lasers are recognized as having a photochemical effect on receptor cells, penetrating the membrane, and being absorbed in the organelles within the cytoplasm. Infrared lasers have a photophysical effect, being absorbed in the membrane, and causing rotational and vibrational changes in the affected atoms. How can

two different processes result in the same effect, since both the HeNe and IR lasers have been reported as being effective in various sectors of laser therapy.

Tiina Karu (Russian Academy of Sciences, Troitsk, Moscow, Russia) has proposed a model for low level laser radiation stimulation of a biological system (i.e. a cell) for visible red light, as shown in Figure 2.58. The receptors are all cytoplasmic, and in particular Karu has pinpointed the components of the respiratory chain within the mitochondria as the primary targets, such as flavine dehydrogenases, cytochromes and cyto-

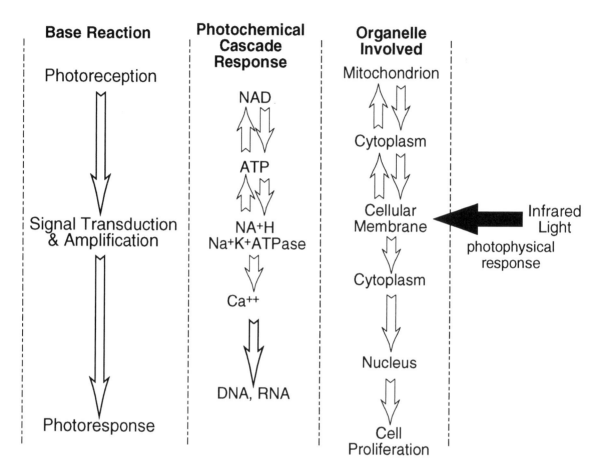

Fig 2.59: *Smith's modification of Karu's model, showing how the photophysical action of infrared light on the cell membrane can have a similar final result as the photochemical action of visible light, even although the reactions are initially dissimilar.*

chrome oxidase. They absorb the energy, and the mitochondria are activated into a higher metabolic state, releasing increased amounts of ATP into the cytoplasm, and altering the redox status of both the mitochondria and the cytoplasm. A photomediated cascade of events occurs within the cell, influencing the transmembrane Ca^{++} flux, which in turn causes even more amplification of the received signal, affecting the nucleus and modulating in some way cell proliferation. This is the basic precept of visible red light photobioactivation.

Infrared energy from an IR laser is instead absorbed in the cell membrane. Kendric Smith (Stanford University, California, USA) thus proposed an adaptation of Karu's mode in which the photoreception occurs at the membrane, initiating the photocascade at a later stage than with visible red light by directly influencing the Ca^{++} membrane flux. This in turn has an effect on the cytoplasm and the mitochondria, initiating the photocascade as in visible light irradiation (Figure 2.59). There is thus an almost doubled effect from IR irradiation. Research from Yamaya, Shiroto *et al* in an experiment on pooled human neutrophils has shown that IR laser irradiation has specific 830 nm receptors existing on the neutrophil membrane which when excited led to an increase in the phagocytic activity of the neutrophil.

Thus both visible and IR laser therapy systems can have similar chain effects in irradiated cells, and ultimately, tissue, despite the fact that under the accepted laws of photobiology they have completely different actions, photochemical and photophysical, respectively. The important fact is that the final result of the biological chain of photoreactions is the same, and both visible light and IR LLLT have been shown to work effectively.

2-2-5 Polarization

As already discussed briefly above, a normal beam of light consists of many individual waves, each vibrating in a direction perpendicular to its path. Normally, the vibrations of each ray have different orientations with no favoured direction. In some cases, however, all the waves in a beam vibrate in parallel planes in the same direction. Such light is described as polarized, that is, to have a single directional characteristic. It may further be defined specifically as linearly polarized light, to distinguish it from circularly or elliptically polarized light.

Light from familiar sources such as a light bulb, the Sun, or a candle flame is unpolarized but can easily become polarized as it interacts with matter. Reflection, refraction, transmission, and scattering all can affect the state of polarization of light. The human eye cannot distinguish polarized from unpolarized light, so objects illuminated by both kinds of light appear the same to it. This is not true of all animals. In fact, light from the sky is considerably polarized, as a result of scattering, and some animals, such as bees, are able to sense the polarization and use it as a directional aid.

Any device that is used to produce polarized light is called a polarizer. Polarizers are often used in laser systems. Most of the methods of producing polarized light involve splitting a beam of unpolarized light according to the direction of the electric vector of the waves and separating the polarized portion from the remainder, such as the simple wire frame polarizer mentioned already. The earliest and simplest method of polarization is to reflect the beam from a nonmetallic surface, or dielectric surface, at a particular angle of incidence, after which the reflected and refracted beams are both polarized. This angle, discovered by Sir David Brewster, is known as Brewster's angle, and is incorporated in the Brewster's window seen in many gas lasers

Certain natural crystals were found to have the property of double refraction, or birefringence in which an incident light beam is split into two linearly polarized beams at right angles to each other. This effect was discovered by Christiaan Huygens in 1678. Because the two emerging beams have little separation, several means of isolating the beams have been devised, such as use of a dichroic filter, which has the ability to absorb light of one wavelength than another.

Linearly polarized light has one electric vector confined to a single plane related to the direction of propagation of the beam. On the other hand, circularly polarized light has an electric vector that remains constant as it rotates, and rotation can be either clockwise or counterclockwise, commonly known as right-handed or left-handed polarization, respectively. A linearly-polarized beam can be found to consist of both right-and left-handed polarized beams, and having a constant phase difference of 90 degrees (1/4 of a wavelength). The beams combine to give a single beam of linearly polarized light. Either circularly-polarized component of the beam can be extracted by use of a thin filter, known as a quarter-wave plate, which can produce either a right-handed or a left-handed polarized beam.

The thickness of the plate is adjusted to give the necessary division of the components.

The importance of polarization of laser light is only now being explored in depth. However, it is obvious from several studies that polarization of monochromatic, noncoherent light in *in vitro* studies radically affects the result. However, for *in vivo* studies, coherence is more important than monochromaticity, polarized or unpolarized. A study demonstrated that the speckle pattern of the HeNe laser contained packets of coherent and polarized light in each speckle. The speckle phenomenon has been demonstrated in HeNe laser energy that has passed through 2 cm of minced meat, thus proving that laser coherence and polarization are not lost in the first few micrometres of living tissue. Polarized laser light has been shown to have a greater effect than unpolarized light, and right-handed or linear polarization are seemingly many times more effective than left-handed polarization. The reasons for this are still being explored, and this subject promises a really fruitful field of research in the near future.

2-2-6 Optical Characteristics of the Skin

Many mathematical models, including the Monte Carlo model, have been proposed to explain or describe what happens to a laser beam of a given wavelength when it enters target tissue. In addition, the extinction length of each wavelength in various homogeneous media has also been calculated, and these data have been published, and are available. From the clinician's viewpoint, this is referred to as the penetration depth of a laser. From the above data, it should thus be possible to give an exact description, wavelength by wavelength, of what will happen to a laser beam when it is aimed and fired at target tissue. Unfortunately, it is not as simple as that. Biological tissue is very rarely homogeneous in its optical characteristics, as it contains blood vessels, which contain blood, and that blood is of a different colour, depending whether it is fresh arterial blood or venous blood. Tissue contains nerves, of different diameters; muscle tissue; lymphatic vessels; melanin granules; and so on. The main target tissue for the laser surgeon in the laser treatment for naevi is the skin, and skin is one of the most complex blends of tissues. It is in fact totally inhomogeneous. As has been already discussed above, the skin has two main layers, the epidermis and the dermis. The epidermis, (first target tissue that any laser must encounter), has itself five different layers, each with its own optical characteristics. It also contains a layer of biological pigment in the granular layer, and the ascending skin cells all contain a cap formation of black melanin granules located over the nucleus (the nuclear cap). The dermis also has different characteristics, due to the type and displacement of collagen fibres, depending on the depth, and also a complex series of blood plexi at certain depths, each with its own absorption characteristics.

When a laser beam is incident on skin, it will react with the target tissue in many ways: it will be reflected, particularly from the diffuse keratinous horny layer; refracted by the clear layer, where it exists, and by the difference in refractive index between the epidermis and dermis at the basal membrane; scattered forwards, and backwards from the cellular components in the epidermis and the multiple fibrous components in the dermis; it will be transmitted through the comparatively unpigmented elements of the dermis, including the ground substance; and it will ultimately be absorbed. Just to complicate matters even further, how much of the beam will fall into which reaction is determined mainly by the wavelength of the beam, and the particular pigment characteristics of the target tissue, as most naevi have an abnormality in colour.

Figure 2.60 shows the absorption spectra for oxyhaemoglobin, haemoglobin, melanin and

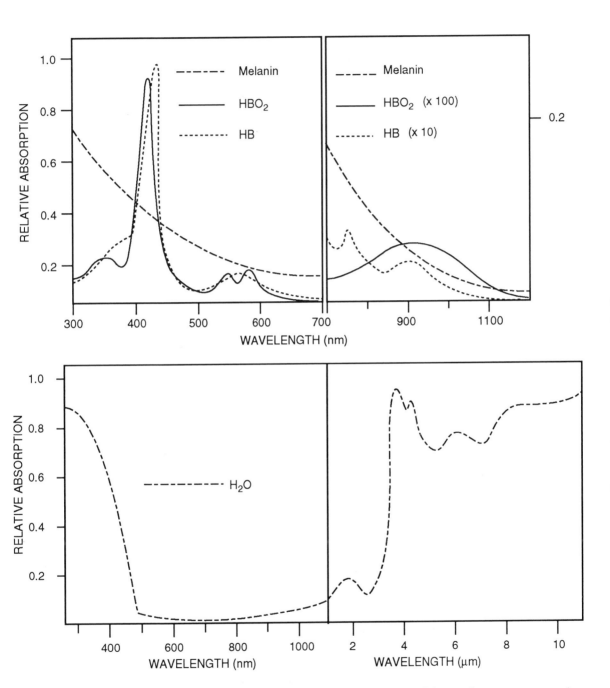

Fig 2.60: *Relative absorption spectra for melanin, oxyhaemoglobin, haemoglobin and water over a wide spectral range. Note the scale of relative absorption in the upper right segment is calibrated logarithmically. (Data compiled from a variety of sources and references: see reference list for this chapter).*

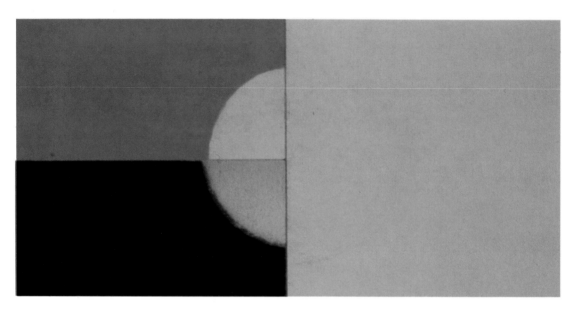

Fig 2.61: *Demonstration of colour selectivity of ruby laser. The target for the ruby laser consists of three pieces of 'footprint' paper (coated paper designed to give a visual indication of laser beam imprint, beam size and homogeneity) joined together: white, black and red. The ruby laser was aimed and fired so that one half of the beam was on the white paper and the other half equally on the red and black. There is no damage to the white coated paper, but homogeneous colour removal of the red and black coating demonstrates the potential of the ruby laser for cell-selective removal of superficial targets in naevi of both the blood vessel (red) and melanin anomaly (black) groups.*

water, for a range of wavelengths from ultraviolet to mid infrared. The wavelengths are shown on the horizontal axis, and relative absorption is shown on the vertical axis. The reader can see at a glance that each pigment component and water has its own particular optimal absorption band or bands. The visible light lasers are comparatively highly absorbed in the biological pigments, but not in water. However even within the visible waveband, there is pigment-dependent absorption, with oxyhaemoglobin more preferentially taking up the yellow light of the dye laser, and the 532 nm green light of the KTP/532 laser, compared with the blue and green wavebands of the argon, for example. There are important differences in the absorption in melanin, which would indicate that the dye laser is the laser of choice where overlying tissue, containing melanin, should be spared, while the blood vessels containing the target erythrocytes are selectively haemocoagulated.

From these data the ruby laser, at 693 nm, might seem to be unsuitable for dermatologic applications with a low absorption rate in haemoglobin, but the actual clinical data only go to show that charts and formulae cannot give the entire picture. The ruby laser, although it is red, is still more preferentially absorbed in red-coloured pigment than in white. Because it has a very short acting time, with extremely high peak pulse power, the pulsed ruby laser, and in particular the Q-switched ruby laser, give an excellent radiant heat effect, with very high cell selective treatment. Figure 2.61 gives a graphic demonstration of the colour-selective potential of the ruby laser. The target is a composite of red, black and white 'footprint' papers, specially-coated paper to give a visual indication of a laser beam imprint and homogeneity. The laser was aimed at the centre of the target and fired. As can be seen, only the red and black coatings were homogeneously damaged, leaving the white coating unharmed.

This is a good demonstration of the ruby laser's cell-selective potential in area treatment of both blood vessel and melanin anomaly group lesions.

More details of the importance of wavelength, colour and colorimetry in the laser treatment for naevi can be found in the next chapter.

It has been suggested that laser energy loses its coherence in the first few micrometres of tissue, and that coherence is therefore unimportant, especially in the low incident power densities used in LLLT. It has also been stated by some who should know better that, from the available mathematical data, incident laser energy cannot possibly penetrate more than a few millimetres into tissue, at most. This is another example of depending too much on formulae, tables of extinction length, mathematical models and *in vitro*-gathered data. The skin defies mathematical models, due to its complexity and inhomogeneous characteristics, and the fact that it is alive. Work from Kato and Nagasawa has shown that there is a great deal of penetration, measurable in centimetres, rather than millimetres, especially at the near infrared wavebands of the GaAlAs diode laser (830 nm) and the Nd:YAG (1064 nm). Using an infrared-sensitive charge coupled device-based video camera (CCD video camera), they have produced videos showing penetration of laser energy of various wavelengths in freshly ex-

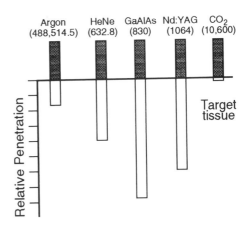

Fig 2.62:
Relative penetration of lasers in comparatively homogeneous biological tissue. (Data compiled from a variety of sources: see Reference list for this chapter)

cised liver, and also for *in vivo* irradiation of gingival tissue. From these data, the relative penetration of selected lasers is shown in Figure 2.62. Please remember that relative penetration is related to absorption *depth*, not *relative absorption*, which is shown in Figure 2.60 above. For deep absorption, the IR beams of the GaAlAs and the Nd:YAG are obviously the most effective, and to an extent, the visible red wavelength of the HeNe, or the new generation of visible light diode lasers now appearing.

2-2-7 Recuperatory and Recovering Power of the Skin

When skin is damaged by incident laser energy, the wound-healing process is activated. This process has two subdivisions. First we must consider the survival threshold of the irradiated cells. If the damage to cells is below their survival threshold, then the cells remain alive, although they have been damaged to some extent. These cells will then spontaneously recover, gradually returning to a near-normal condition without the need for much help with reepithelization. This is referred to by the author as the *recuperatory power* of the skin. On the other hand, if the damage to the cells is beyond their survival

threshold, then cells will turn necrotic, and the damaged area must be reepithelized from the borders of the surrounding undamaged skin, and any skin appendages left intact in the damaged area. The author calls this the *recovering power* of the skin.

In many laser treatments for naevi, the wound is reepithelized by a combination of these two skin healing processes. The recuperatory power of the damaged skin cells will usually be found acting in some of the skin appendages in the treated area and in the borders of the wound between the totally damaged cells and undamaged cells, gradually restoring them to a state where they can assist in the reepithelization process. The recovering power of the undamaged skin cells in the meantime starts the reepithelization process from the outer margins of the wound.

As will be discussed in detail in Chapter 3, the aim of the clinician in the treatment of naevi is to achieve what the author terms the *intact skin condition*, which means skin which is apparently scar-free and normal looking from a macroscopic viewpoint. In order to achieve the intact skin condition, wound epithelization should be complete in 10 days, 14 at the most. However, it is recognized that only 2 mm of new epithel can be produced from a wound margin alone in 10 - 14 days. For complete reepithelization in the maximum 14 day intact skin period from the margins alone, the wound must therefore not exceed 4 mm in diameter or width. However, by using the recuperatory powers of slightly damaged skin cells located in the skin appendages in the damaged area, this wound width or diameter of 4 mm can be extended, and the combined recovering power of the skin appendages and surrounding normal skin ensures that epithelization is complete within the 10-14 day period required to achieve the intact skin condition.

2-2-8 Maximum Intact Dose

By balancing the area and depth of damage caused by a laser impact, reepithelization within the required 10 days can be consistently achieved using the recuperative and recovering powers of the skin, and an intact skin condition can be achieved. In getting the correct balance between depth and area damage, in other words a consideration of 3-dimensional damage volume, the laser dose is a very important factor. The dose required to achieve the maximum effect with the minimum of damage, while still achieving the intact skin condition is termed by the author the *maximum intact dose*, or MID.

Each laser has its own characteristics, depending firstly on the wavelength, and then on the power and energy densities (discussed in detail in Chapter 3-6). The author designed an experiment to compare the effects of argon, Nd:YAG and CO_2 lasers on skin of the nude mouse, using Evans blue exudation (EBE) from the target tissue as a macroscopic marker for having achieved a similar histological effect with the different lasers. The incident power and irradiated area were the same for each laser (3 W and 2.0 mm in diameter, respectively, a power density of 9,548 W/cm^2). Only the irradiation time was changed until EBE was seen in the target tissue. To achieve the same macroscopic and histologic changes, the argon laser required between 0.3 - 0.4 s; the Nd:YAG required between 18.0 and 19.0 s; and the CO_2 laser required between 0.03 and 0.04 s. With the CO_2 laser value normalized at 1, the argon laser thus required a dose 10 times and the Nd:YAG 475 times that of the CO_2 laser to achieve the same macroscopic and histologic effect.

Having established a value for the MID over a range of power densities for the argon laser, for example, it would then theoretically be possible to achieve the same effect with the CO_2 laser at a dose 0.1 times the argon dose, and at a dose 47.5 times the argon dose with the Nd:YAG laser. This is a theoretical consideration, and other factors such as the type of naevus being treated, its area and depth, the site of the naevus and the age, sex and race of the patient must all be factored in when considering the MID. Chapter 3, sections 6 and 7 below will examine in detail the separate factors in choosing appropriate laser parameters to achieve the intact skin condition and arrive at the MID.

2-2-9 Side Effects

At first sight, a side effects-related discussion might not appear relevant in this section. Every patient must be considered as an individual, and many side effects from both laser surgery or laser therapy can be traced to an over-use of the 'cookbook' approach, or to insufficient attention to the patient's history and pretreatment or pretherapy work-up. The 'cookbook' approach is particularly true of laser surgery, where a particular type of lesion or disease is treated with preset parameters in every patient regardless of age, sex, race or the site of the lesion; or where treatment has been carried out without due regard to individual factors such as skin colour, psychological state, patient history or degree of informed education received and understood by the patient.

2-2-9-(A) Side Effects in Laser Surgery

It is important to consider the maximum intact dose (MID), and by adjusting power densities so as to achieve the maximum effect with the minimum damage, using intraoperative technique management, the laser surgeon will certainly help to prevent side effects.

The preoperative patient history work-up, patient education, and postoperative care are also extremely important factors in avoiding side effects. Before using the laser on a patient, many elements must be investigated, including the general physical condition, and particularly the patient's history, and any related familial history relevant to the condition being treated. The patient's psychological state must also be assessed, since a naevus can just as upsetting mentally as physically, often even more so.

The major side effects associated with laser surgery are hypertrophic scar, secondary hyperpigmentation and infection of the wound. Infection is more a part of wound management, and so is dealt with in Section 3-3-2 below. The patient's tendencies towards hyperphotosensitivity, hyperpigmentation, hypertrophy, shock and infection must therefore be carefully assessed. Excessive sun-burn reaction following normal solar exposure may well indicate a condition of excessive photosensitivity. If the patient is suffering from an allergic condition, for example asthma or urticaria, there may well be a tendency towards hyperpigmentation following any injury. The condition of existing scars, such as postoperative scars, smallpox or BCG vaccination marks, will indicate the patient's tendency to form hypertrophic scars or true keloids. If the lesion is prominently visible, for example on the face, or if its presence somehow prevents the patient taking part in normal social pursuits, (a large naevus spilus on the chest wall may make the patient shy of any activity involving exposure), then there is likely to be a strong psychosomatic element in addition to the physical presence of the lesion. This psychosomatic element may well affect, or be affected by, others in the patient's immediate family or social circle.

Although it is over 30 years old, the laser is still comparatively 'new' in its medical application: new enough still to have an aura of mystery and 'high-tech' for the average layman, and also perhaps some feelings akin to fear. It is unfortunately true to say that there are still some clinicians who do not understand fully just how the laser can remove a skin blemish, and why it can do that better than another conventional methodology. In that case how can the medical laser professional expect his or her patient to understand? The answer is the education programme. Before having even the test treatment, advocated as one of the first stages in Ohshiro's Total Treatment Concept, the patient must be enrolled in a well-constructed and informative education programme. This is important from two aspects: first, naturally, is that knowledge of the history, background and basics of the laser, and its capabilities, what it can and (even more important) cannot do in the condition from which the patient suffers, will give the patient a firm base from which to make the decision to proceed or not to proceed with the laser treatment: it will also go a long way to removing any of the misconceptions the patient may harbour about the laser as a 'death ray', and replace the science-fiction with 'science-fact'. Secondly, and of at least equal significance, the education programme brings the patient into contact with his or her clinician, and the support staff: this is the first stage in building up the extremely important patient/clinician rapport on which full understanding of the laser procedure, and its aftercare, really depends. It is this rapport which will help the patient with the psychological problems arising from their condition, and which will also reinforce the necessity of adhering strictly to the basic postoperative wound care procedures: that latter aspect is the one from which the unexpected side effect associated with infection may often spring, from misunderstanding or ignorance of correct wound care management. Without the rapport between patient and clinician, the patient may well sometimes be reluctant to report any unusual symptoms during the course of the wound's healing, which should of course be reported immediately: even if the symptoms turn out to be part of the normal process, the patient should be able to call their clinician at any time. If the symptoms do turn out to be the genesis of an unexpected and unwanted side effect, the earlier they can be dealt with the better. A strong education programme coupled with good patient/staff rapport will help avoid all these hazards.

2-2-9-(B) Side Effects with LLLT

With LLLT systems, wound care management is not a problem. In fact, LLLT is often used to solve problems which occur in postsurgical wound management. By their very nature, dedicated LLLT systems are almost incapable of producing damage of a thermal nature. A possible hazard however is the patient's being photosensitized to the wavelength of the laser being used, which would result in a photochemical reaction of a non-thermal nature, possibly producing severe erythema or vesicular eruptions. Photosensitiza-

tion can be caused by one of the porphyrins, for example, either occurring spontaneously from some physical abnormality in the patient, or by exogenous application, either from a plant or from medication. Even low power densities of 3 W/cm^2 of the appropriate wavelength can then cause a phototoxic reaction in the target tissue. Everyday exposure to normal sunlight will indicate if the patient is already photosensitized to radiation within wavelengths of approximately 320 nm to 2000 nm. Within these wavelengths the spectral irradiance of terrestrial sunlight is capable of producing an abnormal response in photosensitized skin. If the patient has no history of unusual erythema or eruptions following solar or everyday-artificial light sources, it can be safely assumed that the patient is not photosensitized to the wavelength of an LLLT system within the above range. 'Sunburn', for example, is to be expected following lengthy exposure on a bright or sunny day. However, something resembling sunburn following little exposure on a dull day, or to any domestic artificial light source would indicate some form of photosensitization. In every case the author recommends a small LLLT test patch, even when there is no history of polymorphic light eruption.

In some cases, especially in therapy for chronic conditions, a patient's pain may intensify after LLLT: the education programme, however, should have made this clear, and the established patient/therapist rapport will ensure that this is accepted as a natural part of the LLLT healing process. Without that acceptance and the rapport, the patient may well come to believe that in fact the laser has 'made them worse', and that is a potential hazard.

Early reports in the field of laser acupuncture pointed to possible adverse side effects from over-exposure to the laser beam, including nausea, involuntary tonic spasms and vertigo. This was however in the field of acupuncture, where a meridian is being treated: in such cases, the treated portion is often distant from the portion requiring treatment, and overexposure of the acupuncture point often affected the entire meridian. With laser therapy, where treatment is based on an anatomical rather than an acupuncture point network, there have been no reports of adverse side effects which could be traced to overexposure: that may be a hazard in laser acupuncture, but not in LLLT, at least according to the literature and personal communication to the present.

The following examples briefly demonstrate the more common side effects. However, side effects are controllable, provided the clinician, his or her staff and the patient are all working together under the concepts of the Total Treatment Concept. The reader is recommended to study the section on wound healing and wound management in the following chapter, and by applying the concepts contained therein, coupled with the other aspects of the TTC, side effects can be minimized, and controlled.

2-2-9-(B-1) Depressive and Hypertrophic Scar

Scar formation falls into one of two categories: depressive scar and raised or hypertrophic scar.

Figure 2.63 shows a typical example of minor depressive scarring. Depressive scars occur where the defect created by the treatment is too large to heal by first intention. Constant damaging of a normally healing wound by picking off the crust, for example, can also lead to depressive scar formation. Figure 2.64 shows two areas, the larger treated by argon laser, and the smaller by ruby laser. The argon laser has been used to treat the entire lesion in one session, and this has damaged the skin beyond the threshold of its recuperatory power. The result is hypertrophic scarring, together with severe secondary hyperpigmentation. This can be avoided by careful attention to the balance between damage depth and damage volume.

2-2-9-(B-2) Secondary Hyperpigmentation

Figure 2.64 demonstrates secondary hyperpigmentation, as already said. Even the ruby laser treated spot has some secondary hyperpigmentation formation. This side effect is very common, and is in many cases inevitable. However, by careful selection of laser parameters during treat-

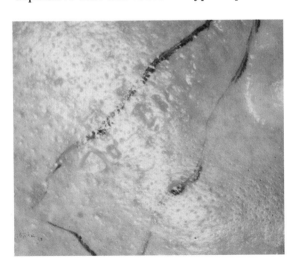

Fig 2.63: *Area of minor depressive type of scarring on right cheek.*

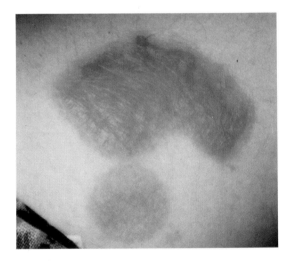

Fig 2.64:
Areas treated by ruby laser (lower, smaller) and argon laser (upper, larger). Both areas have some secondary hyperpigmentation, but the argon treated area also exhibits hypertrophic scarring, because of failure to observe the damage depth/damage volume consideration

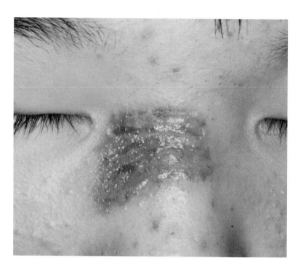

Fig 2.65: *Example of ulceration of laser-treated*
area.

ment, and by use of LLLT coupled with depigmenting ointment after the treatment, secondary hyperpigmentation can be easily controlled.

2-2-9-(B-3) Infection and Ulcer Formation

Infection needs no illustration: infection prevention is part of careful wound management, which is dealt with in detail in the following chapter. The same applies to ulcer formation, which is one of the common sequalae of infection. Figure 2.65 shows an example of an ulcerated wound in its early stages. Antibiotic treatment coupled with good wound care and prophylactic LLLT can control this problem.

CHAPTER 3:

LASER TREATMENT FOR NAEVI

This chapter will combine the physiological basics from Chapter 1 with the basic laser physics of Chapter 2; will explore diagnostic considerations and techniques; will examine all aspects of wound healing, including wound management; will look in depth at the doctor-patient relationship; and will draw the relationship between laser parameters and surgical effect. Following these, the basic concepts of treatment for naevi will be examined, including Ohshiro's Total Treatment Concept. Finally laser safety will be introduced and discussed in detail.

3-1 LOCATION OF NAEVI

The morphological and physiological discussion of the location of the different types of naevus relative to the epidermis and dermis has already been covered in Chapter 1. However, from the point of practical laser treatment for naevi, the location consideration is very important, and classification by depth according to the treatment becomes more important overall than the textbook consideration of the location of a naevus. In Chapter 2, the author discussed the maximum intact dose (MID). From a practical treatment standpoint the MID is that combination of laser parameters which achieves the best clinical result, in other words a macroscopically normal skin condition from the points of colour, configuration and function. The location of naevi classified by depth, by treatment is an important factor in deciding on the MID.

Figure 3.1 is a schematic of the skin, showing the epidermis, dermis and sub-dermal layers. For the purpose of laser treatment, the author has reclassified the normal anatomical terms into zones, as shown in the Figure. Zone I consists of the epidermis: zone II consists of the dermis, and is further subdivided as shown into zone IIa from the dermal papillary processes to the 250 μm depth, and zone IIb from the 250 μm depth to the base of the dermis. The author refers to areas I and IIa as the 'intact zone' since almost any nevus existing there can be easily treated, leaving skin which is macroscopically normal, what I refer to as the intact skin condition (see sections 3.3 and

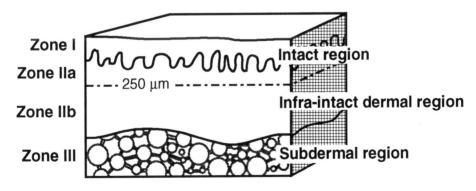

Fig 3.1: *Schematic of the skin, showing conventional anatomical layers, and the author's laser treatment-derived zones.*

3.6 below for a further discussion on the macroscopically intact skin condition). Zone IIb is referred to as the 'infra-intact dermal region'. Zone III is the sub-dermal region, and these are the depth classifications which will be used in this chapter.

From the treatment point of view and the above location classification, naevi can be divided into 7 types: type 1, existing in zone I and type 2a existing in zone IIa, the 'intact' type; type 2, existing in zone IIb, the 'infra-intact dermal' type; type 3, existing in zone III, the 'subdermal' type; type 4 existing in zones I, IIa and IIb, the 'intact/infra- intact dermal' type; type 5, existing in zones I, IIa and III, the 'intact-subdermal' type; type 6 existing in zones IIb and III, the 'infra-intact dermal/subdermal' type; and type 7, existing throughout zones I, II, and III, the 'full range' type of nevi.

As far as the classification of naevi by location is concerned, it can generally be said that the naevi existing in zones I and II must be treated. Concerning the problem of the easily apparent colour, the more superficial the naevus cells or materials are, the more light can be reflected back from them through the skin to the eye of the observer, and thus the more apparent the lesion appears. When a naevus exists in area III only, however, then its colour is usually too deep to be seen through zones I and II. Therefore, unless there is a malignant change of a zone III naevus, or there is a concomitant configurational or functional defect, such naevi can be left untreated.

Examples of some naevi classed under their location types are as follows. Type 1: naevus spilus, naevus spilus tardivus, the junctional type of naevus cell naevus, vitiligo, hyperpigmentation and hypopigmentation. Type 2a: the spotty type of haemangioma simplex, strawberry mark, the superficial intradermal type of naevus cell naevus, and some types of cavernous haemangioma. Type 2; Mongolian fleck, blue nevus, and the deeper intradermal type of naevus cell naevus. Exclusively type 3 naevi do not really concern the clinician for the reasons already stated: they are in fact usually too deep for their

Table 3.1: *Location of naevi by zone*

Type	Location Zone	Examples
1	Zone I	NS, NST, junctional NCN, vitiligo, *etcetera*
2a	Zone IIa	spotty type of HS, strawberry mark, superficial intradermal NCN, some types of CH, *etcetera*
2b	Zone IIb	Mongolian fleck, blue naevus,deeper intradermal NCN, and so on
3	Zone III	(Not usually seen from the surface)
4	Zones (I + IIa) + IIb	Ohta's naevus, HS + CH, HS + Ohta's naevus, strawberry mark + HS, *etcetera*
5	Zones (I + IIa) + III	NS + subdermal CH
6	Zones IIb + III	cavernous haemangioma, *etcetera*
7	Zones I + II + III	full-range HS, Sturge-Weber's syndrome, Klippel-Trenaunay-Weber's syndrome, Tierfel naevus, *etcetera*

Abbreviations: CH = cavernous haemangioma; HS = haemangioma simplex; NCN = naevus cell naevus; NS = naevus spilus; NST = naevus spilus tardivus

abnormal colour to be visible through the overlying dermal and epidermal tissue.

As already discussed in Chapter 1, there are the combination types of naevi, and they are also classified as such under the above location criteria. Type 4 exists in zones I and II, and includes: Ohta's naevus; haemangioma simplex + cavernous haemangioma; and the compound type of naevus cell naevus. Type 5 is found in zones I, IIa and III, so only the components existing in zones I and IIa need to be treated. Type 6, for example cavernous haemangioma, which exists in zones IIb and III only needs the IIb components removed. Type 7 is the full range naevus, existing

in zones I, II and III, and includes amongst others Sturge-Weber's syndrome, Klippel-Trenaunay-Weber's syndrome and some types of the Tierfel naevus: only the zone I and zone II components need treated, unless there are any abnormalities other than colour in the zone III naevus component which can be perceived by an outside observer. Table 3.1 shows the above information in summary. Another important consideration in the depth of the treatment is the skin appendages, which extend down to and beyond the basement membrane: these are of particular importance in treating MAG naevi.

3-2 DIAGNOSTIC CONSIDERATIONS

Before the test treatment with the laser or lasers to be used (for a discussion of the laser test treatment, see 3-10-1 below), other general diagnostic considerations can be applied to help determine which laser or lasers might be best for each patient. These include colorimetry and thermography.

3-2-1 Colorimetry

Colorimetry is the science involving the comparison of colours, using an instrument known as the colorimeter. Before explaining the mechanics and application of the colorimeter, a brief discussion of the concept of colour and colour perception is in order, including the application of colour systems such as the Munsell system, and how different aspects of colour perception can be used in laser treatment for naevi.

3-2-1-(A) Colour and Colorimetry

Colour is an important factor in our lives, but if asked to explain 'colour', the average person could not describe what exactly colour 'is'. Put a single ray of light energy from the sun or from many artificial light sources through a triangular prism, and we can see that they are both composed of a large number of single colours.

When this light, composed of several wavelengths, strikes an object of a particular colour, that object will absorb all other colours except its own and reflect that particular wavelength, or waveband. The reflected light comes back into the

eyes of the observer. The energy reaches the retina, where the frequency of the incident light is transformed from electromagnetic light energy to electrical energy, and relayed to the brain. The brain then recognizes and classifies the light as a particular colour, brightness and vividness.

Light from the sun will have more in the longer wavelength red than the fluorescent tube, which will show a preponderance of shorter wavelength blue light. Because of this difference, certain colours such as in clothing will look 'different' under fluorescent light and natural sunlight.

The color of an object as perceived by the brain depends greatly on the colour reflected from the object being viewed. This eye/brain classification of the colour is referred to as the *sensitive value* of colour. On the other hand, quantification of the actual spectral components of the colour is referred to as the *physical value* of the colour. Accordingly, the clinician uses the sensitive value of the colour of a naevus, reflected back from the naevus to his or her eyes, in the diagnostic study of the naevus: the sensitive value of the naevus colour is also used in assessment of the treatment effect.

The physical value of the naevus colour must be applied for the actual laser treatment of naevi: the physical value is used to determine such parameters as the irradiation dose and the irradiation area. In laser treatment for naevi, the surgeon uses the absorption rate of the physical value of the 'colour' of the incident beam. In these ways, we can recognize the valid application of both the sensitive and the physical values of colour in diagnosis, treatment, and evaluation of the therapeutic effect.

Finally, the clinician can classify colours in such a way that they can be accurately reported, and can be equally accurately recognized by a third party. This medicoscientific classification of colour is embodied in the establishment of the science of *colorimetry*.

3-2-1-(B) The Sensitive Value of Colour

The human eye is capable of perceiving colour. There are many methods of colour classification based on colour perception. The human eye is

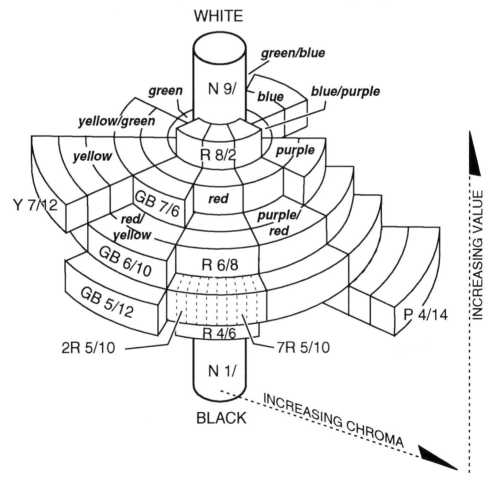

Fig 3.2: *An adaptation of Munsell's 'Colour Tree' from which the classification of colours can be derived. (Adapted from Munsell AH "A Grammar of Color", ed. Birren F: Van Nostrand Reinhold Company, New York USA).*

capable of distinguishing a range of colours from purple to red (400 nm - 700 nm). This is not an absolute range, however, and differs from individual to individual. In photobiology, this range is classed as the visible spectrum. The two main classification systems based on the sensitive value of colour are the Oswald system and the Munsell system. The Munsell colour system is used in the medical field because it has a slightly more 'scientific' basis than the Oswald system. In 1898, Albert H Munsell created his "colour sphere" or "colour tree" which can be used to classify colours accurately and consistently (Figure 3.2, adapted from Munsell A H "*A Grammar of Color*", ed Birren F: Van Nostrand Reinhold Company, New York). Munsell started with a central achromatic core, with white at the top 'pole' and black at the bottom, which he divided into 11 stages with shades of gray in between the two colour poles of black and white. He called this the axis of *value* in his colour classification. He surrounded the achromatic central core with concentric circles of colour. He called these the rings of *hue*, and he divided them into 10 segments, with red, yellow green, blue and purple in between which are the colour mixtures of red-yellow, yellow-green, green-blue, blue-purple and purple-red, giving the standard 10 hues of the Munsell system. As each hue is further divided into 10, this gives a very exact classification for each of the standard hues of 5.0 R, 5.0 YR, 5.0 Y and so on, finishing up with 5.0 PR. Of these concentric rings of hue, the outermost, on the 'equator' of the sphere, are the most vivid, decreasing in saturation towards the central achromatic core. Munsell called these saturation steps the *chroma* of the colour. Figure 3.3 shows the chart for red 5.0 R from the sphere, which shows how the chroma changes horizontally, while the value changes vertically. All colours are classified under the Munsell system by these three components, so a colour is expressed by its hue, value/chroma: a shade of red could thus be expressed as 5.0 R, 6.0/7.0. In this way, Munsell

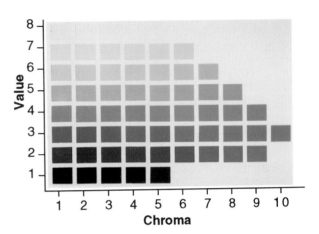

Fig 3.3: *Chart from Munsell classification of colour for 5R (mid value red).*

standardized the classification of colour. These colour charts are still made from the human 'sense', and so we refer to this perception of colour classification as the ***sensitive value*** of colour. Using this colour sphere, one can compare all the colours of nature and classify each colour in a particular and consistent way, which is the expression of the sensitive value of that particular colour.

3-1-2-(C) The Physical Value of Colour

When 'white' light or any mixture of light of different colours is passed through a prism or a diffraction grating, the light is broken up into its different spectral components, each of which occupies a narrow waveband. The resultant spectrum from white light forms the visible spectrum, the colours of the rainbow, from violet to red as already discussed above. When this is extended beyond violet and red into the ultraviolet and infrared components, respectively, it is referred to as the invisible spectrum. The combination of the visible and invisible spectra is called the wide spectrum (Figure 3.4). Special analyzing and recording electronic equipment can produce a visible record of this spectrum: the print out is called a spectrogram, and the equipment used to produce it is called the spectrometer.

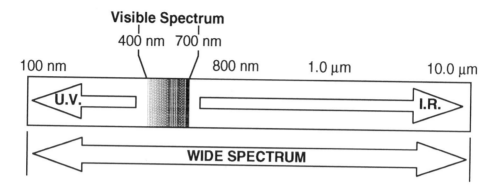

Fig 3.4: *The wide spectrum, incorporating visible and nonvisible elements of 'light'.*

Figure 3.5 shows in schematic form a typical colour computer, or more correctly, a microprocessor-based photospectrometer. The handpiece is connected to the main console by a flexible coaxial cable, which carries the colour-balanced 'white' efferent light from the console light source to the handpiece in the central portion of the cable, and also carries back the information from the receptors in the handpiece through the outer cable to the computer in the console. Both the efferent and afferent cables are of fibreoptic construction. The handpiece is placed over the sample tissue, and the spectrometer is activated. The light source in the system produces a beam of balanced 'white' light, which is first passed through a diffraction grating to separate the light into its spectral components. The computer samples both a reference beam, which is taken from the outgoing light by a beam splitter, and the incoming light reflected from the tissue under test. The spectra of the two beams are prepared, and the computer then draws a plot of absorption against wavelength from 400 nm to 700 nm on a precision pen plotter. The spectrum may also be shown as a colour picture on the unit's VDU (video display unit).

In clinical practice, the computer data are stored on a floppy disk, and entered against the patient's number on their treatment record card, so the data can be located and retrieved at any time. At least two readings are taken, one (or more) from the lesion, and one from the surrounding normal skin. Thus the computer presents the physical value of the naevus pigment in the area of interest and surrounding normal skin pigment for each patient, or for several sites in the lesion in the case of a naevus exhibiting colour changes within itself.

3-2-1-(D) Clinical Application of Colorimetry

As already discussed above, there are two values of colour which can be used in a clinical setting: we can refer to them as the subjective value, which is a component of the sensitive value of colour, and the objective value, based on the physical value of colour. The subjective value depends on reflected light: the photospectrometer depends on the absorption of light to calculate and display the objective, physical value of colour. Patients perceive, see and visibly quantify the difference in colour between their naevus and the surrounding normal skin by using the sensitive value of colour. At the same time, they also use the sensitive value of colour when assessing the postoperative improvement in the colour of the lesion. If the clinician wants a good doctor/patient rapport, then the doctor must use the sensitive value of colour in the diagnosis and treatment assessment, when talking to the patient. The laser beam however is totally objective. The laser beam has no subjective viewpoint, and the reaction

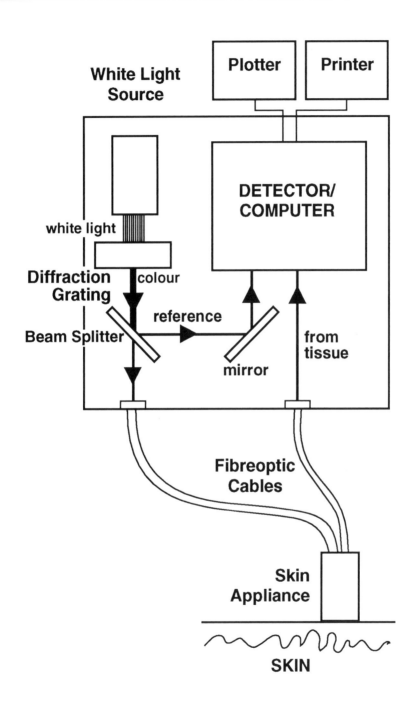

Fig 3.5: *Schematic layout of typical colour computer. See text for details.*

Table 3.2: *Sensitive values for the most representative colour from red, yellow, green, blue and purple colour charts (hue = 5 for all)*

Colour (Hue)	Value/Chroma (Mean of Results)	Value/Chroma (Rounded Off)	Perceptibility Factor
5R	3.8/12.1	4/12	0.65
5Y	8.3/11.8	8/12	1.14
5G	5.2/8.2	5/8	2.4
5B	3.4/8.1	3/8	0.71
5P	2.7/5.9	3/6	0.83

between the wavelength of the incident beam and the pigment in the lesion is governed by purely physical laws: Thus in the case of naevus treatment, the difference in the physical value of the colour of the naevus region and of the surrounding normal skin is very important.

3-2-1-(D-1) Comparison of the Sensitive and Physical Values of Colour

An experiment was designed to assess the difference between the sensitive and physical values of colour. On a slightly overcast but dry day in spring, at 15:00 hrs, 20 informed and consenting passers-by were chosen at random to participate in the experiment. The time of day and weather type were chosen because there was no direct sunlight, but there was a well-diffused neutral illumination level. First each volunteer was checked for green/red colour blindness using the standard colour vision deficiency test cards. The participants were then shown a set of Munsell colour charts (prepared to JIS standard by the Japan Colour Research Institute) for 5R, 5Y, 5G, 5B and 5P, the 'standard' hue for each of the 5 main colours, and asked to choose the value/chroma which represented to them the purest colour, i.e. the 'reddest', 'most yellow', 'greenest' and so on, of the colour samples on each chart. Table 3.2 summarizes the results.

Using a Murakami MICC system microprocessor-based photospectrometer (Murakami Color Research Laboratory, Tokyo, Japan) the mean figures for value/chroma as assessed from the study were plotted for each of the 5 colours. As the Munsell system can only deal with whole numbers, the mean figures were rounded off to give the figures in the third column of Table 3.2. The results of this plot are shown in Figure 3.6, which plots the spectral radiance factor (vertical axis) against the wavelength (horizontal axis).

The first point which can be seen from the physical value of the chosen 'pure' colours (from the sensitive value) is that some of them contain spectral peaks for two or more colours, and so are not physically speaking 'pure' at all. 5P 3/6 has minor peaks in the blue and yellow wavebands, with its major peak in the red. 5Y 8/12 has a peak in the yellow and another in the red waveband. Secondly, it is possible to calculate the 'perceptibility factor' of the chosen colours by relating the value of the colour (its 'brightness') with the percentage points ($\times 10^{-1}$) of the spectral radiance factor of the colour's main peak. Thus we find that green 5G (value of 5 and spectral reflectance, SR, of 2.1) has a perceptibility factor, PF, of 2.4. This is followed by yellow (5Y 8/12, SR 7, PF = 1.14); purple (5P 3/6, SR 3.8, PF=0.83); blue (5B 3/8, SR 4.2, PF=0.71); and red (5R 4/12, SR 6.2, PF=0.65). This scoring is summarized in the last column of Table 3.2. According to this method of calculation of the perceptibility factor, the shade of red chosen by the volunteers in the experiment was the least perceptible colour. This points clearly to the importance of dealing both the sensitive and physical values of colour in both diagnosis and post-treatment follow up in laser

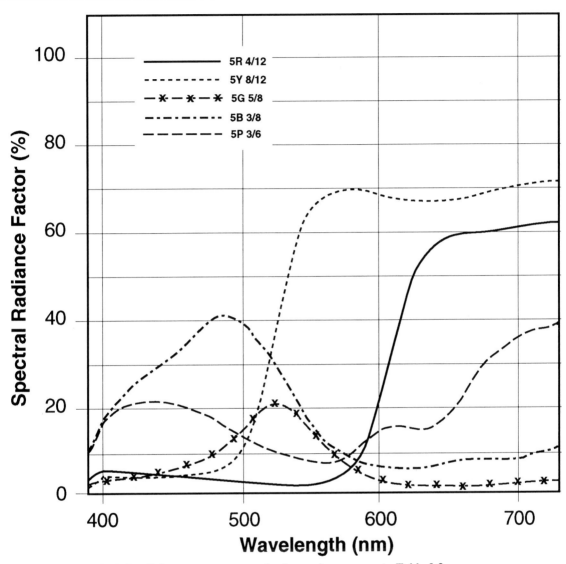

Fig 3.6: *Colour spectrograms of colour values as seen in Table 3.2.*

treatment for naevi.

In the next part of the experiment, the colour computer plotted two sets of figures for each colour. In the first set, the value remained constant while the chroma was altered in steps from the lowest (N = neutral) to the highest reading for that colour on the Munsell scale, and in the second set the value was altered against a fixed chroma. Representative results can be seen in Figure 3.7:a and b for 5Y and 3.7:c and d for 5P. 3.7:a and c

show the fixed value results and 3.7:b and d the fixed chroma. The overall picture is very similar for both colours, and for the others not shown. An increase in chroma results in a wider range of distribution of spectral radiance factor (i.e. spectral reflectance) between the short blue and longer red wavebands with greater differentiation of the component waveband peaks especially in yellow and purple, and an increase in value retains more or less the same spectral distribution curve with a

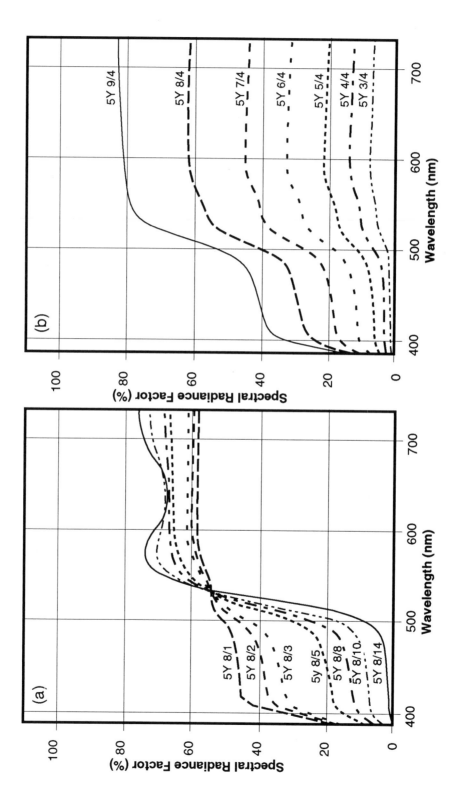

Fig 3.7: *Colour spectrograms of 5Y (a and b, this page) and 5P (c and d, facing page), plotting both with fixed value (a and c)and fixed chroma (b and d).*

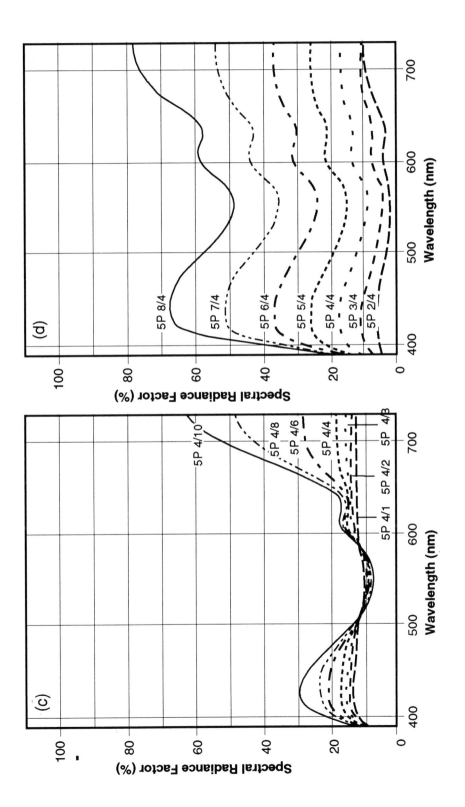

relative increase in the overall reflectance factor.

3-2-1-(D-2) Clinical Application of the Sensitive Value of Colour

The clinician assesses the sensitive value of the colour of the patients' naevi using a set of standard colour charts, from which the hue, value/chroma of the lesion and of the surrounding normal skin can be accurately assessed and entered on the patient's record card. As treatment progresses, the colour change in the treated areas can be compared easily with the original assessed colour.

3-2-1-(D-3) Clinical Application of the Physical Value of Colour

Figure 3.8 shows a typical reflectance spectrogram for oxyhaemoglobin and deoxyhaemoglobin (in solution in pure H_2O). The higher the reflectance, the lower the absorption: the bottom section of the 'block' represents the reflectance values, and the upper area can thus give an idea of wavelength-dependent absorption. From the purely physical value, the short blue light waveband is very highly absorbed in oxyhaemoglobin, but in actual practice the penetration into *in vivo* tissue is highly limited, making this waveband unsuitable for pigment removal. Peaks in HbO_2 absorption peaks can also be seen at 418, 542 and

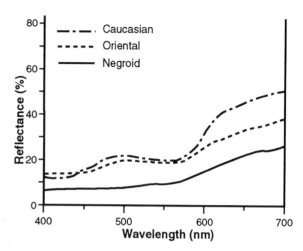

Fig 3.9:
Normal untanned male skin (anterior aspect of the arm) comparing Caucasian, Black and Oriental skin types.

577 nm, but the higher potential absorption at the 418 nm band is offset by poor tissue penetration, making vessels at a depth of greater than 100 μm difficult to reach. This shows how the physics of laser/tissue interaction must also be considered as complementary data to the physical value of HbO_2 absorption as assessed photospectrometrically. Note the lack of similar peaks in the deoxyhaemoglobin curve, due to the colour shift from bright red to purple.

Figure 3.9 shows the spectrogram for normal untanned male skin (anterior aspect of the arm), comparing Caucasian, black and oriental skin types. The HbO_2 peaks are still evident in the Caucasian and oriental curves, but they are filtered out by the overlying tissue, and augmented by the presence of other pigments such as melanin in the stratum granulosum and below, and β-carotene. In the Black skin type, the high concentration of epidermal melanin almost completely flattens out the HbO_2 peaks. Figure 3.10 shows the spectrogram of melanin (DOPA-melanin in solution in pure H_2O). Comparing this curve with the spectrogram in Figure 3.9 above, the influence of the greater melanin concentration in the Oriental and Black skin compared with the Caucasian type

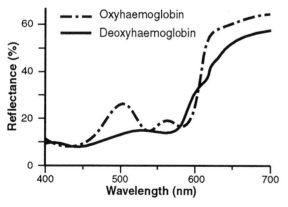

Fig 3.8:
Reflectance spectrogram in visible light range for oxyhaemoglobin and deoxyhaemoglobin in solution in purified H_2O.

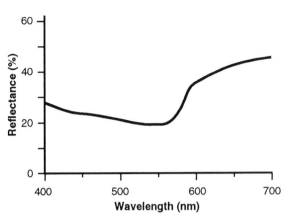

Fig 3.10: *Spectrogram of dopa melanin in solution in pure H_2O.*

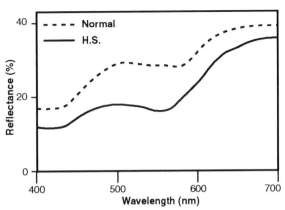

Fig 3.11:
Visible light spectrogram of typical haemangioma simplex compared with normal skin. The degree of difference between the two curves can be used to determine the optimum wavelength for treatment.

is clearly visible, especially at the longer wavelengths on the right of the spectrogram.

3-2-1-(D-3)-(a) Haemangioma Simplex

Figure 3.11 shows the spectrogram of a typical haemangioma simplex (HS) lesion compared with normal skin. The HbO_2 peaks are naturally more clearly seen in the HS curve because of the presence of the haemoglobin-carrying erythrocytes in the ectatic vessels of the lesion. The absorption differential between the two curves is clearly visible across the entire visible light spectrum. Lasers currently used in the treatment of HS are the argon (488 nm, 514.5 nm), KTP/532 (532 nm), copper vapour (511 nm, 578 nm), argon dye (577 nm), flashlamp dye (585 nm, 590 nm) and ruby (694.3 nm) lasers. If we compare the difference in absorption at these wavelengths between the normal tissue and the HS curves, the wavelength giving the optimum absorption differential will be seen. The higher the differential, the better the absorption; the better the absorption, the greater the potential degree of light conversion to radiant heat. For this particular lesion, the yellow-light dye lasers would give the most efficient absorption characteristics. However, it is extremely interesting to note that even the red light

of the ruby laser at 694.3 nm would give a fair absorption differential in the lesion represented by this curve. Thus the application of spectrography to represent the physical value of colour shows a popular misconception stemming from the rules of the sensitive value of colour, namely that any colour will absorb its complementary colour best. Even the red HS lesion will absorb red ruby laser light with a satisfactorily high absorption differential.

From the author's experience, HS on the head and neck can be subdivided into two types by colorimetric spectrography: type 1 is where the absorption differential is greater in the mid-range wavebands, such as the argon, KTP/532 laser, dye and copper vapour lasers, than in the longer red ruby waveband. Type 2 is where the absorption differential is greater at the ruby waveband than in the mid-spectral bands. Statistically, type 1 accounts for 75% of all cases, and type 2 for 25%. If the absorption differential is less than 5%, then that rules out the wavelength or waveband to which it applies: the difference between the absorption characteristics of the lesion and normal skin is too small to guarantee good differential absorption of the laser beam in the target lesion, compared with

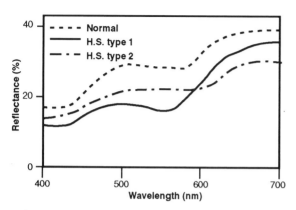

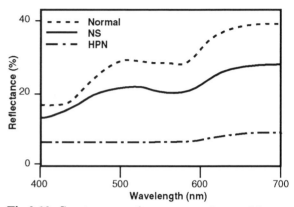

Fig 3.12: Typical spectrograms for HS types 1 and 2.

Fig 3.13: Spectrograms for naevus spilus and hairy pigmented naevus.

the surrounding normal skin. In the early days of the author's clinic, when there was a choice between only the ruby and argon lasers, these typing spectrograms were very important. In the interim, the pulsed ruby laser has fallen somewhat into disuse. At the time of writing, with the large selection of laser wavelengths available, the photospectrometric classification into types 1 and 2 is no longer quite so important. However, with the advent of the pulsed ruby laser, giving an ul-

trashort pulse width measured in nanoseconds, the red end of the spectrogram has once again become available. Figure 3.12 shows typical spectrograms for HS types 1 and 2.

3-2-1-(D-3)-(b) Melanin Anomaly Group

Not to ignore the spectrographic findings in the melanin anomaly group, Figure 3.13 shows typical spectrograms generated from naevus spilus and hairy pigmented naevus, respectively, compared with normal skin. The lighter-coloured nae-

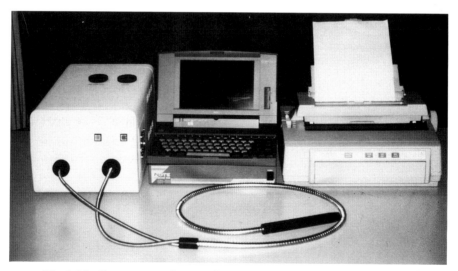

Fig 3.14: Components of new wide spectrum photospectrometric system.

Table 3.3: *Specifications of new wide-spectrum photospectrometer*

Item	Specification
Main Application	1: Physical assessment of abnormal skin colour of a naevus patient for selection of optimal physical wavelength for treatment 2: Postoperative physical assessment of colour change in the treated area
Measurement available	Spectroreflectivity and spectrotransmissivity
Wavelength range	400 nm - 1,100 nm (1.0 nm increments)
Light source	Halogen lamp
Detector	1024 element linear image sensor
Light guide	Quartz optical fibre bundle (50 cm long)
Method of Measurement: Reflectivity	Probe attached to system placed on skin surface or coloured material for measurement
Transmissivity	Specimen placed in 'black box'
Display processing rate	faster than 1 sec
Display peripherals	Graphical colour display on VDU or hard copy on colour plotter. Print-out of graphs in coordinate data. Autocalculation available of data gathered before and after treatment of lesion

vus spilus still demonstrates some of the HbO_2 peak characteristics, which disappear in the darker-coloured hairy pigmented naevus.

3-2-1-(D-3)-(c) New Considerations: Wide Spectrum Photospectrometry

The above spectrograms are all based on the visible light spectrum: in current treatment considerations, many more laser wavelengths have been added, and so the most realistic consideration is to use a spectrophotometer which can display results over a wider waveband, to include especially the near infrared. The author's clinic has just acquired such a prototype system, seen in Figure 3.14. Table 3.3 gives the main specifications of the system, which works on basically the same principle as described above.

Some representative samples will now be presented.

SS-1) Haemangioma Simplex (HS)

The patient seen in figure 3.15.a is a 2.2 year old female with HS of the right cheek. Area 1 is the untreated area, and area 2 is the contralateral normal cheek. Figure 3.15b shows the spectrometric findings. Note the clearly visible 'blood curve' between 500 nm and 600 nm. The pretreatment findings in Figure 3.15a show that this is a fairly mild form of the pinkish, deeper HS, and this is also seen in the spectrogram, showing only small differences in reflection between the normal and untreated lesion skin color.

136

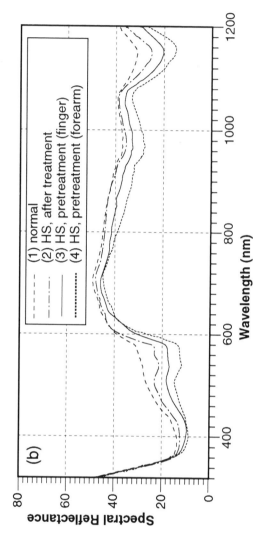

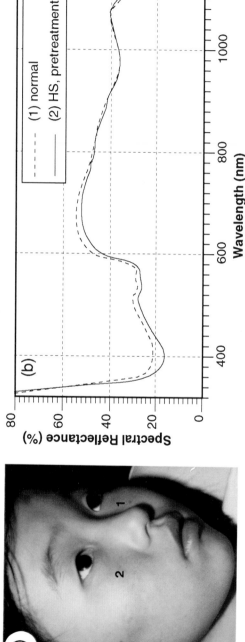

Fig 3.15: **a:** *2.2-year-old girl with HS of the right cheek.* **b:** *wide spectrogram comparing untreated naevus with contralateral normal skin colour. Because this is a comparatively mild case, there is not a trmenedous difference between the normal contralateral skin and the untreated HS.*

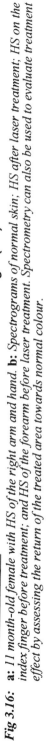

Fig 3.16: **a:** *11 month-old female with HS of the right arm and hand.* **b:** *Spectrograms of normal skin; HS after laser treatment; HS on the index finger before treatment; and HS of the forearm before laser treatment. Spectrometry can also be used to evaluate treatment effect by assessing the return of the treated area towards normal colour.*

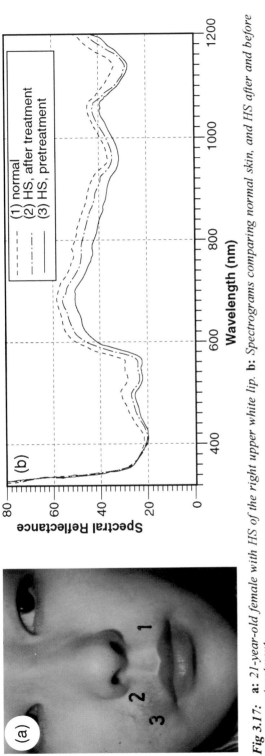

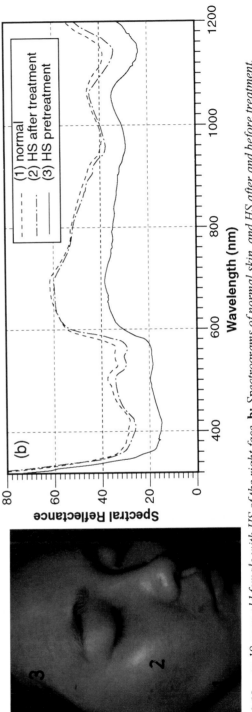

Fig 3.17: **a:** *21-year-old female with HS of the right upper white lip.* **b:** *Spectrograms comparing normal skin, and HS after and before treatment.*

Fig 3.18: **a:** *18-year-old female with HS of the right face.* **b:** *Spectrograms of normal skin, and HS after and before treatment.*

138

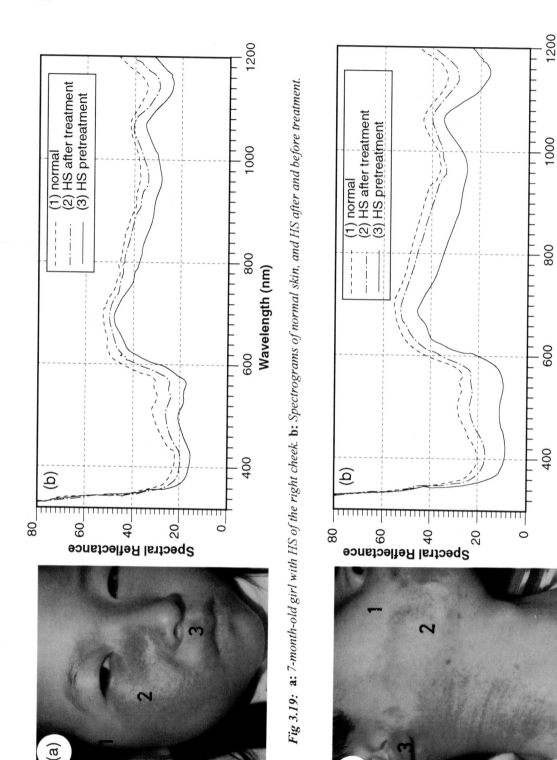

Fig 3.19: a: 7-month-old girl with HS of the right cheek. b: Spectrograms of normal skin, and HS after and before treatment.

Fig 3.20: a: 12-year-old boy with HS of the right neck. b: Spectrograms of normal skin, and HS after and before treatment.

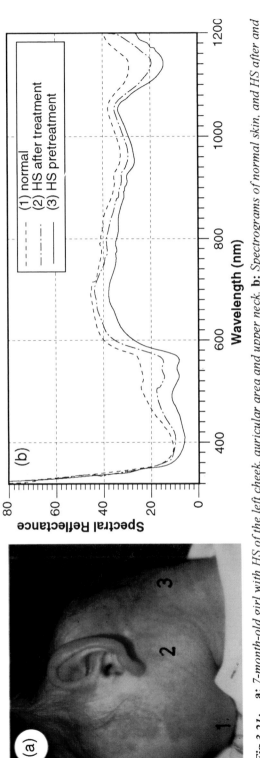

Fig 3.21: **a:** *7-month-old girl with HS of the left cheek, auricular area and upper neck.* **b:** *Spectrograms of normal skin, and HS after and before treatment.*

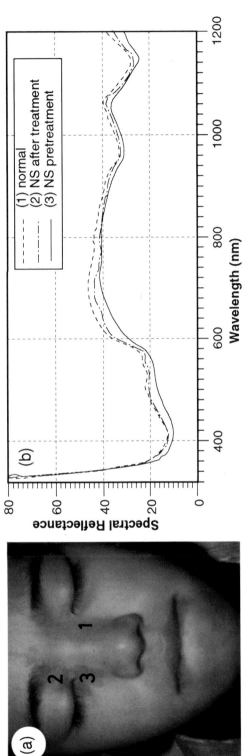

Fig 3.22: **a:** *12.25-year-old girl with naevus spilus of the inner aspect of the right eye.* **b:** *Spectrograms of normal skin, and NS after and before treatment.*

140

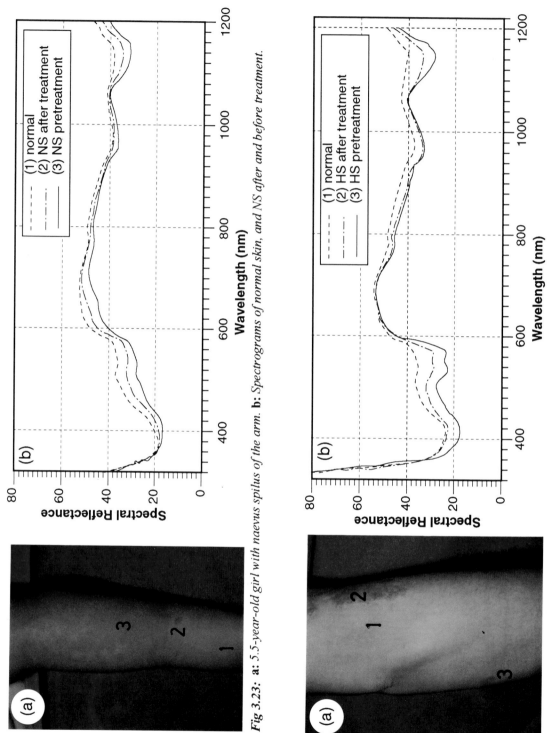

Fig 3.23: **a:** *5.5-year-old girl with naevus spilus of the arm.* **b:** *Spectrograms of normal skin, and NS after and before treatment.*

Fig 3.24: **a:** *25-year-old female with HS of the arm.* **b:** *Spectrograms of normal skin, and HS after and before treatment.*

SS-2) HS

The patient in Figure 3.16a is a 11-month-old girl with HS of the right forearm and hand. Areas 1, 2, 3 and 4 correspond respectively to: normal skin; after treatment; HS pretreatment, index finger; HS pretreatment, forearm. Figure 3.16b shows the spectrometric findings. A difference in the physical value of the HS colour in the index finger and forearm indicates that the lesion on the forearm may well respond better to treatment, as there is a larger difference between that reflectance curve and the normal skin. The curve of the treated area is much closer to the normal colour, showing good colour removal. This is an indication of how colour spectrometry may also be used in treatment assessment.

SS-3) HS

The patient in Figure 3.17a is a 21-year-old female with HS of the right upper white lip. Areas 1, 2, and 3 correspond respectively to: normal skin; after treatment; HS pretreatment. Figure 3.17b shows the spectrometric findings.

SS-4) HS

The patient in Figure 3.18a is an 18-year-old female with HS of the right cheek and forehead. Areas 1, 2, and 3 correspond respectively to: normal skin; after treatment; HS pretreatment. Figure 3.18b shows the spectrometric findings.

SS-5) HS

The patient in Figure 3.19a is a 7-month-old girl with HS of the right cheek. Areas 1, 2, and 3 correspond respectively to: normal skin; after treatment; HS pretreatment. Figure 3.19b shows the spectrometric findings.

SS-6) HS

The patient in Figure 3.20a is a 12-year-old female with HS of the right jaw and neck. Areas 1, 2, and 3 correspond respectively to: normal skin; after treatment; HS pretreatment. Figure 3.20b shows the spectrometric findings.

SS-7) HS

The patient in Figure 3.21a is a 7-month-old female with HS of the left cheek, ear, postauricular region and neck. Areas 1, 2, and 3 correspond respectively to: normal skin; after treatment; HS pretreatment. Figure 3.21b shows the spectrometric findings.

SS-8) Naevus Spilus (NS)

The patient in Figure 3.22a is a 12-year-old boy with NS of the right cheek and forehead. Areas 1, 2, and 3 correspond respectively to: normal skin; after treatment; HS pretreatment. Figure 3.22b shows the spectrometric findings. Note the flattening out of the blood curve in the pretreatment curve compared with the previous haemangioma patients, and the restoration of the blood curve in the post-treatment spectrometric findings, indicating good removal of the naevus spilus melanin pigment.

SS-9) NS

The patient in Figure 3.23a is a 5.5-year-old girl with NS of the left arm. Areas 1, 2, and 3 correspond respectively to: normal skin; after treatment; NS pretreatment. Figure 3.23b shows the spectrometric findings.

SS-10) HS

The patient in Figure 3.24a is a 25-year-old female with HS of the right arm. Areas 1, 2, and 3 correspond respectively to: normal skin; after treatment; HS pretreatment. Figure 3.24b shows the spectrometric findings.

Simply relying on the physical value of colour as shown by colorimetric spectrography to select the most appropriate laser, however, is an oversimplification. Many other factors must be considered. The site of the naevus, the depth of the naevus and the distribution of the naevus by depth are all important factors which must also be taken into consideration. The physical properties of the laser beam must be considered: continuous wave, pulsed and Q-switch pulsed beams all have different potential effects in the target tissue. The complex physics of laser/tissue interaction must also be very carefully examined, when selecting the most appropriate laser, or lasers, to treat any lesion. This manipulation of a large and varied sum of knowledge is part of what sets the Total Treatment Concept apart from the standardized

'cookbook' approach, and has enabled the author to produce consistently good, repeatable, side-effect free results in the laser treatment of naevi.

3-2-2 Thermography

Thermography is a method whereby a pictorial record of heat distribution in the target tissue is obtained using an infrared-sensitive camera connected to a colour digitizer, microprocessor-controlled and enhanced, which takes a series of scans at preset intervals, and displays the digitized colour-coded picture on a CRT which can be photographed using an instant camera for prints or a standard 35 mm camera for slides. The data may also be saved to disk and can thus be recalled at any time. A standard thermographic set-up can usually be set to record patient number, date and time on the thermogramme, in addition to giving other data such as the ambient temperature, and a colour scale matched with temperatures for interpretation of the picture. The scale usually runs from blue (coldest) to red (hottest), and can be set to show colour gradations in fractions of a degree or whole degrees, depending on the range recorded and sensitivity required.

The use of thermography in low reactive-level laser therapy (LLLT) for pain has been well-documented, where it is used to record and diagnose areas of acute pain with local inflammation, seen as areas warmer than the surrounding skin, or chronic pain conditions, usually associated with areas cooler than the norm, especially at the extremities in for example Raynaud's syndrome. An interesting combination is seen in chronic rheumatoid arthritis, where an area of lower temperature contains areas of higher temperature which indicate local foci of acute inflammation, commonly seen in this condition.

3-2-2-(A) Thermography and Naevi

Thermography has possible applications in the diagnosis of naevi, especially those in the blood vessel anomaly group. It is a very good indicator of vessel depth, type and density. Blood acts as the body's cooling system, and so blood vessels

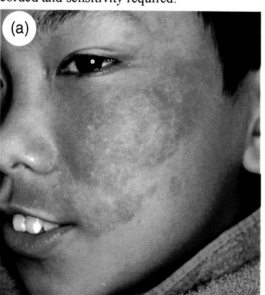

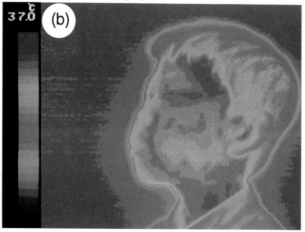

Fig 3.25:
a: *young male patient with preoperative findings of HS of the left cheek.* **b:** *Thermogram of same patient. Cooler area on thermogram can be interpreted as deeper-lying HS.*

nearer the surface will appear warmer on the thermogramme than those situated deeper in the skin. Likewise, veins will appear cooler than arteries. Figure 3.25a shows an example of a thermogramme of a facial haemangioma in an 11-year old boy, compared with the clinical pretreatment findings. Figure 3.25b gives pretreatment findings of the actual lesion. The thermography shows an area cooler than the surrounding skin, so it can be deduced that the haemangioma is situated in the deeper layers of the skin. Appropriate laser treatment is then decided accordingly.

3-2-2-(B) Thermographic Technique

In order to apply thermography with accuracy, it is necessary to have an area dedicated to the taking of thermograms, where the equipment can be left permanently set up. The area should be screened from the surrounding clinic, with, if possible, an attached waiting room. Patients having thermography should be given an opportunity to rest and acclimatize to the room temperature, which should be maintained within as narrow and similar a range as possible. The season of the year and degree of heating or cooling of the clinic will affect the patient's initial temperature, and also how far they have had to walk to get to the clinic: these factors should be considered in deciding the acclimatization period, and this should be taken into consideration when setting the appointment. If disrobing is necessary, this should be done as soon as the patients enter the area, with light gowns provided if necessary to allow for any cooling artifacts resulting in removal of clothing. This will also allow for the normalization of any heating artifacts caused by possible embarrassment.

Several scans should be monitored to see if there are any artifactual changes taking place, before the final scan is frozen on the screen and photographed. The same techniques apply both before and after treatment, if appropriate.

Thermography is a two-dimensional picture of a three dimensional surface, which involves taking several thermograms to cover a large area, and which thus increases the possibility of extraneous artifacts. New techniques have been reported for full-body triaspect thermography, using a system of high-reflectance mirrors positioned so that the three aspects (facial and both lateral) of the patient's face or body can be captured in the one thermogramme. An even more complex system allows for panoramic thermography, in which steady rotation of the patient round their horizontal axis is coupled with a high response real-time thermocamera and a multi-image processor. This provides a continuous thermographic image of the total body surface on the one composite thermogramme. These are developments which might have applications in the future for the diagnosis of large-area haemangioma.

3-3 WOUND HEALING OF THE SKIN

The skin is subject to a large number of wounds of varying degrees of seriousness throughout one's lifetime. These wounds are caused by trauma or by surgical operations. Depending on the wound healing process, the prognosis of each wound will be extremely different. In this section wounds of the skin will be examined in detail, which have a close relationship to laser treatment for naevi.

The authors would like to pay special attention to the process and conditions which can lead optimally to very fine scarring or the macroscopically invisible scar, which is the ultimate goal when removing naevi. Once the skin is injured the injury will inevitably be followed by some form of scarring. It is very difficult to prevent visible scar formation, and it is only in a few cases that an invisible scar can be achieved. If the postoperative scar carries a greater demerit than the original lesion, then that treatment must be labeled as a failure. Such cases are often seen in laser treatment for naevi. The better the abnormal colour removal, and the finer the scar, the greater the merit of the treatment.

The art of laser treatment is to damage the abnormal naevus cells and tissues, but to control the laser/tissue reaction so that damage in the surrounding normal tissue is below the survival threshold of that tissue. The skill to limit damage to the target tissue, while sparing surrounding uninvolved tissue, is acquired only with a lot of practical experience, coupled with theoretical knowledge, as the difference of the reaction to the laser between normal skin cells and abnormal naevus cells is sometimes very small. Even with the greatest skill in the world, however, depending on the original condition of the lesion, it is impossible in many cases to get satisfactory results.

3-3-1 Principles and Basic Mechanisms of Wound Healing of the Skin

There is a number of well-documented basic principles which govern the wound healing process, and an understanding of them will go a long way to helping the clinician achieve the best possible clinical result. An understanding of the mechanisms involved is also important, as it is when these mechanisms go out of control that wound healing is imperfect, and scar formation inevitable.

3-3-1-(A) The Cytological Prognosis of Wound Healing

Wound healing of the skin falls into three phases: the latent phase, the fibrin proliferation phase, and the scar phase.

3-3-1-(A-1) The First (Latent) Phase

This phase lasts from 1 to 4 days following the injury, and is characterized by an acute inflammatory response, during which the permeability of blood vessels in the area of the wound increases, coupled with vasodilation. Leukocytes migrate to the wound area, and the increase in the levels of histochemical mediator and controller amines and polypeptides such as histamine, kinin and prostaglandin all have an effect on the wound healing action and reaction. By three days following the injury, neovascularization is seen at the wound margins with the appearance of capillary buds infiltrating into the wound from the margins. At first fibroblasts and then myofibroblasts are seen in large quantities, together with other mononuclear cells. Granular droplets are also present, as are phagocytic cells which scavenge the wound area removing necrotic tissue, clot fragments, and other wound detritus, and fibroblasts move into a proliferative stage of collagen synthesis.

3-3-1-(A-2) The Second (Fibrin Proliferation) Phase

As the synthesis of extracellular collagen increases, the wound is filled with a layer of granulation tissue, which is rich in newly formed capillaries, fibroblasts, phagocytes, and mast cells. Collagen is rapidly synthesized by the fibroblasts, and the tensile strength of the wound increases remarkably, brought about by the gradual spread throughout the wound of new collagen fibrils, which randomly cross-link to form a strong fibrous matrix across the base of the wound bed. Further fibre-fibre linkage continuously increases the mechanical tensile strength of the wound, until by the fifth or sixth day, interdigitation is seen between the collagen fibres in the wound bed and the collagen at the wound margins.

3-3-1-(A-3) The Third (Scar) Phase

In this phase of wound healing there are alternate sessions of collagen synthesis and collagen lysis, and from the end of the second phase, mature collagenous scar tissue can be seen gradually forming across the wound. The time period of this phase can vary enormously, depending on a large number of factors, some of which will be discussed below: it can take as long as one year or more. The proteoglycans in the ground substance have a very important role in the stabilization of extracellular collagen fibre cross-linkage formation, causing a conjunction between the fibronectin, manufactured by the fibroblasts and present on the cellular membranes, and the intercellular ground substance during cell fusion.

3-3-1-(B) Pattern of Wound Healing

There are two patterns in wound healing: healing by first intention, and healing by second intention.

3-3-1-(B-1) Healing by First Intention

When the wound edges of an incision can be approximated accurately and heal, the healing process results in either a fine linear scar or with varying degrees of hypertrophy. In this case the wound is said to heal by first intention.

3-3-1-(B-2) Healing by Second Intention

When the wound incorporates a skin defect, or if there is a large gap between the wound margins, then the edges of the wound cannot be approximated, and the wound is said to heal by second intention. For the successful cover of these defects, the formation of large amounts of healthy granulation tissue and epithelization are necessary. The epithelial cells gradually advance on the granulation tissue from the wound margins. Thus the wound healing time is delayed, and when the defect is large, formation of a large scar cannot be avoided. In severe cases, involving large areas, the tendency of the wound to contract forms scar contractures, which often lead to deformity and functional disorders in the affected area [see 3-3-1-(C)]. In such cases, the contractures must be corrected, and skin grafting may be used to replace the scar tissue to restore normal appearance and function.

Extensive burn wounds are representative of the most severe cases of scar contracture, and most scars following laser treatment for naevi are included in this type of healing, although usually very mild examples. In the case of a normal burn wound, a lot of the damage is caused by secondary thermal injury due to conducted heat, and can thus be quite extensive. The laser on the other hand causes primarily a radiant heat burn, and is thus usually more limited in depth than other burn injuries. The naevus consists of normal and abnormal coloured cells. Radiant heat is usually more absorbed is usually more absorbed in the abnormal coloured cells than the normal ones, and so selective laser treatment is achieved.

However, whether a wound heals by first or second intention, the basic wound healing mechanism is the same, and the difference in the final result depends on the extent of the wound.

3-3-1-(C) Wound Contraction

The purpose of the wound healing process is to recover the damaged surfaces of the wound by means of new epithel, known as wound epithelization. In case of deep injuries it takes time to create new skin, and the larger the wound, the longer the healing time required. Contraction is one of the mechanisms to aid the epithelization of a wound by reducing the wound area, and thus shortening the time required for coverage. Contraction is not be confused with contracture, although they have the same genesis. Contracture is to be avoided, but proper contraction of the wound is to be encouraged. In animal studies, contraction of the wound by 40% to 80% of the original wound area has been reported. Reasonable contraction of the wound speeds up the healing process, and can help decrease the size of the eventual scar. However, depending on the degree of the injury, the site and extent of wound care and management, over-contraction can lead to scar contracture, resulting in deformity and functional disorders. This is especially true for wounds around the eyes or the mouth, or any of the joints, so wound contraction must be carefully monitored. Some fibroblasts in the healing wound undergo transformation to form myofibroblasts, which have synthesized parallel fibrils resembling smooth muscle which bring about the contraction of the wound.

3-3-1-(D) Epidermal and Dermal Roles in Wound Healing

The function and the role of the dermis and the epidermis in the wound healing process are different. The epidermis consists of a layer of mother cells from which daughter cells are constantly produced by means of cell division, and is thus able to regenerate on its own. On the other hand, the dermis has no such division-based proliferation, and thus has to rely on new materials being delivered to the wound space which eventually change into scar. In other words scar tissue is the material of dermal repair.

However, as the epidermal defect is repaired using its own cell proliferation, the regenerated area can be repaired so that it is almost the same as the surrounding normal skin in some 'special cases'. This 'special case' is the ideal goal of treatment, but is not easy to obtain. Details regarding this skill are dealt with elsewhere in the book.

3-3-1-(E) Epithelization

Within 24 hours after injury to the skin, detachment occurs at the epidermo-dermal junction of the skin surrounding the wound, freeing the epidermis from the dermis. The freed epidermis then tends to migrate into the wound, overlapping the wound margins. At the same time, cell division occurs in the basal layer, increasing the rate of recoverage of the wound, known as epithelization. Migration stops when the margins of the advancing epithelium encounter each other. Epithelization occurs from the wound margins, but even more importantly it also occurs from any epidermal remnants left in skin appendages in the wound area, such as sweat glands, hair follicles and sebaceous glands. Thus there are islands of epithelization advancing outwards from the skin appendages and an inward migration of epithel from the wound margins. In a large wound area, if the damage depth is limited to the papillary process of the dermis, then epithelization from appendage-based epidermis is very helpful and rapid, but it depends both on the concentration of appendages in the wound area, and on the amount of living epidermis left in them. Thus in the case of an extensive, deep dermal defect with no remaining appendages reepithelization is very slow, and wound healing is poor, as only the margins of the wound are producing inward-migrating epidermis. A typical epidermal migration rate is from 0.25 mm - 0.5 mm per 24 hours, depending on conditions in the wound: an overdry wound will slow down the rate. Newly regenerated epithelium on a wound is known as scar epithel. On histological examination, it has no rete pegs, and is easily detached from the dermis. There is an absence of skin ridges and furrows, giving scar epithel its abnormal flattened, lustred or shiny texture.

3-3-1-(F) Cosmetic Aspects of Wound Healing

Following repair after injury, a wound will nearly always leave some form of visible scar, except in a few special cases which appear almost normal. The range of scar formation varies from that invisible to the naked eye (the *macroscopically intact skin condition*), and large keloid formation, with a large variety of intermediate stages. Scar genesis is very complex, but it is very definitely linked to the relationship between the depth of damage, and the total time taken for the epithelization.

3-3-1-(F-1) Relation between Wound Depth and Epithelization

Wound healing is said to have completed the first stage when the area has been covered completely with a layer of epithelium. The faster the coverage, in general, the better the appearance of the scar. The biggest factor affecting epithelization time is the depth of damage to the skin.

3-3-1-(F-1)-(a) Very Superficial Wounds (200 µm)

Wounds with a depth of less than 200 µm are regarded as very superficial. As the epithelium is from 100 µm to 150 µm in depth, damage to the underlying dermis is limited to the superficial part of the subpapillary layer, so most of the skin appendages with their live epidermal component are spared, and can take part in speedy reepithelization. Temporary hyperpigmentation may mark the area of new epithelium, but once that has faded away it is very difficult to distinguish the new regenerated skin from the normal (*i.e.*, the intact skin condition). This type of damage is typical in the case of a superficial excoriation, in the donor site of a thin split-thickness skin graft, or 1st degree and superficial 2nd degree burns. Snowy dry ice application and some laser treatment for naevi also fall into this category.

3-3-1-(F-1)-*(b)* Superficial Wound (<250 μm)

There is a clear difference in the degree of fineness of the collagen fibres above the 250 μm depth, and below that depth. At 250 μm, there is still enough epidermis in the appendages to give assistance to reepithelization of the wound, although it will be slightly slower than for the very superficial wound. The macroscopically intact skin condition may still be possible with wounds of this depth depending on the site of the wound and management, but they usually leave a slight scar.

3-3-1-(F-1)-(c) Medium Wound (250 μm ~ 300 μm)

Wounds at this depth still reepithelize fairly fast, and usually mild scarring occurs.

3-3-1-(F-1)-(d) Deep Wound (300 μm ~ 400 μm)

At this depth, if the wound is wider than 2 mm - 3 mm, scarring will definitely occur, and the greater the wound area, the more hypertrophic the scarring is likely to be. Some deep 2nd degree burns fall into this category.

3-3-1-(F-1)-(e) Very Deep Wound (400 μm)

Unless the wound area is very small, damage at this depth will take a long time to heal and result in severe scarring, the so-called hypertrophic scar. Deep second degree and third degree burns are examples of wounds in this category.

3-3-1-(F-2)Wound Volume and Epithelization

The above considerations will alter on a site-by-site basis, and will be influenced by the thickness of the injured skin, the site, the race, sex, age and physical condition of the patient, and so on. The above-mentioned data on depth/damage classification was compiled from studies on split-thickness skin graft donor sites where the depth of damage is known accurately. In case of a burn it is not easy to assess immediately the damage depth. However, it is clear that there is a strong relationship between the depth of damage and the area of the wound: in other words, the wound volume. Large areas with superficial damage will usually epithelize very well: deep wounds with small surface area will also epithelize well: there is a point where a volumetric constant can be almost be taken as an indication of the outcome of wound healing. In laser treatment for naevi, under the Total Treatment Concept, this relationship between damage depth and damage area is carefully monitored, and has led to specific treatment types, such as spotty, lineal or area treatment, bearing in mind the need to get as invisible a scar as possible for the final result. This will be dealt with in detail later in this chapter. The wavelength of the laser must also be taken into account, and the total damage after laser treatment will depend also on the degree of radiant heat effect confined to the target cells or materials and the width of the band of secondary conducted heat effect damage.

3-3-1-(F-3) Importance of Epithelization Period in Second Intention Healing

There is a direct relationship between speed of epithelization and final result, so the actual period of reepithelization can be used as a yardstick by which the final result can be judged, in the case of wounds which heal by second intention. In the case of laser treatment, when epithelization is complete in seven days, then the result is usually excellent, and can be nearly always be classed as the macroscopically intact skin condition. If reepithelization is complete within 10 days, the result is generally still very good, and can be classed as almost intact. If the period of epithelization passes the 14th day then the possibility of visible scarring, and even hypertrophic scarring, must be taken into consideration. If the epithelization period is over 21 days, a hypertrophic scar will almost certainly be the outcome, and skin grafting should be considered as a preventative alternative.

3-3-1-(G) Inhibiting factors in Wound Healing

There are many factors which can inhibit wound healing, and if they are not taken into account, then there may well be a very poor result as far as wound healing is concerned. Inhibiting factors can be subdivided into local and general factors.

3-3-1-(G-1) Local Factors

Some of the local factors are endogenous and environmental, and others are indigenous to the body itself.

3-3-1-(G-1)-(a) Infection

Infection is one of the most common and troublesome complications, and is a major enemy to the wound healing process. Infection favours collagen lysis and retards collagen synthesis. In these conditions, the wound can actually increase in both area and depth: healing time is prolonged, and the scarring is usually very bad. If infection occurs even in the case of a well-designed treatment to prevent possible scarring, scar formation is nearly always inevitable.

In these circumstances, for patients who were having a naevus removed for cosmetic purposes, if infection occurs the result is often worse in appearance than the untreated naevus.

For infection, prevention is really better than the cure. Foreign bodies must be kept out of the wound. Local and systemic antibiotics should be given prophylactically, and special attention must be given to the local circulation to ensure a good blood supply to the wound. Haematoma formation will sometimes lead to haemosiderin toxicity, delaying wound healing even more.

3-3-1-(G-1)-(b) Local Circulatory Disturbance

Too tight and too fine sutures, unsuspended limbs, tight bandage or very strong pressure dressings can lead to local oedema and an ischaemic condition in the wound area. The wound is then deprived of the necessary blood circulation, retarding the progress of the wound healing process, with occasional marginal ischaemic wound necrosis.

3-3-1-(G-1)-(c) Operative Technique

Operative technique is one of the important factors in wound healing. It is important to avoid inhibiting factors in any surgical handling. The essential point is that the tissue should always be handled gently, atraumatically, not to cause additional iatrogenic trauma and not to over-operate.

3-3-1-(G-2) General Factors

There are many general factors affecting wound healing, but their effect on the final result is not as direct as those local factors.

3-3-1-(G-2)-(a) Age

Younger people tend heal faster than those of advancing years. It has been reported that sutured wounds made on foetuses of small animals heal without scar by regeneration of new tissue.

3-3-1-(G-2)-(b) Disease

If the patient has a disease such as anaemia, diabetes mellitus, malignancy or malnutrition, and so on, or has suffered severe trauma, wound healing is liable to be complicated by infection, and the entire wound healing process tends to be delayed. These diseases can be a contraindication to laser treatment for naevi for cosmetic reasons.

3-3-1-(G-2)-(c) Vitamins

Vitamins A and C are known to activate collagen synthesis: vitamin B_2 affects tissue metabolism; and vitamin K, the clotting factor, stops bleeding. All of these have potential effects on overall wound healing in patients on a course of these vitamins, or deficient in them.

3-3-1-(G-2)-(d) Medication

Steroid and other anabolic agents taken over a long period at high dosages have a retardative effect on wound healing.

3-3-1-(G-2)-(e) Immobilization of the Wound

Insufficient wound immobilization, especially in areas of the body prone to movement like the joints, allows continuous movement which can cause bleeding, exudation and oedema, with subsequent disturbance of the wound healing process.

3-3-1-(G-2)-(f) Moisture

Too much moisture is bad from the point of view of providing a culture medium for bacteria: however, too little moisture in a wound will slow down the speed of epithelization by up to half the normal rate.

3-3-1-(H) Promoting Factors in Wound Healng

As mentioned already, vitamins C and A in reasonable doses will have a good effect on collagen synthesis. Some other oral drugs, non steroid anti-inflammatory agents (NSAIDs), for example, and some local physical therapy are reported to have very good effects on wound healing. The use of NSAIDs to promote wound healing is not widely known, but is effective. In addition, any therapy which can reduce local oedema and increase circulation and lymphatic drainage has beneficial effects on wound healing rate and final result. Low reactive-level laser therapy, LLLT, has proved very useful in this aspect of wound healing promotion.

3-3-1-(I) Clinical Process of Wound Healing

So far the morphological and histochemical aspects of wound healing have been discussed. In this section, I would like to describe especially the process and nature of scar over the long period of repair.

3-3-1-(I-1) Scar Formation Process

When an operation has been carried out in a reasonable manner, and the wound has been accurately sutured, on the fifth postoperative day there is almost no swelling, and the suture line looks well-closed. At that stage, most of the sutures can be removed, because the tensile strength of the wound is rapidly increasing by the fifth day, and spontaneous dehiscence is unlikely. The earlier the sutures can be removed, the less the formation of suture marks. However, the patient must be warned not to stretch or scratch the wound, because it could still be physically disrupted at that early stage. At 14 days postoperatively, the tensile strength is pretty high, and by three weeks after surgery, even direct force to the wound borders will probably not cause it to reopen.

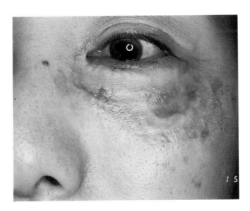

Fig 3.26: *Immature scar, showing shiny, lustred surface.*

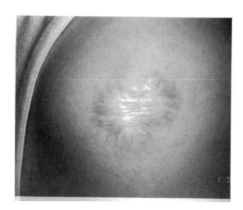

Fig 3.27:
Capillary invasion from the scar margin into surrounding normal areas as a prelude to true keloid formation.

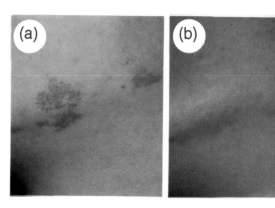

Fig 3.28:
Example of well-healed, mature scar demonstrating the intact skin condition following ruby laser area treatment.

On the other hand, at 14 to 21 days after surgery, hardness in the tissue around the suture line, one of the harbingers of hypertrophy, may start to appear. In some cases, a fine, linear scar can be seen. The time of appearance and the grade of the scar are quite different depending on each case.

In the very best of cases, there is no enlargement, spread or thickening of the scar, and after 6 months the very fine suture line will be practically invisible. In some cases, however, the suture line will noticeably thicken or spread, finally forming in the worst case a large and unsightly keloid. Between the two extremes of best- and worst-case scarring there is a large variety of degrees of scarring, ranging from normal scar, to hypertrophy, to large hypertrophic keloid formation, with no really clear border between each category.

As said before, the basic wound healing mechanism in second intention healing is the same as in healing by first intention. In the course of maturation, the chroma of the colour of the growing scar is high, bright red, with a shiny, lustred surface, occasional tenderness and itching. (Figure 3.26)

Another important sign which indicates the prognosis of a scar lies along the scar margin.

When a scar has a clear margin, then the scar usually stops cleanly at the margin, and does not tend to spread into surrounding normal skin. Capillary invasion from scar into the surrounding normal areas leads to progressive scar growth invading these areas. (Figure 3.27)

There is still controversy over the clear distinction between a hypertrophic scar and true keloid. However, it is usually accepted that the growth of a hypertrophic scar is limited to the original scar line. A true keloid, on the other hand, invades the surrounding normal tissue. In the time course, the hypertrophic scar will stabilize and mature, losing the bright red colour, and becoming soft and white. The true keloid, on the other hand, tends to continue to grow despite many types of treatment.

3-3-1-(I-2) Colour and texture of Regenerated Skin

Considering the wound healing process following a superficial second degree burn, once epithelization is complete the affected areas are often accompanied by hyperpigmentation, but that usually spontaneously fades to give normal skin colour and texture, in 6 to 12 months. (Figure 3-28).

On occasions, scar epithel is accompanied by hypopigmentation or total depigmentation, but unlike hyperpigmentation, these conditions more rarely regress spontaneously.

In the case of healing by second intention, there is a large range of variations in the colour, texture and thickness of the scar, giving a completely different range of final results. In any event, including wounds healing by first intention, control of the wound healing process, and control of any adverse side effects, must be in the hands of the clinician and managed under the Total Treatment Concept.

3-3-1-(J) Factors Affecting Scar Formation in the Third Phase

As has been noted, except for rare cases which leave no visible scar, it is almost impossible for a wound to heal without forming some kind of scar. However it is possible to exert influences on the healing wound to control scar formation. That is the basic principle which underpins postoperative wound care and management. The early stages of wound healing are fraught with so many inherent inhibitive factors, but the most important phase where external control can have an effect is in the third phase, because it lasts much longer than the other two, and therefore gives much more opportunity for exogenous control factors to be applied. Some of these factors are inherent in the patient, and some are applied by the clinician.

3-3-1-(J-1) Race

There is a great difference in the wound healing response comparing the Caucasian and Oriental races. The Oriental skin, although much more resilient to the sun has a much higher tendency to hypertrophic scarring after injury.

3-3-1-(J-2) Scar Predisposition

Even in the same race, there can be a large difference in each patient's propensity to form hypertrophic scars or keloids. If a patient has a known hypertrophic-forming tendency, as seen from previous wounds, inoculation marks and patient's history, then any operation for cosmetic purposes should be performed with great care.

3-3-1-(J-3) Tension on the Scar

There is usually tension exerted on a scar from the surrounding skin. This tension can result in enlargement of the scar, and possible hypertrophy. Approximation of wound margins by suture against tension usually results in high tension on the wound. The scar may appear normal on removal of the sutures, with a fine, lineal mark. Because of the tension, however, it will soon start to expand and thicken, and hypertrophy will probably be the final result. In severe cases, this may be accompanied by scar contracture. In this situation, some form of incision designed to release the tension is required. On the other hand, in cases of severe scar contracture, release of tension by means of skin transplantation can be remarkably effective, with very rapid regression of the scar hypertrophy.

3-3-1-(J-4) Scar Formation and Wrinkle Lines

The wrinkle lines of the skin are also related with the factor of tension, and represent the lines of least resistance within the skin to the forces imposed on it. A surgical incision which follows these lines will therefore have more chance of natural healing with an excellent result, than an incision made at right angles to the wrinkles, and thus at right angles to the muscular or other forces acting on the tissue. When planning the direction of an incision in lined skin it is better to consult the natural wrinkle lines of the skin, also known as the cleavage or Langer's lines. (Figure 3.29, following page.)

3-3-1-(J-5) Wound Instability

The degree and frequency of movement in a healing wound are important factors in the cause of possible hypertrophic scar formation. For wounds in the region of joints, fixation of the joint is thus often necessary to help ensure the best possible treatment result.

3-3-1-(J-6) Sites Prone to Hypertrophy

There are several sites on the body known for their hypertrophic tendency, compared with other areas. The skin over the sternum and shoulders, for example, is susceptible to hypertrophic scar formation. Areas around the mouth and jaw, be-cause of the motion factor, are also danger zones.

There are on the other hand areas where hypertrophy does not often occur: these include amongst others the inguinal region, skin of the scrotum, the labia minor and major and the upper eyelid.

3-3-2 Wound Management

The stage of postoperative wound care and wound management is also of great importance: after leaving the clinic and before returning for the next appointment, how the patient looks after the wound has a very large influence on the final outcome of the wound healing. Good wound management is thus an essential part of the patient education programme and forms a major element in the doctor-patient relationship. The manage-ment of wounds can be classified under two main time-related headings: the pre-epithelization and the post-epithelization periods.

3-3-2-(A) Wound Treatment

Loss of dermis with or without inflammation can be classed as an ulcer. Normally, most of the wounds created by laser treatment for naevi are not primarily ulcers, but may become ulcers if infection occurs. The period before epithelization is therefore a very important stage in wound man-agement to achieve the optimum result.

3-3-2-(A-1) Pre-epithelization Stage

There are many causes for the appearance of skin defects: trauma, burns, or surgical procedures are amongst some of them. In many mild cases, the skin defect will heal in several days, without scarring. In some cases, however, there is retar-dation of the healing process, and the wound remains open even after many treatments over a long period of time. This can be referred to as a nonhealing ulcer. Between these two extremes there are many intermediate stages, which mostly depend on the depth of the wound. The local blood circulation and lymphatic drainage are also very important factors. The purpose of treatment is to control any pain and to protect the wound against infection and wound exudation. The goal of the surgeon is to achieve epithelization in as short a time as possible. Treatment methodology usually changes depending on the depth of the wound. In cases involving local circulatory dis-turbance, special care must be taken to encourage improvement of the circulation, in addition to the other factors influencing wound healing.

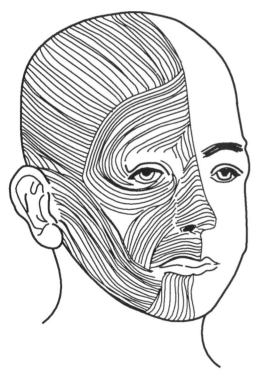

Fig 3.29:
Cleavage (or Langer's) lines of the face. Any incision or linear type of laser treatment must be planned to follow these lines as closely as possible, in order to

3-3-2-(A-1)-(a) Superficial Wound

Superficial burns (1st degree or mild 2nd degree burns), donor site for thin split thickness skin grafts, laser treatment for naevi or snow dry ice treatment: these can be classed as superficial wounds. If the wound healing is uncomplicated by infection, these wounds will usually heal rapidly with a slight but noticeable scar. Maintaining the sterile condition of the wound is very important to protect against infection. There are two techniques of wound management: dressing the wound and the open treatment.

3-3-2-(A-1)-(a-1) Wound Dressing

A dressing is designed to cover the wound. This is done with a variety of sterile dressings. Gauze is one of the most common materials, but care must be taken to prevent the gauze adhering to the wound. New epithel is very fragile, and is easily removed when changing the dressing if the dressing has adhered to the wound. To avoid this the author usually uses silicon gauze with an ointment directly on the wound. There are two types of silicon gauze: the woven type and the fine mesh type. In the case of the woven type there is a tendency for newly forming epithel to penetrate into the weave of the gauze. When the gauze is removed at changing time, it can therefore remove new epithelium from the wound. This can result in the deepening of the wound, and may cause ulcer formation. The mesh type of gauze on the other hand tends to repel new epithelium, and will usually spontaneously detach from the new epithelium after epithelization is complete. This is the best result.

Wound exudation is absorbed in a layer of cotton gauze placed over the silicon mesh gauze. When changing the dressing, normally the cotton gauze can be removed easily and replaced with fresh gauze, leaving the mesh silicon gauze in contact with the wound. In cases of minimal exudation, dressing changes are not required. In these cases the dressing can be left as it is for several days.

Moisture control of the dressing is very important. Too much moisture offers a good culture medium for bacteria. If the patient cannot attend the clinic regularly to have the dressing checked and changed, then they are instructed to control moisture by blowing cold air through the dressing using a hair-drier set to 'cold'. This is a particular problem in the summer in Japan, or any subtropical or tropical country where the humidity is very high. There is the opposite concern of over-dryness which may delay wound healing. This is however preferable to infection of the wound.

The ideal ointment should have a high oil content, with little water, which is much better for successful wound management than the opposite. In the authors' institute 'Eksalve'® ointment is used from the Maruho Pharmaceutical Company, Limited. This ointment contains a suspension of a small amount of inactivated bacteria in a hydrocortisone base, and has been proved to be effective against infection and over-fibrosis of the wound. Because of these properties, this ointment can be used even on infected ulcers.

3-3-2-(A-1)-(a-2) Open Treatment

When no gauze is used to cover a wound, it is referred to as the open treatment. The wound is deliberately left open to the air, mostly as a measure to prevent moisture build-up and subsequent infection. This method is used on wounds on the face, or breasts. Cracking of the wound crust surface may occur because of over-dryness of the wound. This method is employed on inpatients, because of the carefully controlled environmental ambient humidity and temperatures found in hospitals.

3-3-2-(A-1)-(b) Deep Wounds

A deep wound is almost impossible following laser treatment for naevi or other conventional methodologies such as snowy dry ice, except in exceptional cases. For deep wounds, epithelization usually takes longer, depending on the wound area: the volume consideration (the relation between area and depth) has already been discussed above. Dressing, using the mesh type of silicon gauze covered with absorbent cotton gauze, is best suited for these wounds. For deeper wounds, it is the practice to change both the cotton and silicon gauze, because of the tendency of the silicon gauze to become involved with the granulation tissue. In superficial wounds, the silicon mesh gauze tends to be lifted by the newly-forming epithelium, but in deeper wounds, the lack of epithel tends to allow the granulation tissue to involve the gauze.

3-3-2-(A-1)-(c) Infected Wound, and Ulcer Formation

In very large and deep wounds, such as a severe and extensive decubitus ulcer, the infection may spread to the underlying bone. These cases are sometimes the result of what started out as a superficial wound, but became infected, seriously delaying the epithelization period. This leads to enlargement and deepening of the wound, turning it into an ulcer. An ulcer is characterized by the simultaneous presence of pus, necrotic tissue, clots and crusting. This purulent wound offers ideal culture for bacteria. The first step in management of this unfortunate condition is to depress the bacterial population by removing all the necrotic tissue and to expose healthy tissue: this is called debridement. Major debridement of large wounds should be done in an operating theatre: minor debridement can be safely undertaken in an outpatient clinic or in the ward for inpatients. Debridement should be done as gently as possible, using scissors and forceps. Extensive debridement is necessary in some cases and some degree of haemorrhage may be inevitable.

If the patient complains of pain during the debridement, surface anaesthesia can be applied to the wound surface using gauze swabs impregnated with a high concentration of local anaesthetic. Bathing and washing the wound in warm water with a bacteriocidal agent such as Hibitane® is very useful for assisting in the control of the bacterial population. Dressings must be changed more frequently than usual to remove the infected exudate. If after three weeks epitheliza-

tion has not taken place, skin grafting must be considered as a preventive measure against hypertrophic scar formation, which will almost inevitably occur.

The above is an extremely severe condition, and is very rarely seen following laser treatment for naevi: this information has been added only as a precaution in case deep ulceration should occur.

3-3-2-(A-2) Post-epithelization Period

There are many types and extents of scar formation following wound healing. Many of these scars will have some degree of hyperpigmentation, hypopigmentation or depigmentation, which appear after complete epithelization. From the histological viewpoint the process of wound union is now almost complete, and nothing more need be done. From the point of cosmesis these disorders must be controlled.

3-3-2-(A-2)-(a) Hyperpigmentation and Hypopigmentation

After epithelization is almost complete, hyperpigmentation can appear in the new epithelium, even though the wound may otherwise exhibit all the characteristics of almost normal recovery. These examples of secondary hyperpigmentation have many points in common with post-inflammatory hyperpigmentation, (the common suntan, following sunburn). The value of the colour tends to be low, with a deepening of pigmentation. In the majority of cases, secondary hyperpigmentation will spontaneously fade away in one year or so.

Especially in the case of laser treatment for naevi in the melanin anomaly group, the clinician must differentiate between recurrence of the naevus pigment and secondary hyperpigmentation. The appearance of the pigment in hyperpigmentation tends to be homogeneous, but inhomogeneous in cases of recurrence of the naevus.

Secondary pigmentation can be controlled. Exposure to sunlight, or even other artificial light sources, must be kept to a minimum: a total UV suncut cream can be applied in tandem with covering the area with clothing, where appropriate.

Vitamin therapy, such as vitamin C or vitamin A can be indicated, or the topical application of a depigmenting ointment containing hydroquinon and a corticosteroid such as hydrocortisone. It is the author's policy always to do a test patch for any ointment or cream, including UV suncut preparations. The test patch is applied, and the patient returns after 48 hours for assessment. If there is no adverse reaction, such as oedema, blister formation or itching, then the cream or ointment can be used.

Hydroquinon-based depigmenting ointment depends for its effect on the chemical's antioxidizing properties. Hydroquinone, p-dehydroxybenzine, acts on the oxidation stage of melanin synthesis in which the melanosomes turn black as the tyrosine in the melanosomes is oxidized by dopa (3,4-dyhydroxyphenalalanine). The hydroquinone acts as a dopa block and the corticosteroid assists in this by accelerating epidermal penetration and absorption of the ointment. Because of the normal precautions concerning excessive and prolonged application of any ointment containing a corticosteroid, application of hydroquinone depigmenting ointment is limited to the night, before sleeping. In the morning the area is carefully cleaned to remove all traces of the ointment and an antisteroid preparation may be applied. There is thus approximately a 1:2 ratio for the application to the resting periods (8 hr to 16 hr). The antisteroid preparation is applied, followed by the suncut cream or ointment, and finally a normal cosmetic is applied over that. This gives three or four layers of extra protection against further photoactivation of the secondary hyperpigmentation process.

3-3-2-(A-2)-(b) Scar, Hypertrophic Scar, Hypertrophic Keloid and True Keloid.

There are many treatments available to prevent hypertrophy after it has started to appear. These include drugs, pressure dressings, irradiation techniques using long wavelength 'soft' X-rays and LLLT. These can be used individually, or in combination.

3-3-2-(A-2)-(b-1)α Oral Drugs

Rizaben (anthranilic acid) was used originally as a treatment for asthma or for collagen diseases including atopic dermatitis. Hypertrophic scar is also a collagen abnormality, coming from a breakdown of the normal collagen synthesis - collagen lysis mechanism which results in oversynthesis of basically immature, loosely formed collagen fibres. The indication of oral anthranilic acid acts on the chemical mediator which has caused the original synthesis/lysis imbalance, and blocks its action thus restoring normal balance.

3-3-2-(A-2)-(b-1)β Steroid Injection

Injections of the glucocorticoid triamcinolone (9a-fluoro-16a-hydroxiprednisolone) into the body of the scar are effective, at a concentration of under 20 mg/ml. Care must be taken not to allow infiltration of the drug into normal tissue. Depending on the case, one injection per week of 0.5-1.0 ml is given, with three or four weeks regarded as a course. Courses may be repeated. Atrophy and softening of the hypertrophic scar is an indication that the therapy is working, but if the injections are stopped before the scar flattens or turns white, the tendency for recurrence is very strong. Other steroids seem to be less effective than triamcinolone, possibly because of the large macromolecular composition of that particular glucocorticoid. The combination of pressure dressings with steroid injections has also proved to be very effective, and give excellent results.

Because of the potential side effects from prolonged steroid use, there is a limit to the total number of injections which can be given. If the scar is extensive and large, then triamcinolone injection on its own is an inappropriate therapeutic method.

3-3-2-(A-2)-(b-1)γ Topically Applied Drugs

Members of the corticosteroid group are usually used for topical application, but the effect is low compared with the injection method. Topically applied steroids are useful to control itching of the scar and work well in the occlusive dressing technique using a patch of clear kitchen film (e.g. Saran-Wrap®, Dow-Corning). It is taped over the wound area overnight to increase the penetrative power of the ointment. Prolonged application should be avoided, because of the possible side effects including redness of the skin, atrophy, capillary ectasia, and so on.

3-3-2-(A-2)-(b-2) Pressure Dressing Techniques

This is a very effective therapy which can be used by the patients in their own homes. It is particularly effective for the younger scar, but when the pressure is removed, the tendency for the scar to grow again is very strong. Accordingly, this is a very long-term therapeutic technique, and must be carefully monitored in order to prevent recurrence of the hypertrophic condition.

Usually a 1 cm thick sponge dressing is used, but there are many thicknesses and degree of elasticity. The sponge is cut to match the shape of the scar, is placed on the scar, and firmly compressed in place with an adhesive tape bandage. After bandaging, the sponge tries to revert to its original thickness, so exerting a steady pressure on the scar beneath it. In the case of an immature hypertrophic scar, care must be taken to prevent any of the tape adhesive surface from coming into contact with the scar surface, because of the sensitivity of the scar epithelium to such stimuli as the chemicals found in dressing adhesives. This well may result in undesirable side effects such as redness, itching and so on, and delay the successful compression of the scar.

In the case of a large scar, it is very difficult to make a uniform contact between the sponge and the entire surface of the scar. In these cases an aluminium backing plate is used in conjunction with the pressure sponge, to give added support to compression of the sponge over the entire area of the scar.

In some scars located on a curved surface over a bony protuberance, uniform compression cannot be obtained using the usual method. To overcome this, an aluminium backing plate

shaped to follow the contour of the protuberance is very useful.

3-3-2-(A-2)-(b-3) Low reactive-Level Laser Therapy (LLLT)

Among treatment methods introduced in the past few years, low reactive-level laser therapy (LLLT) has been described in the literature as affecting both the physical and the chemical factors which are also found in hypertrophic scar and keloid formation. LLLT has also been applied in cases of slow-to-heal or nonhealing ulcers, infected ulcers, enhanced bone fusion and tendon healing and for general prophylaxis against scarring.

LLLT has been shown both experimentally and clinically to activate and blood and lymphatic vascular flow is when it is not active, and at the same time the levels of the chemical inflammatory mediators are topically decreased. With the depression of the inflammatory response and increased lymphatic drainage oedema is also removed. Taking these factors into consideration, it could be expected that LLLT might have a good effect as a noninvasive therapy for hypertrophic scars and keloids. The author has successfully applied LLLT, alone, and in combination with some of the conservative techniques already discussed above, or with nonconservative surgical intervention, and the results have been very promising.

Conservative methodology alone gives poor results, and requires a very long treatment time as mentioned above. Nonconservative surgical intervention, with conventional scalpel or laser excision and vaporization, also generally has a poor record, with recurrence a major problem. As for nonconventional techniques, pure LLLT alone is often insufficient, giving an unsatisfactory result over a very long time course.

In order to offset these possible detracting points, LLLT must be applied as an adjunctive therapy. LLLT applied together or alternately with conservative methodologies has proved effective, and LLLT applied after a nonconservative surgical procedure helps control postoperative pain and the inflammatory response. The GaAlAs infrared diode laser, with a continuous wave (c/w) output power of 60 mW at 830 nm, has been used in contact or noncontact mode with very good results. In addition, the continuous wave 1064 nm Nd:YAG laser can also be used, with low output powers and a large spot to give appropriately low incident power densities. The use of LLLT as a completely noninvasive adjunctive therapy following surgical intervention, in tandem with conservative pressure therapy, drug therapy or a combination of all of these is completely within the precepts of Ohshiro's Total Treatment Concept (TTC).

Patients with hypertrophic scars and keloids suffer not only the physical aspects of the lesion, but also the psychological effects. Both the psychosomatic and somatopsychic aspects of these lesions, in keeping with the TTC, must be recognized and incorporated in the therapeutic regime on an individualized basis, patient by patient. This is another aspect of Ohshiro's TTC at work in clinical practice, not just specifically for hypertrophic scars and keloids, but for almost every aspect of wound control and management.

3-4 DOCTOR-PATIENT RELATIONSHIP

Some important considerations in the doctor-patient relationship have already been covered in some detail in Chapter 1-1-3, *(Psychological Aspects of the Naevus)*, and the reader is requested to review that section again. In this section the author would like to expand on some of the points dealt with in that earlier section, and go on to examine some others not covered specifically there. The doctor-patient relationship can be divided broadly into two main areas: inside the clinic and outside the clinic.

3-4-1 Inside the Clinic

Within the clinic, the doctor-patient relationship naturally has as its main subdivision the actual physical and mental relationship between the doctor and his or her patients, but additionally the relationship with the laser nurse, the laser therapist, the design and running of the clinic environment, the relationship between the patients and their family and the handling of laser safety and the patient are all important factors which must be taken together and work to create a strong doctor-patient relationship. The importance of a coherent and cohesive doctor-patient relationship is one of the key points in the author's Total Treatment Concept.

3-4-1-(A) Doctor/Patient Rapport

In any clinical situation the rapport between the patient and the clinician treating him or her is an important element in assuring the success of the treatment. In laser treatment for naevi, this rela-tionship becomes even more important, because of the nature of naevi, the laser treatment and in particular the postoperative care of the laser wound.

The rapport between doctor and patient is essential for several reasons, all of them connected with both the successful physical removal of the lesion and the mental attitude of the patient. Patients must come to and return from their treatment sessions confident in the following points. The patient, or their family where appropriate, must feel that the clinician and clinic staff fully understand the clinical, physical and mental aspects of their particular problem. They must come to understand as fully as possible for themselves the nature of the naevus, so that the naevus becomes simply another type of disease which is capable of some degree of improvement. They must understand that the removal of the abnormality of configuration and colour, and restoration of normal appearance, is clinically feasible to a greater or lesser degree, depending on a combination of factors including their own care of the postoperative wound. A strong patient education programme must therefore be part of the initial consultation, which will carry forward into the actual treatment itself and will help with the points already mentioned. The patient must have a reasonably accurate expectation of the chances and degree of successful removal of the naevus. In the case of the young child, this is especially true for the family rather than the child, as already covered in detail in Chapter 1-1-3. Patients must have total confidence in the clinician and the support staff, so that all instructions regarding wound aftercare will be followed exactly. Patients must feel able to report quickly any unusual symptoms in the course of the healing of the wound. If the patient is a little afraid of upsetting the doctor, then reports of unexpected symptoms are sometimes delayed, resulting in adverse side effects which could have been avoided.

We must never forget that there are two sides to the doctor-patient rapport. In addition to the psychological considerations for the patient and their family, the mental approach for the physician is important. The clinician also needs to have a clear idea of the treatment course, be able to make a realistic assessment of the outcome, and be able to communicate this in confident terms to the patient. The doctor must also work well with his or her nurses so that the patient has confidence in the entire medical team, not just the doctor. In order to accomplish this, as has been said before, the laser clinician requires a large range of interdisciplinary skills in both the psychological, physical and medical sciences, so that he or she can sustain and maintain the clinician's side of the important rapport between doctor and patient.

3-4-1-(B)   The Laser Nurse

The laser nurse is very important in the naevus clinic. Patients tend to see more of the nursing staff than they do the doctor who actually treats them, and so the importance of the nurse as a

go-between for the patient and the doctor is immediately evident. From the very early stages of their relationship with the clinic, patients see a great deal of the laser nurse.

After the initial consultation, which is the start of the rapport between the doctor and the patient, it is the laser nurse who should explain again to the patient what the test treatment will involve, and so she or he must be able to answer any of the patient's questions on the naevus or the lasers to be used. The laser nurse therefore requires a thorough grounding in the physiology and pathology of the different naevi groups and the naevi themselves in addition to the usual medical and clinical skills and knowledge required of a nurse. She or he must learn the basics of laser physics, laser-tissue interaction, the mechanics of the different systems employed in the clinic and of course the specific mechanics and concepts of wound healing and wound management which apply to laser-created wounds. Having obtained all that knowledge, the nurse must be able to communicate it to the patient, so good communication skills are required.

It is the nurse who has to comfort the younger patients before and after laser treatment, which may sometimes be painful but is always a little frightening for the younger child, so the nurse has to be able to handle and soothe upset children gently but firmly. Other children, or even other adults in the waiting room will always tend to react to a crying child by building up psychological barriers against the possible pain that the child has obviously suffered to make him or her cry that way. In fact, the 'fright factor' in laser treatment is much higher than the pain factor, especially with the pulsed systems, as these produce a sudden powerful laser shot which is to a greater or lesser extent accompanied by noise, a bright flash (even through goggles) and the tangible sensation of the laser impact on the tissue all of which can shock the younger patient into crying. The nurse must be aware of this, and be quick to distract the attention of the child after the laser treatment to take their mind off what they have seen and felt, so that it does not build up an association in the child's mind between the clinic and fear. The foregoing does not only apply to the younger patient, however, and the nurse must recognize when a patient requires a little extra reassurance and be able to give it.

The nurse is responsible for applying and changing dressings, and must therefore have a full understanding of the range of creams, ointments and dressing techniques. She or he has the responsibility for reinforcing the written wound care instructions which patients should receive to help then care for their wound at home, between visits to the clinic. The preceding section (3-3-2) on wound management has already stressed the importance of good wound care on the successful outcome of a laser treatment: the nurse is an important figure in impressing this on the patient.

In addition to dealing with the patients, the nurse must also be able to work well with the doctors in the clinic, so that there is a harmonious atmosphere in which everyone knows their job and is able to carry it out smoothly and competently. This in turn is communicated to the patient as a well-run and efficient clinic, which reinforces the doctor-patient relationship and gives the patient confidence in the clinic, its staff and all aspects of the treatment and post-treatment wound care.

3-4-1-(C) The Laser Therapist

Low reactive-level laser therapy (LLLT) is now being used more in clinics especially in Japan, China and Europe. Because of this changing trend, a new clinical specialist has evolved, the laser therapist. As it is a noninvasive therapeutic technique, it is not necessary to be a qualified medical doctor to give this treatment, and with an increasing patient population in the laser therapy field, it is important that other qualified medical professionals take over LLLT applications to free up the physicians for tasks which require their special skills and training. It should not be easy to become a laser therapist, however. In the author's

clinic, which is being used by other clinics in Japan as a model, laser therapists have to go through a three-year training scheme, in which they progress from junior therapist to senior therapist and finally therapist instructor. During this training the student therapists must study amongst other subjects basic laser physics and laser-tissue interaction; basic anatomy, physiology and pathology; pain and its aetiologies, oriental medicine; pharmacology, and laser system management. There is also a comprehensive in-service hands-on training programme under the guidance of physicians and qualified therapist instructors.

Therapist instructors hold either grade A, B or C. Grade A instructors teach at junior and senior therapist levels, and grade B instructors can teach additionally at therapist instructor level. Both grades A and B teach nationally. Grade C instructor therapists can teach at a therapy clinic overseas, under the auspices of the International Laser Therapy Association (ILTA), and must therefore be proficient in one or more foreign languages.

This comprehensive training programme is very important, in the author's view, as laser therapy has suffered in the past from a bad reputation as a second rate semi-paramedical treatment carried out by untrained or poorly-trained nonmedical individuals. A large proportion of the patients at the author's clinic attend for pain therapy or other LLLT applications, and so first-class treatment and full clinical back-up is essential to achieve a good therapy result. This result is very much dependent on the rapport between the therapist and the patient, and in turn between the therapist and doctor, which are important aspects of the overall doctor-patient relationship.

3-4-1-(D) The Clinic Environment

Of equal importance as the clinic staff to the patients' well-being and feelings of comfort and security is the actual environment of the clinic itself. The disease-related streaming in the authors' clinic has already been mentioned. This means that patients with the same condition tend to be in the clinic at the same time, and so form a strong mutual support group. A comfortable and tastefully-decorated waiting area is essential, with adequate seating. A video system on which information videos can be played is a good addition to the waiting room, as is some form of relaxing background music when the video system is not in use. The intention of the clinic environment and design is to reassure and relax patients, so that they can go in for their treatment with the minimum tension possible. If space permits, a recovery room or area is a valuable asset, allowing patients, especially the younger ones, to recover from their laser treatment session where that is necessary.

3-4-1-(E) The Patient and Family

In many cases the patient will attend the clinic together with a family member: in the case of young children this is always the case. It is extremely important that the accompanying family are as aware of all aspects of the disease and its treatment as the patient, even in the case of the adult patient. In the case of the young child or mentally-impaired adults, the family are the ones who must make the decisions regarding treatment and who are responsible for the postoperative wound care, so it goes without saying that they must understand the nature of the disease, its treatment and the aftercare necessary to ensure a good treatment result. This understanding does not come from the doctor alone, but must be assisted by the laser nurses and all of the other clinical staff. If this rapport exists, the family will provide strong support for the treatment and help in the conditioning of the patient to accept both the treatment and its aftercare. Chapter 1-1-3 goes into this relationship in detail.

3-4-1-(F) Laser Safety and the Patient

The subject of laser safety as a whole is covered in 3-12 below, but there are some aspects of safety with laser treatment which are part of the doctor-patient relationship, and should be considered here. Association is a powerful psychological effect, and for the impressionable younger patient (and some of the older ones) it is very important that some of the aspects of laser safety are not associated with unpleasant experiences. All surgical laser applications require eye protection of one kind or another. Goggles or glasses are the most common. It is extremely important that the younger patient does not associate the putting on of the goggles with possible discomfort, otherwise the treatment becomes an ordeal even before the laser is used. Most safety goggles are tinted, which changes the wearer's perception of his or her surroundings: this can be applied to positive effect with the younger patient, if they are encouraged to enjoy the change of colour of everything and everyone in the treatment room. One or two acclimatization sessions without laser treatment might well be very rewarding. It helps if everyone in the treatment room wears the goggles: this should always be the case, of course, but very often ancillary staff or observers on the periphery of the area do not bother, or there are not enough goggles to go round.

Other aspects of laser safety can be a little intimidating for the first-time patient of any age, at the test treatment for example: the antireflective decor of the treatment room; windows blacked out or nonexistent; hazard warning signs and illuminated warning lights; central locking for the treatment room doors, which engages with an audible 'clunk'; and the protective eyewear as already mentioned: these are all very necessary for good laser safety, but if not explained beforehand, they can induce a feeling of uncertainty in the patient which is particularly counterproductive when associated with a painful treatment session. Comprehensive patient education will help to eliminate this problem, with a tour (actual or on video) of the facilities including the treatment room, and all its accessories. A good explanation of why these safety features are required with a positive approach to the welfare of the patients themselves should be included. With this approach, laser safety becomes another reinforcing factor for the overall doctor-patient relationship.

3-4-2 Outside the Clinic

In its largest perspective and scope, the doctor-patient relationship is not confined to the clinic itself: there are other aspects of the relationship which extend beyond the walls of the clinic into the outside world, and which can have an effect on how the patient perceives the clinic and the doctor. These include the mass media, communication between the doctor and laser manufacturer and the local and local or national health authorities.

3-4-2-(A) Doctor-Mass Media

There is no doubt that this is the age of mass media. Laser surgery and laser therapy are still new and 'high tech' enough to be of interest to the mass media, and practitioners and patients are sometimes asked for television, radio or press interviews. This in itself need not be a problem, in fact it can be advantageous to the image of laser surgery. The problem comes with the patient who has had an unfortunate experience, whether through their own doing, the clinic's or a combination of both, and an interview with an unhappy patient will obviously not be a good piece as far as public relations (PR) for the clinic and for the concept of laser surgery as a whole are concerned. The way to avoid unhappy patients has already been detailed in 1-3-3 and in the preceding section (3-4-1). Even with an unhappy patient, the doctor-patient relationship should be such that the problem should never have to go beyond the clinic, but be capable of solution by discussion and explanation between the patient and the clinic staff.

Another problem in this area is over-enthusiastic claims carried by the mass media by laser physicians who should know better. All aspects of the doctor-patient relationship must be considered, and although such claims may well benefit clinics concerned in the short term, long-term disillusionment will inevitably set in, and we will have the 'unhappy patient' syndrome already mentioned above. It is very tempting to exaggerate the effectiveness of laser surgeries and treatments, even slightly, to paint a better picture, but truthful and restrained reporting of treatments and results will be much better for all concerned, and are a necessary constraint of a good doctor-patient relationship.

3-4-2-(B) Doctor - Manufacturer

Laser surgery and laser therapy are constantly evolving as new procedures are developed and old ones are perfected and refined. This process occurs first between the laser physician and his research and development staff, and of course secondly between the doctor and the patient, on whom the new techniques are finally tried. In order for this process to improve the care of the patient, there should be a constant dialogue between the doctor and the laser manufacturer, so that any problems inherent in the system can be quickly resolved, and any new techniques which require modification of an existing system can be quickly and safely carried out. Manufacturers must be prepared to recognize beneficial changes to equipment design and implement them rapidly to keep pace with the safe development of laser surgery and medicine, which is another aspect of the overall doctor-patient relationship.

3-4-2-(C) Doctor - Local and National Health Authorities

In many countries, laser surgery is regulated by local and national health authority regulations, especially as to what laser systems can be used, and the procedures for which they are safe and appropriate. In order to preserve a good doctor-patient relationship, laser clinicians should not try out new procedures on patients except under the guidelines allowed by the requisite authority. In general, research and development of new equipment and techniques requires approval following analysis of data from animal tests before clinical trials can be started on humans. After the clinical trials are complete and the data analyzed for safety and efficacy, then approval of the technique is issued. By following this timetable of procedures the laser physician will always be able to offer the patient laser treatment which is completely within the guidelines of the appropriate authority, and which is proven safe and effective. An effective treatment result then depends on many other aspects of the doctor-patient relationship, including the individual clinician's skill, the unity of the clinical staff and the patient's following completely the guidance for postoperative wound care.

3-5 LASER TREATMENT PARAMETERS AND THE CONTROL OF SURGICAL EFFECT

In this section, we will gradually move away from theory and start to explore the clinical significance of the different reactions between laser energy and tissue. Much of what has been discussed in Chapter 2 above will be related to the clinical effects resulting from laser/tissue interaction. In particular the important relationship between the selection of laser parameters and the surgical effect will become evident.

Laser parameters are bound by physical laws: some of the parameters cannot be changed, the inherent parameters. Others are completely under the control of the clinician. It is by selection of the inherent parameters and altering the controlled parameters, that a whole range of biologic effects can be achieved in the target tissue. The inherent parameters of a laser are its wavelength and beam type, i.e. continuous wave or pulsed; long or short-acting: these have already been discussed above in Chapter 2 under the characteristics of light and photothermal reactions, respectively. This section will thus concentrate on the parameters selected by the surgeon, and how they can be used to control the surgical effect. The main parameters under the surgeon's control are the laser power incident on target tissue, the area of the target tissue irradiated by the laser, and the length of time for which the tissue is exposed to the laser beam. The combination of these parameters offers the laser surgeon a controllable range of surgical effects ranging from nonphotothermal activation to total tissue photodestruction.

3-5-1 Output Power

The output power of a laser system is measured in watts. There are two points where this power may be measured: where the laser beam emerges from the system, and the point at which the beam is incident on the target tissue. In the case of a laser aimed at tissue without any form of delivery device, the loss of power between the laser aperture and the target tissue will be comparatively small. However in the case of a laser using some form of delivery device, such as an articulated arm or fibreoptic cable, then the beam incident on the tissue will be noticeably less than the beam at the proximal end of the delivery device, the actual difference depending on the efficiency of the delivery device. Many surgical laser systems will indicate an output power on some form of display screen: this is usually the power *at the laser*, however, and not the power *at the tissue*. The laser surgeon should always check the actual incident power with some form of external power meter, and will then know exactly how much power is being delivered to the tissue, since it is the power of the incident beam which will help determine the laser/tissue reaction. It is obvious that this is a fairly important parameter, and the more watts a laser can generate, the more powerful it obviously is. The output power of a laser taken on its own, however, is not a solid indication of the ultimate reaction of the beam when it is absorbed by the target tissue.

3-5-2 Irradiated Area

A laser beam incident on tissue illuminates or irradiates a certain area, which in most surgical lasers is roughly circular in shape. This two-dimensional area is referred to as the irradiated area, and is usually expressed in square centimetres. Because the area (a) of the laser spot on tissue is calculated by using the formula $a = (\pi r^2)$ cm^2, where π is the constant 3.142, and r = the radius (one-half the diameter) of the laser beam at the tissue, even a slight change in the spot size will mean a dramatic change in the irradiated area. A beam spot size with a radius of 2 cm has an area of 12.6 cm^2: a spot with double that radius has an area of approximately 50.2 cm^2, not double, but 4 times the former spot. Making the radius ten times smaller will decrease the irradiated area by a factor of 100. It is thus much more easy dramatically to alter the irradiated area of a laser than it is to alter its output power. Even in a 100 W laser, for example, the difference between 1 W and 100 W is only two orders of magnitude, but it is the entire controllable range of output power.

Altering the irradiated area is most easily accomplished by using a focusing lens system, and by moving the beam into or out of focus. Different focal lengths of lens will give different beam patterns. A short focal length will give a point of focus nearer the lens, with a rapid divergence of the beam beyond the focal waist. A longer focal length will give a point of focus further from the lens, with less divergence of the beam. The greater the divergence of the beam, the more the irradiated area is altered relative to the focal point with comparatively small movements of the delivery device in and out of focus.

3-5-3 Power Density and Spatial Beam Distribution

By combining the output power of a laser in watts, and the size, or more strictly the area of the incident beam on the target in square centimetres, one of the most important parameters to the laser surgeon can be calculated: the power density, or irradiance, of the incident beam. More than any other parameter, the power density will give the user an idea of the actual power delivered to the target, rather than the output power of the laser alone.

The power density (PD) is found by dividing the incident power by the area of the beam at the tissue, according to the formula:

$$PD = \frac{W}{\pi\, r^2} \ (W/cm^2)$$

where W is the power in watts, and πr^2 is the area of the spot in square centimetres

The power density can thus be controlled within a large margin simply by moving the delivery device up to or away from the point of focus. Figure 3.30 (following page) illustrates the control a laser surgeon will have over the actual power at the tissue from a laser beam with a constant output power of 2 W. At the point of focus, with a spot size of 100 μm, the power density at the tissue is over 25,000 W/cm^2. Depending on the wavelength, this power density will certainly cut most soft tissues. Doubling the spot size to 200 μm cuts the power density by one quarter, to over 6,000 W/cm^2. At a spot size of 1 mm, the power density is approximately 250 W/cm^2, and increasing the spot size to 1 cm cuts the power density to approximately 2.5 W/cm^2, associated with laser therapy applications rather

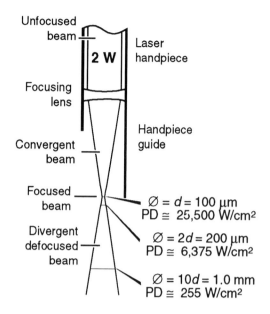

Fig 3.30:
Relationship between power density and beam focus or divergence. The same 2 W beam could thus be used to incise, coagulate, or for haemostasis simply by moving the handpiece nearer or further away from the focal point on the target tissue.

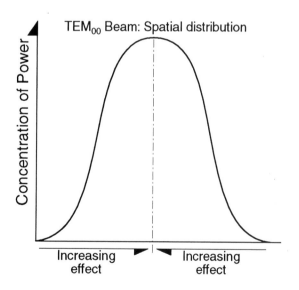

Fig 3.31: *Typical Gaussian curve of TEM_{00} single mode laser beam.*

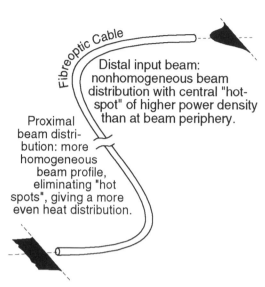

Fig 3.32:
Multimode beam from distal end of fibreoptic gives more homogeneous distribution of power, compared with 'hot-spot' at proximal end: good for homogeneity of pigment removal.

than laser surgery. So without touching the laser output power, the surgeon can manipulate only the focus of the beam to increase or decrease the power density by several orders of magnitude, depending on the position of the delivery device handpiece relative to the tissue and the focal length of the lens. Depending on the wavelength, that range of power densities will provide the power at the tissue to cut, vaporize and coagulate living tissue, all with the one beam and the one output power.

Spatial beam distribution is referred to as the beam mode. The beam mode is the term correctly used to describe the longitudinal cross-sectional distribution of power in a laser beam, (transverse electromagnetic mode, TEM). The most common single-mode beam in surgical lasers is the Gaussian mode, TEM_{00} (pronounced tee-ee-emm zero zero). Power distribution can be shown schematically as a Gaussian curve, with the greatest concentration in the centre, lessening towards the periphery, as seen in Figure 3.31. This gives an inhomogeneous beam with a higher power density at the centre than at the periphery. When a laser cavity imposes a single mode on a laser beam, it is referred to as mode-locking. Putting a mode-locked beam into a fibreoptic-based delivery device, however, destroys the mode-locking, and the beam emerges from the distal end of the fibre as a multimode beam, giving a much more homogeneous distribution of the power across the beam (Figure 3.32). For incision, the Gaussian beam has advantages, while for homogeneous removal of abnormal coloured cells or materials, the more even spatial distribution of the multimode beam is superior.

3-5-4 Irradiation Time

The surgeon can also control the irradiation time measured in seconds, the period for which the laser beam irradiates the target tissue for a given laser 'shot'. This is also referred to as the exposure time. The longer the irradiation time, in general the greater the damage effect in tissue, and the less specific it becomes, as already mentioned under the discussion on the radiant heat and conducted heat effect. The rate of linear motion of the beam on the target tissue relative to the irradiation time will also affect the clinical result.

3-5-5 Inter-Irradiation Interval

The inter-irradiation interval is the period in between laser 'shots' during which the laser is not incident on the target tissue. It is often ignored, but it has at least almost as much bearing on the final tissue effect as the irradiation time. If the inter-irradiation interval is too short, then the heating effect in tissue is greater for each consecutive exposure, and a high level of nonspecific coagulation, or tissue cooking effect, can result in the irradiated area. A longer inter-irradiation interval will allow a greater cooling effect from the blood flow in the target tissue, which may assist in achieving a more tissue-specific effect by sparing more of the surrounding tissue in the target area.

3-5-6 Energy, Total Energy and Energy Density

The incident energy of a laser beam is calculated by the product of the incident power in watts and the irradiation time per exposure in seconds, expressed in joules (J). By multiplying the exposure time per shot by the total number of shots, the total irradiation time is calculated, which in turn can give the total energy delivered, often seen in the literature as the 'total joules'. When the spot size is added to the calculation, the surgeon can work out the energy density, or radiant flux. If the power density can be compared with a medicine prescribed, the energy density can be looked at as the dose. However, as every pharmacist is aware, if the medicine is not correct, altering the dose will not usually help. The energy density is expressed in joules per square centimetre (J/cm^2) and is found by the formula

$$ED = \frac{W \times T}{\pi r^2} \ (J/cm^2)$$

with the same values as the formula for calculating the power density as given above, and where T is the irradiation time in seconds.

The output power and irradiated area, giving the power density, can be thought of as a mainly two-dimensional effect, governing the photon density of the incident beam at the target tissue: the potential power which can regulate the area of tissue damage or surgical effect. In order to move the two-dimensional area consideration into the third dimension of damage depth and volume, the fourth dimension of time must be added to the equation to bring in energy and energy density. The laser surgeon in the treatment of naevi must always consider the three-dimensional aspect of the disease being treated, and so the combination of output power, irradiated area, exposure time per shot and total exposure time becomes critical when considering a specific required tissue effect.

3-5-7 Scanning Parameters

Some naevi exist over a large body area. Especially when treating the superficial abnormal coloured cells or materials a 'painting' of the area with laser is required. For very large areas, this can be extremely tiring for the surgeon, and so some manufacturers have developed scanning devices which move the laser beam in predetermined patterns over the target tissue. These range from the simplest mechanical devices, capable of covering simple rectangular geometric patterns, to complex computer-controlled systems, which can irradiate irregular areas, usually delineated with a guide beam controlled by a joystick. The computer then scans the beam to and fro within the set pattern.

The speed of the scan is an obviously important parameter, as is the laser output power. If the power is insufficient, the clinical result will be unsatisfactory, with not enough removal of the target cells or materials. If the scan rate is too slow, then the damage volume will be greater than anticipated, with the possibility of slow wound healing and scar formation.

The other important consideration is the configuration of the area being scanned. For an area like the middle of the back, the distance from the scanner head to the target tissue will remain fairly constant, thus assuring a homogeneous delivery of laser energy to the target tissue. If the area requiring treatment extends over an irregular surface, then some areas will be nearer the scanner than others, meaning that they will get a different power density and dose compared to the areas further away. The most complex scanners are designed to compensate for this, with cross-reference multiple target beams giving the computer the information to plot and alter the required height for the scanner head. However the problem still exists of keeping the scanned beam as much as possible perpendicular to the horizontal plane of the tissue being treated, to achieve the most efficient laser/tissue reaction, so no matter how complex the system, the use of scanners would appear to be limited to superficial colour removal, and only on selected areas of the body.

3-5-8 Pulsed Beam Parameters

As already discussed, a pulsed beam has totally different characteristics compared with the continuous wave beam, and a different set of parameters. The main pulsed beam parameters depend on the type of pulsing used, normal, or Q-switched, and whether the laser is fired in a single pulse, or a train of pulses.

3-5-8-(A) Peak Power and Pulsewidth

The original pulsed ruby laser was capable of producing a maximum of one pulse every minute. To try and produce more pulses than that would have very quickly damaged the cavity components, because of the stress imposed on them by the massive amount of power needed to produce the single pulse. The ruby laser could produce a pulse of one millisecond (1 ms) in width, with a peak power of from 10,000 to 40,000 W (10 kW - 40 kW). The power is measured at the very tip of the pulse, hence the term peak power. The use of kilowatts as a parameter is not really practical in clinical applications, and so the pulsed ruby laser output was usually described in joules. Compared with the switched continuous wave laser, which could produce at the shortest bursts of from 10 to 100 ms with a power range of 2 W to around 100 W absolute maximum, the original pulsed laser systems appeared very short acting. However, the pulse produced was inefficient, with a comparatively slow decay from the peak of the pulse producing a number of ragged sub-peaks of lesser power. In order to improve the quality of the pulse, the quality of the cavity had to be increased, and Q-switching was applied to the laser cavity, already explored in Chapter 2, Section 2-1-6.

3-5-8-(B) Q-Switch Parameters

With improved Q-switching technology and better designed components, it became possible to produce many more pulses of much higher peak power and in a shorter period than with the normal pulsed laser, and the ultra-short acting beam was introduced to laser surgery, with peak powers in megawatts and pulsewidths measured in pulsewidths of nanoseconds or even picoseconds. By using extremely rapid Q-switching, a train of high peak power Q-switched pulses is produced, with a comparatively large interpulse interval. The mean effect of this series of high peak power pulses in tissue, however, is very similar to a continuous wave beam, and with the large interpulse interval the average power of the laser at the tissue was reduced to values from 2 to 20 W, similar to the output from continuous wave systems. This train of pulses is known as quasi-continuous wave, and is the basis of the so-called 'superpulse' facility seen on some CO_2 laser systems.

The benefits of this type of laser generation lie in the comparatively improved electrical efficiency of the cavity, and there are clinical advantages to the quasi-continuous beam in the target tissue, with less thermal spread into surrounding tissue and less charring of the target area compared with a continuous wave beam of similar power.

3-5-9 Configuration and Colour Control

The main aim of the laser surgeon in the treatment of naevi is control: control of shape, and control of colour. If the naevus consists only of an abnormality in colour compared to the surrounding normal skin, then the surgeon has to control only the colour. If there is also abnormality of configuration, then the surgeon must treat or control the configurational abnormality before controlling the colour problem. Both types of control are based on manipulation of the parameters discussed above.

3-5-9-(A) Configuration Control

The building blocks of our body consist of collagen of one type or another. Collagen type I is the main building block of soft tissue, and so it is this type of collagen which the laser surgeon has to deal with mostly, and control, when there is an abnormality of shape. Some configurational abnormalities, such as pedunculated soft tumours, can be easily excised at the pedicle: in these cases, configurational control is comparatively easy, and requires only excisional capabilities such as the CO_2 laser, contact Nd:YAG or higher powered visible light lasers are capable of. When the configurational abnormality is not easily excisable, as in a sessile tumour, then the surgeon must use the most appropriate laser parameters to control the shape. Collagen is a protein, and when heated enough, protein shrinks: on the other hand when heated too much the protein will completely dry out and eventually burn. Laser parameters must then be chosen which offer precise control of this capability of shrinkage. In Chapter 2, the effects of radiant and conducted heat were discussed. For configuration control, the conducted heat effect must be balanced with the radiant heat effect to give the correct degree of 'cooking' as a result of which shrinkage will occur. After controlling the abnormal configuration, the abnormal colour control can then be considered.

3-5-9-(B) Colour Control

For colour control, specific cellular or material targets must be damaged or destroyed in order to restore the abnormal colour to the normal condition, compared with the surrounding normal tissue. Power density, the combination of the incident laser power and the irradiated are of the laser beam, offers a two-dimensional capability for colour control. However, biological and other pigments do not often exist uniformly at one single depth in the target tissue, and there may even be a combination of different colouring agents, such as haemoglobin and melanin, at a range of depths and concentrations. Colour control is therefore much more precise than configu-rational control, requiring cell- or material-selective treatment parameters.

Colour and configurational control have a common treatment denominator. For both configuration and colour control, the surgeon must have a firm grasp of the three-dimensional treatment concept, playing damage area off against damage depth to give the overall damage volume. The three laser parameters of power, exposure time and irradiated area have thus to be carefully balanced with beam mode and type to obtain the desired range of selective damage. The following section will explore the various considerations of this overall parameter management which allows control of both configuration and colour.

3-6 LASER TREATMENT

In Section 3-3, wound healing was discussed, The relationship between damage depth and damage area was stressed, from the aspect of achieving what Ohshiro has referred to as the intact skin condition. No matter how well a wound heals, there is always some scar formation even though it may only be visible under light or electron microscopy. As argued in Section 3-3, when a treatment wound heals to present macroscopically a normal skin colour, texture and configuration compared with the surrounding normal skin, that is the intact skin condition, more correctly referred to as the macroscopically intact skin condition. In Section 3-5, the parameters available to the laser clinician were discussed from a prac-tical viewpoint. The purpose of this section is to combine the practical knowledge from Sections 3-3, 3-5 and elsewhere with the theoretical considerations of laser generation and physical characteristics of laser energy already discussed in Chapter 2, to obtain an insight into how the laser is actually used in clinical practice for the treatment of naevi to achieve as much as possible the intact skin condition.

Laser treatment can be subdivided into two main considerations. Surgical laser treatment, or high reactive-level laser treatment (HLLT), and therapeutic laser treatment, or low reactive-level laser therapy (LLLT).

3-6-1 Surgical Laser Treatment (HLLT)

Surgical laser treatment is defined as a treatment method, using high incident power densities of appropriate laser energy, to remove or irre-versibly alter tissue structure or architecture to correct an abnormality in colour, texture, configu-ration or function. Most but not all laser treatment for naevi falls under the category of surgical treatment, which is based on a photothermal pho-todestructive reaction. The temperature in the irradiated tissue depends on the combination of laser parameters already outlined above: the output power of the laser, the spot size and the time for which the laser energy is incident on the target tissue. The range of photodestructive reactions associated with the laser tissue reaction is temperature-dependent.

R-1) Protein Denaturation (40°C ~ 55°C).

Although protein denaturation is a photothermal response, it is reversible, and therefore requires a separate section outwith the photodestructive reactions. All connective tissue in the body is composed of collagen. Collagen is a complex proteinous substance composed basically of a triple α-helix polypeptide chain. In dermal collagen, these polypeptides are produced by fibroblasts, in the form of procollagen, a collagen precursor The gelatinous proteins form the α-helical chain called procollagen; the terminals at each end of the chain are enzymatically cleaved, and the chains are crosslinked internally and to each other by fairly fragile hydrogen bonds, which are extremely heat-sensitive, breaking down and delinking at temperatures in excess of 40°C. The procollagen chains group into bundles of collagen filaments, which in turn group and crosslink to form bundles called fibrils, which then crosslink in bundles to form fibres. In soft tissue, collagen fibres then form random bundles to make up the collagen matrix. In tendon tissue, the collagen matrix is much more polarized in its layout, with a greater order to the way in which the fibres lie to make up the matrix, compared with the comparatively random structure in dermal collagen. Muscle matrix organization lies somewhere in between dermal and tendon collagen.

The dermal collagen matrix is composed of cable-like bundles of collagen fibres in a viscous liquid called the ground substance, randomly interwoven to give great tensile strength. At temperatures of 40°C to 53°C, the procollagen and individual fibril hydrogen bonds are broken, and the collagen denatures, or 'melts', to its parent gelatinous form. At this stage the overall matrix still more or less retains its form, but now there are some denatured procollagen chains and fibrils with broken but still viable bonds. When the tissue temperature drops to below 40°C, these bonds will reunite, but not necessarily with their previous partner.

Some rearrangement of the matrix therefore takes place, but with very little cellular damage, if any, and consequently little or no need for the repair mechanism. That is protein denaturation.

R-2) Protein Degradation (55°C ~ 63°C).

The collagen matrix depends on comparatively fragile hydrogen bond interlinking between procollagen chains and collagen fibrils to form fibres, and further crosslinkage between individual fibres to form thicker and thicker cable-like bundles, randomly oriented to each other as described above. Temperatures in excess of 40°C will break the comparatively fragile hydrogen bonds between the fibrils, and the smaller fibres, but leave the bonds viable (protein denaturation). Temperatures from around 55°C begin to destroy the viability of the bonds, including the cross-linking in the larger fibre bundles, and the complex structure of the matrix collapses or degrades, allowing the ground substance to infiltrate individual fibre bundles, which then collapse on each other: the higher the temperature, the more complete the degradation. Lowering the temperature will not completely restore the matrix, and some cellular damage results, so this change is at least partly irreversible, and is the first of the photodestructive changes.

Protein degradation appears in histological specimens as an increased transparency in hematoxylin-eosin (H-E) staining of superficial dermal tissue following laser irradiation, accompanied by a slight pyknotic change in the epidermal and superficial dermal cellular nuclei.

R-3) Coagulation (63°C ~ 85°C)

At temperatures in excess of 63°C, in addition to denaturing then degrading the collagen protein in the affected tissue, with a resulting infiltration of ground substance, the heating effect causes the loosely infiltrated mass to contract, coalesce and form a tighter-knit, firmer mass of degraded collagenous material with a smaller volume than the original tissue, forcing the ground substance out as it contracts. This effect is called coagulation. Coagulation is typified in H-E stained histological specimens by a homogeneous appearance in affected tissue. The normal, irregular cellular interstices and random collagen matrix architecture disappear, replaced by a regular, tighter-knit mass. Basophilic and pyknotic changes are clearly seen in the epidermal and dermal cell nuclei. When blood is present in the mass of coagulum, coagulation is aided by the presence of fibrin, an insoluble fibrous protein, which is histochemically altered to form a tough, net-like structure through the coagulated mass, binding it together.

R-4) Vaporization (>100°C)

At temperatures around 95°C the intra-and extracellular fluids at first begin to form small bubbles or vacuoles in the tissue, clearly seen in histologic specimens. At 100°C the fluids instantly vaporize, and the dramatic rise in pressure caused by the steam in tissue literally blows the target tissue apart, thus removing some of the tissue in the form of minute particles which can be aspirated along with the steam. Vaporization also causes a certain amount of heat conduction to the underlying

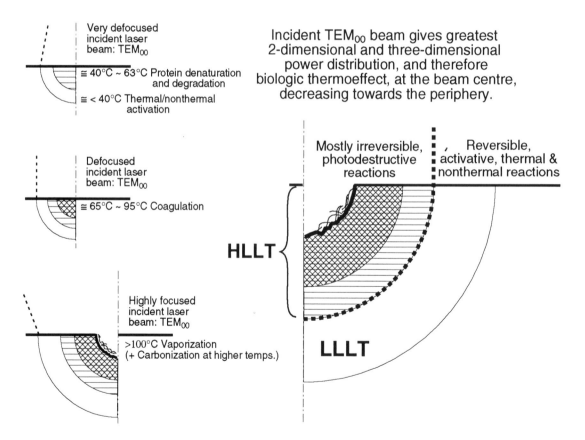

Fig 3.33: *Schematic representation of the range of biologic photothermal laser/tissue reactions, and demonstration of the possible simultaneus occurrence of these reactions. Control of the incident power density through alteration of the spot size is the most important single parameter for efficient reaction control, although wavelength and irradiation time must also be taken into consideration.*

and surrounding tissue causing some coagulative necrosis in the nearest tissue layers and protein denaturation in the farther layers. This tissue heating will lead to more tissue necrosis in the farther layers as the healing process starts. The greater the degree of radiant heat effect, as discussed above, the less will be this wave of secondary thermal damage, and *vice versa*.

In the healing process, degraded collagen is partly macrophaged, and partly restructured, coagulum is macrophaged and replaced by a more fibrotic matrix. Carbon char particles represent foreign body material, and excite more macrophage cell activity to ensure their removal or encapsulation. In all of the above photobiologic reactions with the exception of protein denaturation, at least some tissue is destroyed, and has to be replaced. The tissue architecture, even in protein denaturation, is altered in some way. The author would therefore like to class all of these reactions as photodestructive, and falling under the umbrella of HLLT.

Figure 3.33 (previous page) demonstrates on the left the range of thermal-dependent biologic pho-

toreactions, controlled by use of appropriate laser parameters. It is possible, as seen in the right of the figure, to have the whole range of reactions almost simultaneously, from vaporization, carbonization and burn-off at the centre of the target tissue to thermal and nonthermal photoactivation at the target area periphery. In other words, in the model as illustrated, LLLT occurs in the peripheral zones simultaneously with HLLT reactions in the more central parts of the target tissue.

In order to limit the tissue damage to the effect required, a number of methodologies are available to the laser surgeon, but they all share the common base of laser parameter manipulation and interdependence.

3-6-1-(A) Spotty, Lineal and Area Treatment

200 μm - 250 μm is the critical depth in connective tissue on which depends good wound healing and the macroscopically intact skin condition. Damage below this depth is much more likely to lead to a prolonged reepithelization period, and to visible scar formation. The area of the damage is also important, as 2 μm is recognised as the average reepithelization from the wound margin

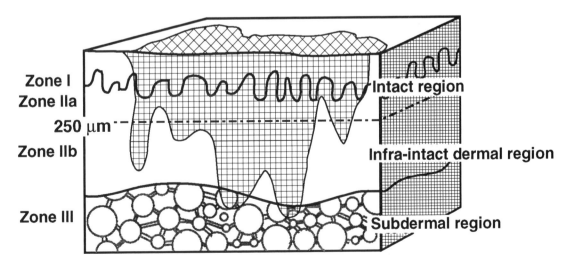

Fig 3.34: Schematic representing a multi-layer naevus, from superficial to subdermal regions.

Laser in Area Treatment

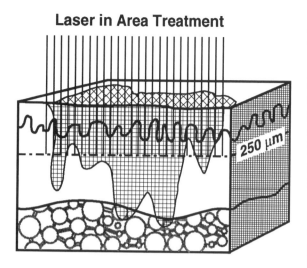

Fig 3.35: *Area treatment method is used to 'paint' superficial-lying naevus.*

alone in a 10-14 day period, which is the preferred reepithelization period to achieve the macroscopically intact skin condition. Taken together, the damage depth and area lead to the volume consideration discussed in the previous section,

and from the damage volume consideration the author has evolved his spotty, linear and area treatment methodologies.

In Figure 3.34 a naevus is seen which exists in several layers, from the superficial to the deeper dermal regions. If this naevus were to be removed in a single laser treatment session, the resulting damage depth would be well below the 250 μm line and the damage area would be large, giving an excessive damage volume. Reepithelization would take considerably longer than the 10-14 day period, and visible scar formation would be inevitable. Under the author's damage volume control methodology, the superficial regions of the naevus, existing above the 250 μm line, can be treated simultaneously (Figure 3.35). This is the area treatment method. As already mentioned in Section 3-3, superficial damage above the 250 μm line will normally reepithelize within the 10-14 day period, giving the macroscopic intact skin condition.

Once the wound has reepithelized, and the epithelium has matured, a second treatment is carried out for the intermediate regions of the

Linear Treatment
(defocused beam)

Residual naevus materials in deeper layers

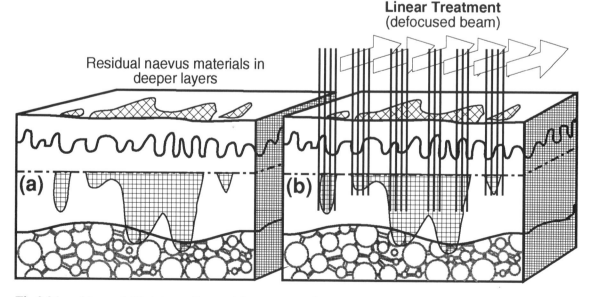

Fig 3.36: a: *Naevus left in intermediate and deeper areas after area treatment.* **b:** *Laser is applied in Ohshiro's linear 'zebra' method for intermediate pigment.*

Spot Treatment
(slightly defocused beam)

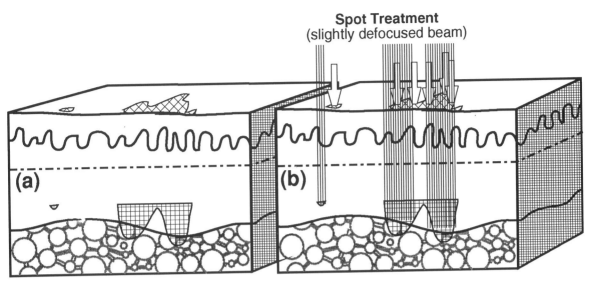

Remaining pigment is too deep to reflect incident light back out of the skin, is thus not seen from outside, and so need not be removed.

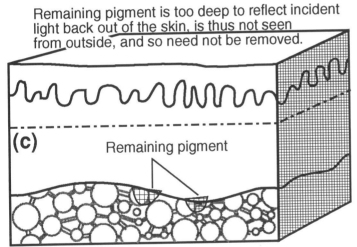

Remaining pigment

Fig 3.37:
a: *Naevus remaining in deeper layers after zebra treatment.*
b: *Laser applied in spotty method for deeper pigment, with damage limited to each spot.*
c: *Pigment remaining in subdermal layers is too deep to be seen, and therefore need not be treated.*

naevus (Figure 3.36). For treatment of this region, the author developed the linear method, in which the laser is applied in a repeat-shot mode, each laser shot slightly overlapping the one previous, in a linear pattern. The maximum lateral size of the treated area is 4 mm, so that even although the critical 250 μm damage depth is exceeded, reepithelization can take place from the wound margins within the 10-14 day period.

After the treated areas have successfully reepithelized, and the new epithelium has ma-

tured, the remaining deeper areas can be treated in the defocused spotty method, where deeper damage, well below the 25 μm line, is limited to the diameter of a single laser exposure (Figure 3.37). Although the damage depth is comparatively large, the actual damage area is extremely small, and reepithelization easily occurs within the 10 days period.

If the clinician remembers the 250 μm 'danger zone', and adjusts the treatment parameters to limit the damage volume based on a suitable area for realistic epithelization following the spot, line and area consideration, then even for extensive lesions treatment can be carried out which will eventually achieve complete macroscopic removal of the lesion with macroscopically intact skin condition. The 250 μm line referred to above is the average value in the Oriental skin. For Caucasian skin, it can be increased on average to around the 300 μm mark.

Finally, the important factor of laser wavelength absorption characteristics has not been mentioned above, but it must also be taken into account in choosing the most appropriate laser for each particular naevus or area in the naevus.

3-6-1-(B) Pinhole Treatment

An extension of the defocused spotty treatment method involves the application of a single focused laser spot. The average minimum spot size of a focused CO_2 laser beam is 100 μm in diameter. With visible light lasers, even smaller spots can be achieved. The increase in incident power density caused by the decrease in the spot size has been discussed above (3-6-3). A 2 W laser with a 2 mm spot delivers an incident power density of approximately 64 W/cm². With a 100 μm spot, the power density is over 25,400 W/cm² (refer back to Figure 3.30 above). This gives a very deep damage effect with efficient tissue vaporization but minimum peripheral damage, depending also on the irradiation time and wavelength characteristics, and is called by the author the pinhole treatment. Pinhole treatment is suitable for removing very deep isolated spots of coloured naevus cells or materials which may remain after the area, linear and spot defocused treatment has been completed. The pinhole method is also very good for the treatment of comedos or pimples.

3-6-1-(C) Incision and Excision

Laser incision or excision is an extension of the pinhole treatment, applied with a continuous focused beam in a linear fashion, which gives in effect a precise linear vaporization, thus incising or excising tissue. Because the laser/tissue inter-

action is thermal, as the laser cuts through tissue small blood and lymphatic vessels in the incised margins are sealed. This gives the advantage of a dry field which is particularly helpful in highly vascularized tissue. The sealing of small vessels will also help prevent the dissemination of viral cells from excised tissue. The CO_2 laser has been the laser of choice for laser incision, but the new higher-powered visible light lasers, 20 W argon (488-514.5 nm) and KTP-532 (532 nm), can actually produce smaller spot sizes for greater precision, and are much more haemostatic than the 10,600 nm CO_2 laser beam. The other advantage of laser cutting is the simultaneous low reactive-level laser therapeutic effect (simultaneous LLLT) which occurs at the periphery of the laser-irradiated tissue. This has accounted for beneficial side effects for laser surgery compared with the conventional scalpel, such as less postoperative oedema, pain and improved early stage wound healing.

3-6-1-(D) Defocused Beam Spotty Treatment

Already mentioned above is the point-by-point application of the defocused laser beam, the spotty treatment method. In practical treatment of naevi, the clinician will very often have to group these individual defocused spots in particular areas of deeper-situated naevus cells or materials. The author calls this treatment methodology the 'leopard' technique, and is very effective for treatment of deeper-lying Ohta's naevus pigment, or for the deeper naevus cells in the spotty type of naevus cell naevus.

3-6-1-(E) Defocused Beam Linear Treatment

The maximum distance which can be effectively reepithelized from the margins of a linear wound in 10 days is approximately 4 mm (2 mm from each margin). In order to use this in effective laser treatment of larger intermediate depth naevi, such as haemangioma simplex, the author developed a multilinear treatment using the defocused laser beam. Treated areas of a maximum of 4 mm in width are separated by untreated areas. The ratio of treated to untreated tissue can be varied depending on the individual lesion being treated. Reepithelization of the treated areas then takes place from the margins of the remaining untreated normal skin. Once this new epithelium has matured and stabilized, the remaining untreated areas are treated, which are in turn successfully epithelized from the new epithelium covering the previously-treated areas. The author calls this the 'zebra' technique, and has used it with consistent success in the treatment of extensive haemangioma simplex lesions.

3-6-1-(F) Laser Coagulation

Laser coagulation is a photothermal destructive reaction in which the irradiated tissue is virtually cooked. In this reaction, the collagen coalesces into an amorphous mass of coagulated tissue, and in doing so, shrinks. Some coagulation will occur simultaneously with laser vaporization in the wound margins, especially with laser having a high conducted heat effect. Excessive coagulation leads to tissue necrosis and is usually minimized by selecting appropriate laser types and parameters.

In some cases, where there is a configurational problem in tandem with the colour problem of a lesion, the effect of coagulation can be deliberately but carefully applied for the correction of the configuration problem, before dealing with the colour removal. Application of a high conducted-effect laser, such as the defocused argon laser beam, with longer irradiation times will produce a shrinking effect in the target tissue, thus helping to restore normal configuration. Naturally, this effect must be carefully controlled to avoid excessive damage to the treated tissue. The clinician must balance the destruction with the recuperative and recovering powers of the skin, as discussed earlier. This is a good example of the 'accelerator and brake' control developed and practised by the author, essential in achieving the desired treatment of maximum effect with minimum damage.

3-6-1-(G) Laser Abrasion

Some lesions require layered removal of excess or affected tissue. This is abrasion, and can be done mechanically with a dermatome, a high-speed revolving burr or chemically with specially-designed compounds. Laser energy can also be used for tissue abrasion. In particular the CO_2 laser, with its precise control and minimal penetration, can remove irradiated tissue by tissue-selective vaporization with a partially-defocused beam. Advantages of laser abrasion over conventional methods are less postoperative bleeding or seeping from the treated area and the beneficial side effects associated with simultaneous LLLT. Disadvantages are that it is possible to over-irradiate the area, producing excessive coagulation in the remaining tissue with the possibility of visible scar formation.

3-6-1-(H) Laser Epithelial Peeling

Treatment for purely epidermal naevi, such as naevus spilus and senile fleck, often involves removal of the epithelium alone followed by some form of cleaning the excess pigment off the exposed dermis. Epithelial removal, or peeling, involves rupturing the dermoepidermal attachment at the basement membrane, after which the epidermis is easily peeled from the dermis in a single sheet. Rupturing the basement membrane can be accomplished with application of dry ice or snowy dry ice, which causes serum-filled blister formation, rupturing the membrane and detaching the epidermis by a combination of physical (cryotherapy) and mechanical reactions.

Another laser application which requires epidermal removal uses the formation of an epidermal 'window' to allow more efficient penetration of the laser into deeper dermal tissue.

In addition to conventional methods, carefully-selected laser parameters can also separate the epidermis from the dermis. For cases of epidermal melanin anomaly group naevi, parameters which will limit laser absorption to the melanin granules in the area of the epidermis between the granular layer and the basal layer will give a very effective epidermal detachment over a large spot size, with minimal photothermal damage in the dermis. Shorter-acting lasers are very effectively applied in this indication. The CO_2 laser, because of its water-absorption characteristics, can very effectively generate enough heat in the epidermis alone to detach it cleanly from the dermis in a non colour-dependent reaction, with a large spot size. Full understanding of laser-tissue reaction and careful parameter selection are essential in this application of the laser.

3-6-1-(I) Laser Microsurgery

Laser energy can be delivered through a variety of delivery devices, some of which offer the capability of coupling the laser to an operating microscope. Those lasers which use flexible fibreoptic-based delivery systems are naturally more easily used in combination with the microscope, because of ease of motion and the ability to site the laser well away from the microscope and a possibly sterile field. The minute spot sizes offered by focused laser energy give the microsurgical specialist a precise photosurgical tool capable of irradiating single cells, or even subcellular organelles.

3-6-1-(J) Laser Tissue Welding

Collagen fibre bundles, which form a major part of dermal tissue architecture, are held together by cross-linking hydrogen bonds. These bonds are susceptible to heat, and at temperatures in excess of $40°C$ they break down. On cooling, the bonds reform, although recent reports suggest this is noncovalent rebonding. With careful temperature control, two blocks of tissue can in theory be joined by this denaturation-renaturation process by a weld of living collagen tissue. Reports on tissue welding for sutureless microanastomosis were appearing in the literature in 1980, followed by laser welding of neural tissue and finally of cutaneous wounds. Recent studies have shown that cutaneous tissue welding can be enhanced by application of a topical photosensitizing dye. Simultaneous LLLT may also have a role in the

success of such welding applications. Although laser anastomosis and reanastomosis has been demonstrated in neural tissue and for reconnection of fallopian tubes and vas deferens transected for purposes of sterilization, widespread applications of laser tissue welding in laser treatment for naevi are a consideration of the future.

3-6-1-(K) Combined Laser Treatment for HLLT

Each laser wavelength has its own laser-tissue reactions, and there is no one laser which can be used for everything, although careful parameter selection as already discussed can increase the range of utility of any one laser. There are areas of overlap between the CO_2 and the argon laser, for example, but it is the areas in which they are unique which make each laser system particularly suited to a fairly narrow filed of application. The most logical extension of this line of argument is to apply a number of lasers in combination for the treatment of naevi. As an example, for the treatment of a full-range haemangioma simplex, the Q-switched pulsed ruby laser is well-suited to remove the superficial lesion components: the argon and KTP-532 lasers are applicable in defocused mode for the coagulation of blood vessels in the intermediate tissue, and in focused mode for the deeper vessels. Longer irradiation times with a slow-acting visible light laser can be used to correct tissue deformity by shrinkage, before the colour abnormality is treated. Deep and extensive coagulation of tissue can be done with the Nd:YAG, if that is required. Deep nests of naevus cells can be precisely targeted with the focused CO_2 laser in the pinhole technique.

The principle of Combined Laser Therapy (CLT) has been advocated and practised by the author for more than 15 years, and has given his clinic a consistent success rate in the removal of many different naevi.

3-6-1-(L) Laser Selective Treatment

In addition to the pigment-dependent selectivity inherent in the wavelength of the laser, the concept of cell- and tissue selectivity depending on the exposure time of the laser beam has already been discussed in Chapter 2. There are four basic treatment categories: ultrashort acting laser treatment; very short acting laser treatment; short acting laser treatment; and long acting laser treatment.

3-6-1-(L-1) Ultrashort Acting Laser Treatment

When it is necessary to destroy target tissue selectively, that is to say, a combination of normal cells and abnormal cells or materials, it is better to use a short irradiation time with a high powered light beam having the characteristic of a high absorption rate in the naevus cells and materials. In that combination of circumstances, the radiant heat effect is very high: radiant heat occurs through the instantaneous conversion of light energy to heat energy. By obtaining as much of the radiant heat effect as possible, the clinician can control the amount of secondary conducted heat, and prevent damage to surrounding tissues from the secondary, more slowly moving thermal wave of conducted heat. In this situation, the blood vessels in the target tissue act like a car radiator, and remove conducted heat by absorption in the blood, transferred to the blood stream, and dissipate the heat throughout the body. By using a laser beam with a very high absorption rate for the target tissue, delivered in a very short Q-switched pulse, i.e. microseconds or nanoseconds, a very highly cellular selective treatment effect is possible.

There is a question of balance, however. With ultrahigh-power pulses, which can be measured in megawatts (MW), even with the shortest possible irradiation time, measured in microseconds (1 $\mu s = 1 \times 10^{-9}$ s) or even nanoseconds (1 ns = 1 $\times 10^{-9}$ s), the incident power and energy can destroy all cells in the target area, in other words, the cell selectivity factor becomes too low, as the cells in the target tissue have all been damaged over their survival threshold. In such a situation, the energy per pulse must be controlled to below the survival threshold of the target tissue of the

normal cells, and the treatment must then be divided up into several sessions, so as to treat the lesion in successive layers, allowing enough time between sessions for the recovering power of the skin to do its work. By this method, although the total treatment time is longer, the laser energy is selectively targeting the naevus cells or materials in each layer, while sparing the overlying normal tissue, and the end result is much better, than if the whole depth range of the lesion is targeted in one immensely powerful pulse.

3-6-1-(L-2) Very Short Acting Laser Treatment

With standard pulsed lasers, such as the original ruby, the irradiation time per pulse was in the approximate range of from $10^{-4} \sim 10^{-2}$ sec.. This gave a comparatively high radiant heat effect, with little conducted heat damage, and enabled fairly high cell-selective treatment.

The cells and materials destroyed or damaged by the laser in the ultrashort and very short acting treatment sessions are removed from the skin surface in the wound crust, or those in the deeper areas are macrophaged by the natural process of phagocytosis, removed by the blood and lymphatic networks, and excreted normally from the body.

3-6-1-(L-3) Short Acting Laser Treatment

When using a switched continuous wave beam, such as the argon or carbon dioxide laser, and short exposure times of ≤0.1 s, the cell selectivity becomes less, and the amount of secondary thermal damage to surrounding normal cells by conducted heat becomes greater. This gives the clinician a comparatively cell-selective treatment and is useful for treating naevi in the intermediate or deeper layers.

3-6-1-(L-4) Long Acting Laser Treatment

Long acting laser treatment (≥1.0 s) is used for laser incision or excision, and gives tissue selective treatment, where the target tissue is removed en bloc. Coagulation is accompanied by shrinkage of the coagulated tissue, and long acting laser treatment can therefore be used deliberately to cause shrinkage in a naevus with both a colour and configurational problem, as discussed above in configuration control (3-5-9).

3-6-1-(M) Practical Laser Treatment for Naevi

This section will offer an overview of the author's experience in his acquisition of different laser types since the mid 1970's, and will then examine some of the practical applications of the laser in the treatment of naevi.

3-6-1-(M-1) Author's Historical Perspective

In the decade after the laser's first successful firing, Fran L'Esperance in ophthalmology, and Leon Goldman and David Apfelberg in dermatology started to publish data on laser applications on human patients. By the mid 1970's the author had become very interested in the possibility of laser applications in the treatment of abnormally coloured skin lesions, and so went to the University of Cincinnati and studied there with Professor Leon Goldman, the recognized pioneer of dermatological applications of the laser. Since then, the author has compiled a large group of different laser systems, each with its own characteristics, advantages and disadvantages. An outline of the development of the lasers currently found in the author's clinic now follows.

3-6-1-(M-1)-(a) Ruby Laser

On his return to Japan from Cincinnati, the author introduced the first ruby laser which he modified for clinical applications in dermatology in Japan (wavelength, 694.3 nm, deep red). This was a 'cannon' type system manufactured by Korad Inc, USA, and was a basic industrial system, which the Japan Medical Laser Laboratory modified for clinical use. Figure 3.38a shows the system with the cover on, 3.38b with the cover off, and Figure 3.38c shows the ruby (upper) and neodymium glass (lower) rods, both of which could be used in this system to give visible red (694.3 nm) and near infrared (1063 nm) laser energy, respectively. The ruby rod was capable of pulses of 160 J, and the Nd:Glass, pulses of 250J.

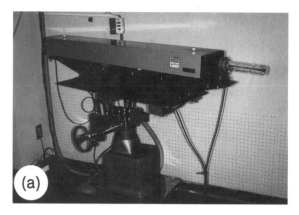

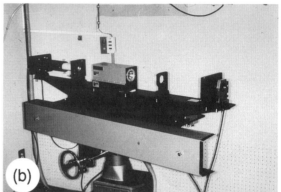

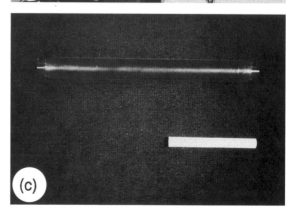

Fig 3.38:
Korad 'canon' type ruby laser adapted by Ohshiro's group for dermatological use.
a: *system with cover on.*
b: *System with the cover off.*
c: *Close-up of ruby rod used in the Korad system and Nd:glass rod in the 'space gun' system to give pulsed output at 694.3 nm and 1063 nm, respectively.*

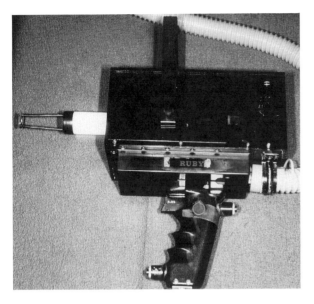

Fig 3.39: Japan Medical Laser Laboratory's 'space gun' ruby laser.

From this system, the author's laboratory moved to design and develop a smaller, more easily used ruby laser, which is seen in Figure 3.39, resembling a 'space gun'. This also used ruby and Nd:Glass rods, and was capable of pulses of 40 J. Despite a lack of popularity elsewhere, the author has continued to use these systems with great success in the treatment of the more superficial skin lesions, such as some types of haemangioma simplex, naevus spilus and naevus cell naevus.

One of the latest developments is the introduction of the Q-switched pulsed ruby laser, with ultrashort nanosecond pulses, which has opened new possibilities in cell-selective treatment for abnormally coloured skin lesions with high peak powers coupled with ultrashort acting time giving a highly efficient

Table 3.4:   Comparison of Q-switched pulsed ruby lasers

Item	SPECTRUM	NSEC
Manufacturer	Spectrum, Inc, USA	Nippon Scientific Engineering Co., Ltd, Japan
Model	RD 1200	none as yet
Wavelength	694.3	694.3
Output energy	4 J max. (however, use at anything over 2 J will shorten lifetime of optical components)	1 J
Pulse width	20 ns	40 ns
Spot size (diameter) (Max. energy density)	5 mm (10 J/cm^2) 6.5 mm (7.5 J/cm^2)	5 mm (5 J/cm^2) 4 mm (8 J/cm^2) 2.5 mm (20 J/cm^2)
Repetition rate	0.5 Hz (one shot/2 sec)	1 Hz (one shot/sec)
Aiming beam	none	semiconductor laser (red)
Main consumable system components	Flashlamp, pockells cell, rotating mirrors (used in the multiple articulated arm), handpiece lens	flash lamp, front mirror
Moisture control	none: it is therefore necessary in conditions of high humidity to lower room humidity, or reconstruct the system	main optical components are sealed in air-tight compartment
Special features	High cell selectivity with ultrashort acting time and high peak powers, but the lifetime of optical components is very short	High cell selective treatment. Three different spot sizes can be selected, with good range of control. Long lifetime of optical components.

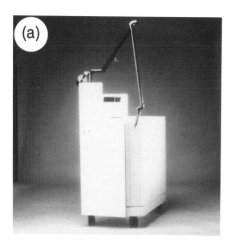

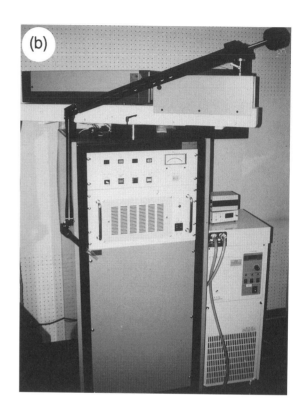

Fig 3.40: Q-switched ruby lasers. **a:** Spectrum RD 1200 and **b:** NSEC system.

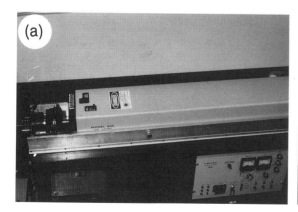

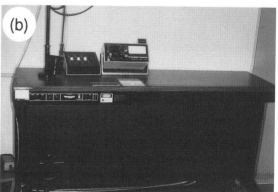

Fig 3.41: Argon lasers. **a:** Lexel model 295 and **b:** Coherent model 2000.

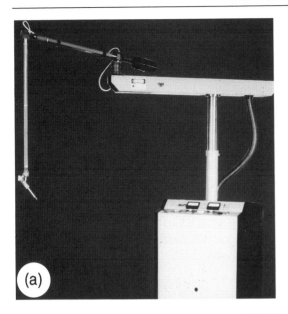

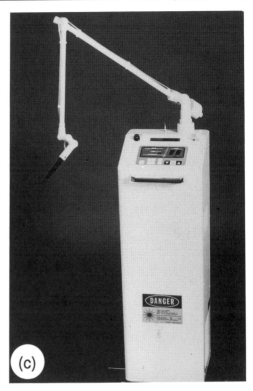

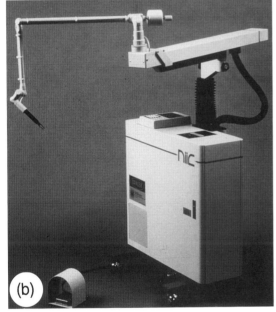

Fig 3.42:
*CO_2 lasers: **a:** Sharplan 791; **b:** NIIC 30Z; and **c:** NIIC IR101.*

Ruby lasers have been somewhat limited by the difficulty of positioning the patient against the fairly immobile system, although the author's space gun design and the articulated arm of the Spectrum system helped to solve that problem.

3-6-1-(M-1)-(b) Argon Laser

The argon laser (main bands, 488 nm, 514.5 nm, visible blue and green, respectively) was adopted by both ophthalmology and dermatology very early on because of its blue/green beam's comparatively high colour selectivity in red pigments, such as haemoglobin. The author has two argon systems, the Coherent 2,000 (Figure 3.41a) and the Lexel Model 295 (Lexel, Inc., USA), which is an industrial system modified by the Japan Medical Laser Laboratory (JMLL) for clinical use (Figure 3.41b). The Coherent system can give output powers of 4 W maximum, while the Lexel

radiant heat effect (see discussion 2-2-2-a above). At present, the author has two such systems, the SPECTRUM RD 1200, from Spectrum, Inc, USA, and a system manufactured by the Nippon Scientific Engineering Company, Ltd, which has as yet no model name. Table 3.4 gives comparative details of the two systems, seen in Figures 3.40a and 3.40b.

is capable of much higher output wattages, 15 W or more. Another advantage of the argon laser is the ability to deliver the power through a flexible fibreoptic cable. This enabled the Lexel system, laser generation and control components to be housed in a completely different room from the treatment room, and controlled by a specially-designed remote console. This has obvious advantages as far as space, environmental (heat, noise) and safety considerations are concerned.

3-6-1-(M-1)-(c) Carbon Dioxide (CO$_2$) Laser

The CO$_2$ laser (10,600 nm, mid infrared) quickly became the workhorse of the small treatment centre, because of its ability to offer precise tissue vaporization or debulking, reasonable haemocoagulation, and comparatively efficient electrical/laser light energy conversion compared to the ruby and argon systems. It also offered multispecialty applications. The author has had three systems: the Sharplan 791, NIIC (Nippon Infrared Industrial Corporation) 30Z and the NIIC IR101, the last of which offers both a CO$_2$ and Nd:YAG beam from the same system (Figure 3.42 a, b and c, previous page). Current CO$_2$ systems work on the basis of a long-life sealed RF (radio frequency) excited tube, obviating the need for the

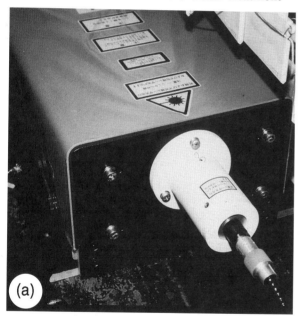

(a)

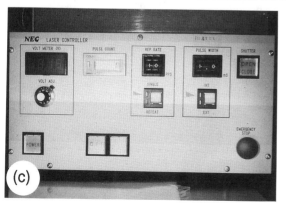

(c)

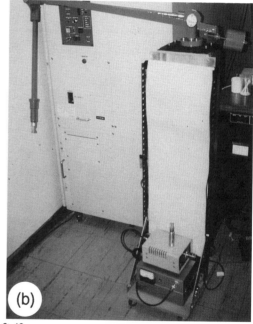

(b)

Fig 3.43:
Nd:YAG lasers:
a: *Control Systems YAG laser.*
b: *Prototype Q-switched Nd:YAG system designed and built by JMLL.*
c: *Example of treatment room remote control console for remotely sited YAG laser.*

bulky gas cylinders seen in earlier models, and reducing both size and cooling requirements.

Although flexible fibres for the CO_2 are currently in development, none is yet readily available (see the section on CO_2 fibres in Chapter 2), and the large majority of systems still use the articulated mirrored arm to deliver the laser energy from the system to the target tissue. This restricts the positioning of the system to near the operative field, and requires special adaptors for operating microscopes, but the most recent designs of articulated arm are much improved both from the point of need for realignment of the mirrors to ensure accurate targeting, flexibility, ease of use and weight.

3-6-1-(M-1)-(d) Neodymium-Yttrium-Aluminium Garnet (Nd:YAG) Laser.

The Nd:YAG laser (1064 nm, near infrared) was initially used in both neurosurgery and urology, where its deep coagulating beam appeared to offer haemostasis of large, well-vascularized tumours. Because of its ability to work well in clear physiological fluids, it could also be used under water irrigation for tumour or polyp removal in the bladder, using specially-designed endoscopes based on the fibreoptic delivery system offered by the Nd:YAG wavelength. In dermatology, the focused beam is useful for deeper-sited pigments, and the defocused beam has found applications in the revision of hypertrophic scars and keloids. The author has two Nd:YAG systems: a continuous wave system, based on an industrial Control Systems (USA) YAG laser (Figure 3.43a) and a prototype Q-switched YAG designed and built by the JMLL (Figure 3.43b). The C/W system has fibreoptic beam delivery, and so can be sited remotely from the treatment room with specially designed flexible delivery systems and remotely-mounted control consoles (Figure 3.43.c).

3-6-1-(M-1)-(e) Copper Vapour Laser

At one stage the author was selected by an Australian pioneering laser manufacturer, Metalaser, as the trial site in Japan for Metalaser's prototype

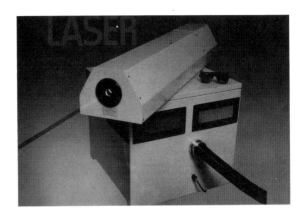

Fig 3.44: *Metalaser copper vapour laser, Dermalase.*

copper vapour laser system (Figure 3.44). This offered the choice of a green or yellow beam, or an admixture of them. The significance of the wavelength was in the high absorption specificity of the two different colours in biologic pigments. With the addition of a dye cell or an alexandrite crystal, this system was also designed to be capable of producing red light for photodynamic therapy (PDT) applications.

Unfortunately, in general the ambient environment is totally different in Japan and Sydney, Australia, and there were many problems over contamination of the copper vapour tube by condensation in the high humidity found in Japan, compared with Australia. Japanese customs officers insisted on opening up the carefully sealed and dry 'box' containing the central components of the system, and it was impossible thereafter to coax the laser into giving a continuous steady output. The project had therefore to be regretfully abandoned. However, the author understands the latest of the company's metal vapour laser systems perform extremely well.

3-6-1-(M-1)-(f) Flashlamp Dye Lasers

Another comparatively recent newcomer to the ranks of practical dermatological lasers is the flashlamp-pumped dye laser [wavelengths from ultraviolet to near infrared, depending on the dye

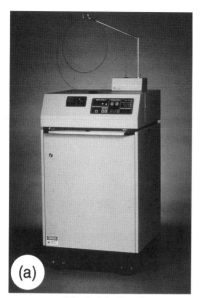
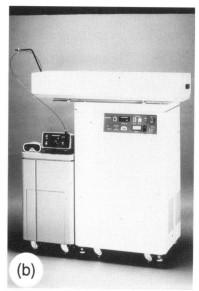

Fig 3.45: *Dye lasers:* **a:** *Candela SPTL1; and* **b:** *NIIC DO 101.*

Table 3.5:   *Comparison of flashlamp-pumped laser systems*

Item	Candela (USA)	NIIC (Japan)
Model	SPTL1	DO 101
Wavelength	585 nm	590 nm
Beam mode	multimode	multimode
Pulse delivery	single pulse	single pulse
Energy density per shot	10 J/cm^2	12.5 J/cm^2
Spot size (diameter)	5 mm	2.5 mm, 5 mm
Pulse width	450 μsec	300 μsec
Peak power	22 kW	50 kW
Pumping method	flashlamp	flashlamp

used: see 2-1-4-(C) above]. The most popular wavelengths in dermatological application are in the visible yellow waveband, and the two systems the author has operate at that colour. The Candela SPTL1 (Figure 3.45a) and the NIIC DO 101 (Figure 3.45b) are the two systems currently in the author's clinic. The wavelength is ideally suited to penetrating through overlying normal tissue selectively to coagulate pigmented lesions, especially in the blood vessel anomaly group, while causing minimal damage to the overlying tissues. Table 3.5 compares these two systems

3-6-1-(M-1)-(g) Laser Therapy (LLLT) Systems

Finally, the author would like to describe the LLLT systems he has been involved with, since there are good indications for LLLT in dermatology. The systems are mostly limited to diode laser-based systems, at a wavelength of 830 nm, although he has also used at times defocused Nd:YAG and CO_2 beams (adapted from surgical systems with appropriate parameters), and also a variety of HeNe systems (632.8 nm), both specifically designed as LLLT systems or adapted from commercial systems by the JMLL.

In the latter part of the 1960's, when L'Esperance and Goldman were announcing their successes in early laser surgical applications, Professor Endre Mester in Budapest, Hungary, published the first results on the application of laser therapy, using doses of low incident energy from a ruby laser, to achieve healing in torpid vasculogenic ulcers of the lower extremities in humans. Almost a decade after that, the author discovered by chance that laser treatment for a haemangioma simplex lesion on the sternum of a female patient not only successfully removed the colour, but also incidentally seemed to have removed the pain of the patient's post-herpetic neuralgia, which had been really severe. Coupled with the results coming in from Mester's group, the author turned the attention of the JMLL to developing a dedicated laser therapy system.

A variety of pilot experiments pinpointed the wavelength of 830 nm as being an ideal all-round wavelength, and so designs were started on an 830 nm LLLT system. Figure 3.46 shows the first prototype, model MEL 01. This was a single channel 15 mW laser based on a gallium arsenide

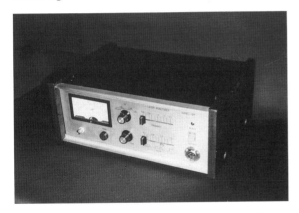

Fig 3.46: *Prototype diode laser, 1980: model MEL 01.*

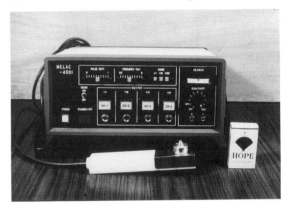

Fig 3.47: *MEL 02 diode laser, with 4 treatment channels.*

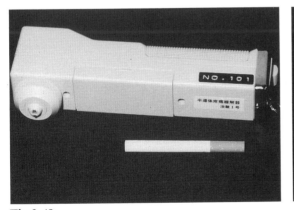

Fig 3.48:
Battery-operated GaAlAs diode laser system, jointly designed by JMLL and Matsushita Electric Company (1981).

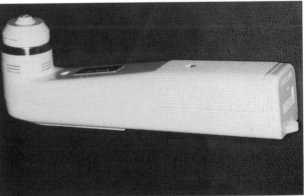

Fig 3.49:
Improved version of battery-powered system.

(GaAs) diode laser, at a wavelength of 830 nm. This system first appeared in 1980. This was followed by MEL 02 (Melac 4001) (Figure 3.47) which delivered the same output power, but had 4 treatment channels. Very early on, the author and the JMLL established good relations with Matsushita Electric Company, better known for their National Panasonic brand of consumer electronics. In 1981, JMLL and Matsushita pooled information and produced the first battery-operated systems, delivering 15 mW at 830 nm, but

using a gallium aluminium arsenide (GaAlAs) laser diode, which gave better stability and energy conversion ratios. This system (Figure 3.48) was announced at the 4th meeting of the International Society for Laser Medicine and Surgery, held in Tokyo in October 1981. It was followed by an improved version (Figure 3.49), again produced in cooperation between the JMLL and Matsushita. Both of these systems, although battery operated, were sophisticated designs, having touch sensors to detect when the probe was in

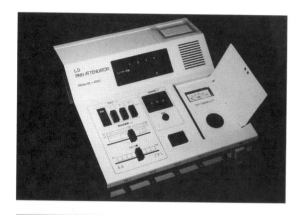

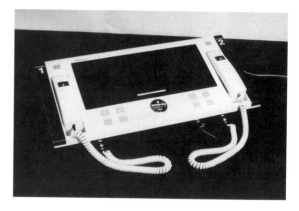

Fig 3.50:
(Above, left) Panalas 4000, Matsushita Electric Company.

Fig 3.51:
(Above) Panalas 4000 DeLuxe: 60 mW GaAlAs system with Japanese Ministry of Health and Welfare approval.

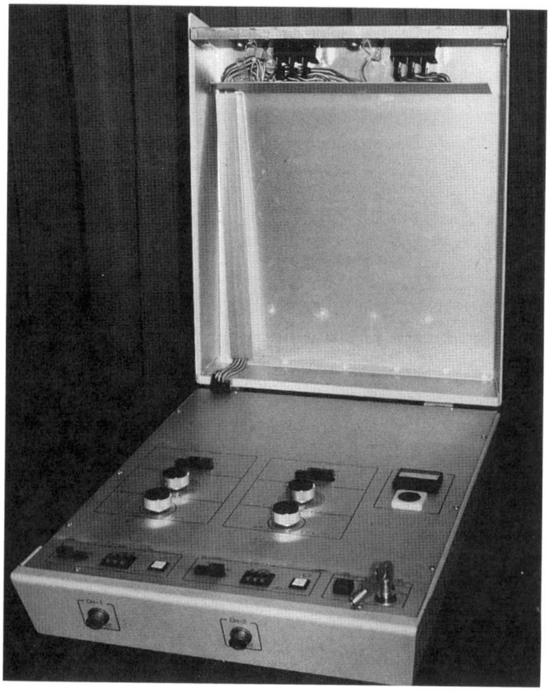

Fig 3.52:
(Left) JMLL GaAlAs prototype system, MEL 03.

contact with target tissue, warning LEDs (light-emitting diodes) and also an audible emission indicator. Matsushita then produced a console-type LLLT system, the Panalas 4000, seen in Figure 3.50. This had all of the features of the previous handy-types, but delivered 60 mW output power, which was found to be more efficient than the 15 mW of the earlier systems. Matsushita refined that further and finally came out with a second-generation model, the Panalas 4000 De-Luxe, seen in Figure 3.51. All of these systems were designed for use with the probe in contact with the target tissue.

At the same time as Matsushita were working on the Panalas, the JMLL were also designing a console-type system, and the first prototype, MEL 03, is shown in Figure 3.52. This delivered 60 mW of 830 nm laser energy generated by GaAlAs diodes, with a twin probe system. Figure 3.53 shows the MEL 04, a further design improvement, still with two probes. This evolved into the MEL 05 system, seen in Figure 3.54, with a single probe, giving 60 mW at 830 nm, continuous wave. MEL 05 was followed very shortly by MEL 06 and MEL 07: they differed externally from the MEL 05 prototype only in the colour of the case, but incorporated advances in the microprocessor-based automatic power control (APC) and better designs of the internal 'watch dog' safety features to ensure exact output power levels.

Following this, JMLL unveiled the commercially-available OhLase-3D1 LT 2001 laser therapy system (Figure 3.55), a third generation of microprocessor-controlled LLLT device. For the first time, the probe head incorporated an antire-

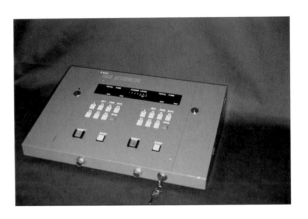

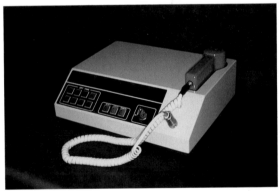

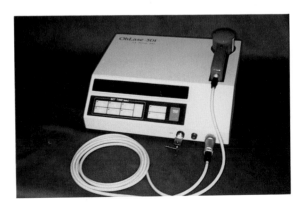

Fig 3.53:
(Above, left) MEL 04, further design improvement on MEL 03.

Fig 3.54:
(Above) MEL 05, single probe system, evolved from MEL 03 and MEL 04.

Fig 3.55:
(Left) OhLase-3D1 LT 2001 GaAlAs third generation microprocessor-controlled laser therapy system, with Japanese Ministry of Health and Welfare approval.

flective window over the laser aperture. This meant that with pressure, blood in the upper microvasculature could be removed, allowing more efficient penetration of the beam. The window also removed a problem found with earlier probes, which had an open aperture. On pressure, skin under the probe would tend to swell into the aperture, and fill with blood by the process of reverse osmosis: this left a number of unsightly red spots on the treatment area, which would however disappear in time. In addition, the Oh-Lase-3D1 probe head had contoured skin sensors, in comparison to earlier pointed ones, which were found on occasions to injure the treated area. The system could also be used in both contact and noncontact modes.

The OhLase-3D1 was designed with the overseas market in mind, with easy maintenance modular construction, so that failure of one component would not necessitate sending the whole system back to the manufacturer. It was in addi-. tion built to comply with existing European and American regulations, and like the Panalas 4000 DL has full approval of the Japanese Ministry of Health and Welfare.

There are now many types of dedicated laser therapy system available, offering a variety of designs, output powers and wavelengths. HeNe systems are available on their own, or combined with an infrared beam. Other systems offer a 'cluster probe' with a wide range of monochromatic super-LED's and laser diodes combined to give a multiwavelength output. Continuous wave (C/W), frequency-modulated C/W (often erroneously called 'pulsed'), or pulsed outputs can be found. In the author's experience, the simple unmodulated C/W output of the GaAlAs 830 nm systems at 60 mW offers treatment efficacy for a wide range of pain complaints, but can also be used for treatment of naevi, amongst others: the removal of abnormal colour or restoring normal colour; correcting abnormalities of configuration; modulating autoimmune response; in prophylactic applications to help prevent scar formation after conventional or laser surgery; and in expe-

diting wound healing to give the intact skin condition. Section 3-6-2 below will deal with some of these aspects in more detail.

3-6-1-(M-2) Laser Treatment for Naevi

In this section the author will present some examples of laser treatment for naevi from his case reports. First however, it is necessary to review some of the basic principles of laser-tissue reaction as they appear in practical laser clinical use.

3-6-1-(M-2)-(a) Bioreactions in Photobiodestructive Treatment

Laser treatment is divided into photobiodestructive and photobioactivative reactions, classed under HLLT and LLLT, respectively (refer back to Figure 3.33 and accomapnying text). Before going on to look at clinical case reports of patients and their treatment, the basic HLLT reactions will be reviewed in specific disease types.

3-6-1-(M-2)-(a-1) Carbonization.

Figure 3.56 shows a patient who had cavernous haemangioma of the lower lip plus haemangioma simplex (HS) of the lip and face. The focused beam of the CO_2 laser was used to excise the cavernous haemangioma, and this is the immediately postexcisional finding. The high photothermal destructive reaction of the focused CO_2 beam is easily capable of excision, and in the wound can be seen traces of carbonization, vaporization, haemocoagulation and protein denaturation, with simultaneous LLLT in the periphery of the irradiated area. Note the lack of active bleeding, even in the highly vascularized haemangiomatous tissue

3-6-1-(M-2)-(a-2) Haemocoagulation and Protein Denaturation

The patient in Figure 3.57 has HS of the left cheek. The ruby and argon lasers have both been applied in test treatment patches. The upper circular area was treated by the ruby laser with a 1 millisecond irradiation time. Haemocoagulation can be seen in the treated area as the areas of black change in the superficial photocoagulated blood vessels, because of the high cell selectivity of the short-acting beam. The lower right rectangular

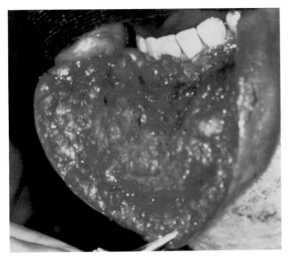

Fig 3.56:
Immediately postirradiation finding of patient with cavernous haemangioma of the lower lip. CO_2 laser excision of haemangioma leaving a clean, dry field.

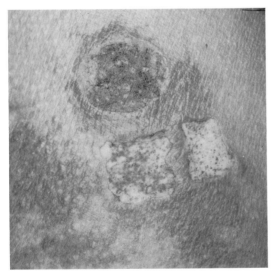

Fig 3.57:
HS on left cheek. Upper circular area was treated with pulsed ruby laser (irradiation time 1 ms). Black change of selective haemocoagulation clearly seen. Lower right rectangular area is immediately after argon laser treatment, with white change of protein denaturation and haemocoagulation. Rectangular area on lower left is some minutes after argon treatment: white change replaced by return of red colour caused by redilatation of thermally constricted vessels.

area is immediately after argon laser treatment, with the typical white change over all the treated area caused by haemocoagulation and protein denaturation following the slower-acting argon laser treatment: compare that with the selective black change in the blood vessels in the ruby-treated area. The rectangular area on the left is some minutes after argon treatment, and the red colour has returned following redilatation of the thermally-constricted, uncoagulated blood vessels in the treated area with cooling of the area.

3-6-1-(M-2)-(a-3) Haemocoagulation and Vacuolization: Dye Laser

Figure 3.58 shows HS on the neck, shoulder and upper arm of this patient treated with the dye laser in the linear zebra method. In this case, immediately after radiation, a grey change can be seen in the treated stripes. This is caused by a combination of haemocoagulation and vacuolization. The vacuolization occurs at the basement membrane, which gives a white change, and the haemocoagulation of the target vessels gives a black change: thus the combination of the white and black changes gives the grey change in the skin characteristic of the dye laser.

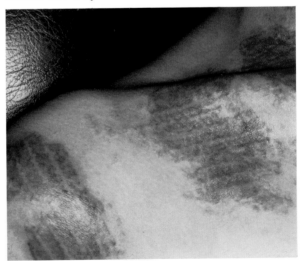

Fig 3.58:
'Grey change' typical of dye laser treatment of HS, caused by a combination of haemocoagulation and vacuolization.

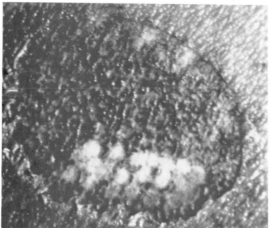

Fig 3.59:
Laser epithelial window over an HS lesion created by ruby laser, with localized argon laser treatment and white change.

3-6-1-(M-2)-(a-4) Laser Epithelial Window

An example of a laser epithelial window over an HS lesion is seen in Figure 3.59. In this case the ruby laser was used to create an area of deepithelialized dermis. The white spots are caused by

treatment with the argon laser directly onto the capillaries, and the white change can be clearly seen, with attachment of the endothelial walls of the targeted vessels.

3-6-1-(M-2)-(b) Practical Treatment Considerations: Case Reports

Using these and other biological photoeffects alone or in combination, with one or more lasers with or without conventional surgical techniques, the author has been treating naevus patients since June of 1975. From then until February of 1994, 19,099 naevus patients have passed through the author's clinic. Of these, by disease type, haemangioma simplex has accounted for 20.5% (3,927); Ohta's naevus for 14.9% (2,847); naevus spilus for 10.9% (2,079); chloasma for 8.4% (1,610); naevus cell naevus for 6.2% (1,177); hairy pigmented naevus for 5.1% (972); lentigo for 4.2% (799); and the remaining 29.8% is composed of miscellaneous others. These data are shown in Figure 3.60. When looking at the totals broken down by the main sections of the blood

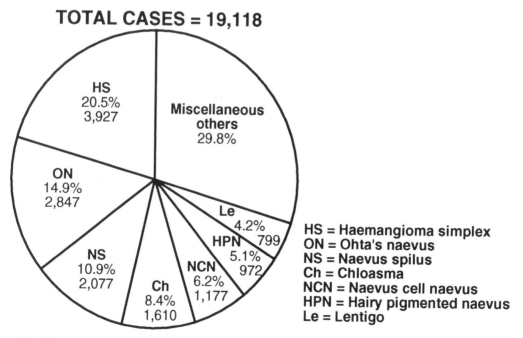

TOTAL CASES = 19,118

HS = Haemangioma simplex
ON = Ohta's naevus
NS = Naevus spilus
Ch = Chloasma
NCN = Naevus cell naevus
HPN = Hairy pigmented naevus
Le = Lentigo

Fig 3.60: *Breakdown by disease of total cases (19,118) in the Ohshiro Clinic from 1975 to 1994.*

TOTAL CASES = 19,118

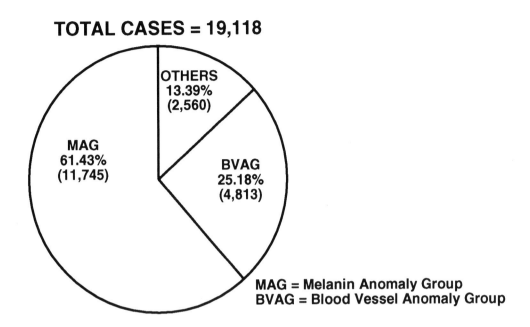

OTHERS
13.39%
(2,560)

MAG
61.43%
(11,745)

BVAG
25.18%
(4,813)

MAG = Melanin Anomaly Group
BVAG = Blood Vessel Anomaly Group

Fig 3.61: Distribution of 19,118 cases by main disease anomaly group.

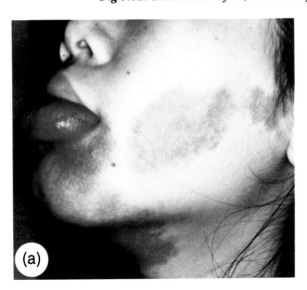

(a)

Fig 3.62:
Haemangioma simplex plus cavernous haemangioma.
a: *Preoperative findings in 12-year-old girl with extensive cavernous haemangioma of the lower lip together with HS of the lip, chin and neck.*

vessel and melanin anomaly groups, 25.2% (4,813) were in the BVAG, 61.4% (11,745) were in the MAG, and the remaining 13.4% (2,560) fell into other miscellaneous groups (Figure 3.61).

The author will show some case histories illustrating these effects used in clinical practice.

3-6-1-(M-2)-(b-1) HS plus Extensive CH

A 12-year-old Hong Kong girl came to the author's clinic with cavernous haemangioma (CH) of the lower lip plus extensive HS of the lower face (Figure 3.62a). Figure 3.62b shows the inner aspect of the lip, mucosa and oral mucosa, with the planned design of the CO_2 laser excision seen by the purple line drawn on the lip. Figure 3.62c is the immediately postoperative finding, demonstrating a dry field in the area of the excision. 3.62d shows the condition 2 years after the operation. Having removed the configurational problem, the remaining areas of HS are now being treated.

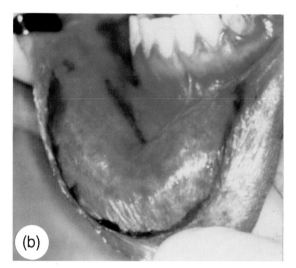

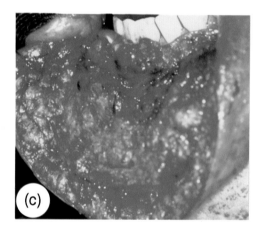

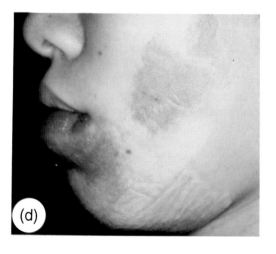

Fig 3.62 (Continued)

b: *(left) Planned excision for CH.*

c: *(Left, centre) CH component successfully excised with CO_2 laser.*

d: *(Left, bottom) Final result 2 years postoperatively.*

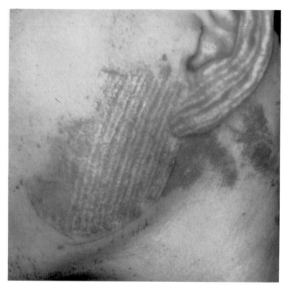

Fig 3.63: *Zebra treatment method for HS, 1:1 ratio.*

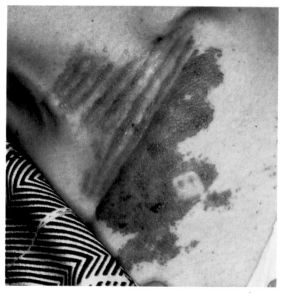

Fig 3.64: *Zebra treatment method for HS, 2:2 ratio.*

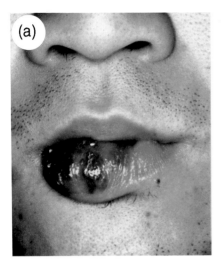
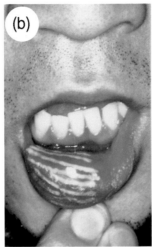
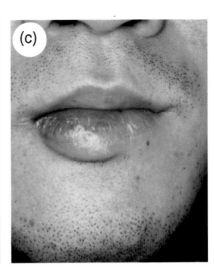

Fig 3.65:

a: *CH plus HS in lower lip.*

b: *Soon after treatment with the argon laser in the zebra method. Longer irradiation time used deliberately to induce shrinkage of the treated tissue.*

c: *Result 7 months after first treatment. Although the author was not satisfied with this result, the patient was.*

3-6-1-(M-2)-(b-2) HS Treated by the Zebra Method

The two HS patients in Figures 3.63 and 3.64 demonstrate different applications of the author's zebra method, already explained above. Figure 3.63 shows the 1:1 ratio of zebra treatment with the argon laser on an HS of the cheek and ear in a 41-year-old male, giving equal linear areas of treated and untreated lesion which gives this technique its name. Figure 3.64 shows an HS on the upper right sternum of a 56-year-old female, also treated with the argon laser, but at a 2:2 ratio. The difference between the treated and untreated areas is clearly visible.

3-6-1-(M-2)-(b-3) HS plus CH

(Figure 3.65a) This is another example of the preoperative finding in a case of CH plus HS in the lower lip of a 25 year-old male, although not as extensive as Case 1. Figure 3.65b shows the condition soon after argon laser treatment in the zebra method. For treatment involving a configurational plus colour abnormality, the configuration is treated with the argon laser at a long irradiation time, usually continuous wave, and an output power of 1 W, in order to use the shrinking characteristic of collagen coagulation. Figure 3.65c shows the condition 7 months after the first operation. The patient was treated 6 times, once per month. While the author was not satisfied with the result, the patient was, and so no further treatment was carried out. This shows the different levels of expectation that can be found from patient to patient and between patient and clinician, but as long as the patient is pleased with the result, that is surely the most important factor.

3-6-1-(M-2)-(b-4) HS plus Configurational Abnormality

Figure 3.66a shows the pretreatment finding of HS with some small soft tumours on the right upper white lip of a 53-year-old female. The area on the patient's right was treated with the ruby laser, with the characteristic black change, while the small tumours were treated with the argon laser, followed by the white change (Figure 3.66b). Figure 3.66c is the result 6 months after the first treatment, with the configurational prob-

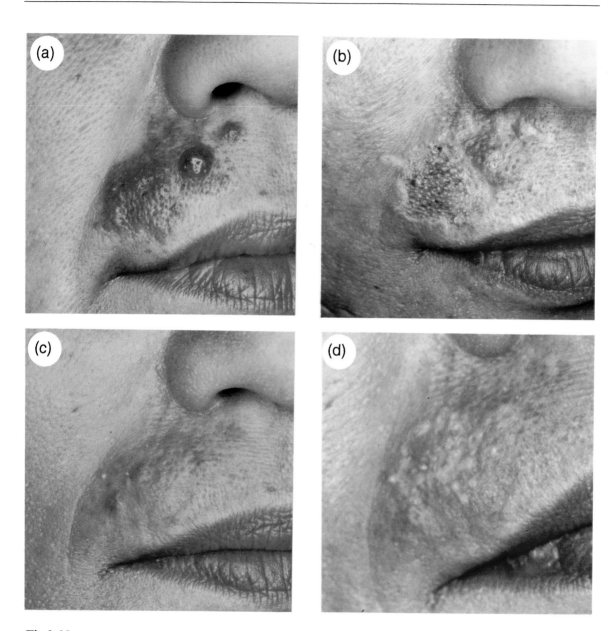

Fig 3.66:

a: *Pretreatment findings of a case of HS with small soft tumours on upper white lip.*

b: *Area on left treated with ruby laser (black change of selective haemocoagulation), and tumours in right area treated with argon laser.*

c: *Result 6 months after 1st treatment: The majority of both configuration and colour problems successfully treated in the first stage.*

d: *Argon laser applied in final modification treatment: note the typical white change of protein denaturation and localized coagulation.*

lem removed. Some areas of abnormal colour remain, and so they are treated with the argon laser in the spotty method to give the white change as seen in Figure 3.66d.

3-6-1-(M-2)-(b-5) HS Treated by Combined Laser Therapy

The 36-year-old male seen in Figure 3.67a has HS plus one big and several small soft tumours together with the HS. The big tumour was excised using the focused beam of the CO_2 laser, (Figure 3.67b), and 1 month later the ruby laser was used to vaporize the small tumours (Figure 3.67c). Figure 3.67d shows treatment of the remaining colour problem with the argon laser in the zebra method, 3 months after the first treatment session. Therefore in this patient the CO_2 and ruby laser were used for volume control, after which the argon laser was used for colour control. This is an example of the author's concept of Combined Laser Therapy.

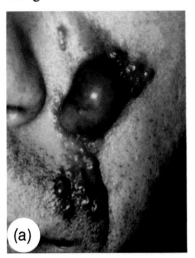

(a)

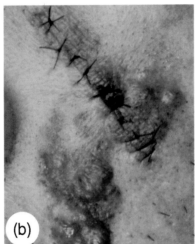

(b)

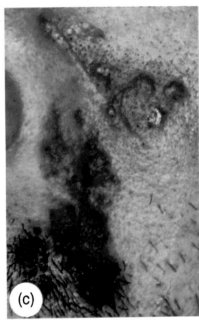

(c)

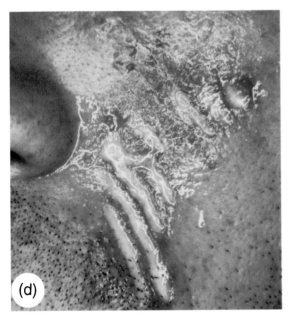

(d)

Fig 3.67: Case of soft tumours combined with HS.
a: Preoperative findings.

b: Large tumour excised using CO_2 laser, wound sutured closed and LLLT applied using diode laser.

c: Ruby and argon lasers applied to small tumours.

d: Treatment of the remaining colour problem using argon laser in the zebra method. A good example of combined laser treatment.

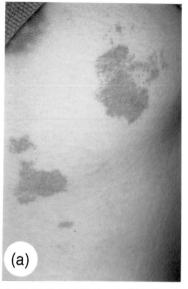

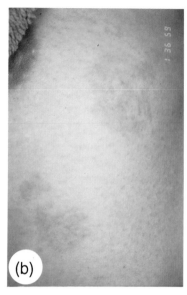

Fig 3.68:
a: *HS on left breast.*
b: *1.5 years after first treatment session using the dye laser: slight hyper-pigmentation remains in treated areas despite application of hydroquinon depigmenting ointment.*

3-6-1-(M-2)-(b-6) HS Treated by Dye Laser

Figure 3.68a is the pretreatment finding of HS on the left breast of a 25-year-old female. In this case, the dye laser was selected as most appropriate. When using the dye laser, usually areas of depigmentation can be found after treatment, but even with the ruby laser, secondary postirradiation hyperpigmentation can occur, and Figure 3.68b shows the condition 1.5 years after the first irradiation. The HS lesions have been removed, but slight hyperpigmentation remains in the treated areas, despite the application of hydroquinone depigmenting ointment.

3-6-1-(M-2)-(b-7) Rosacea

Figure 3.69a is the pretreatment condition of a 60-year-old male with capillary ectasia, a form of rosacea, on the tip of his nose. The argon laser was used to treat the vessels, and the condition in Figure 3.69b shows the result after 5 treatment sessions. Although the argon laser was used in

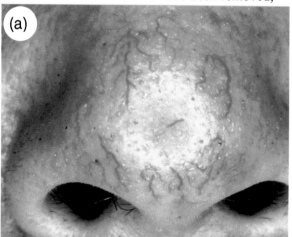

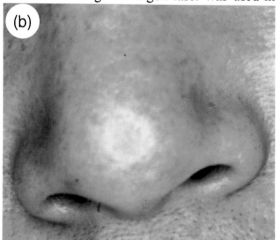

Fig 3.69: **a:** *Capillary ectasia on the tip of the nose, pretreatment findings.* **b:** *Result after 5 argon laser treatment sessions in spotty defocused treatment method.*

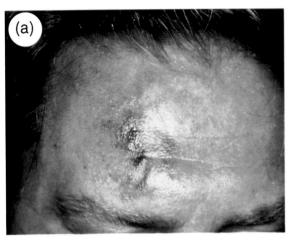

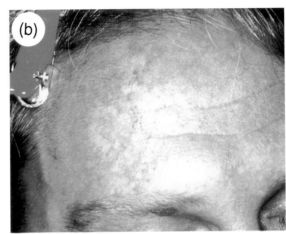

Fig 3.70: *Example of laser/tissue reactions by race of the patient.* **a:** *HS lesion on brow of Caucasian patient.* **b:** *Result after treatment with the ruby laser at 90 joules. Normally, with Japanese patients, the maximum treatment energy is 30 J/cm².*

this patient, the CO_2 laser can also be used, depending on the type of rosacea. For vessels of a larger diameter, the argon laser is the system of choice: for smaller vessels, the CO_2 laser is used. Both lasers are applied in the spotty defocused type of treatment.

3-6-1-(M-2)-(b-8) HS, Caucasoid Skin

There are important differences when treating different skin types, race by race. The 34-year-old Caucasian male seen in Figure 3.70a has an HS lesion on his right forehead, seen in the figure immediately after treatment with the ruby laser at 90 J/cm². The black change is clearly visible all over the lesion, but despite that high power, the result as seen in Figure 3.70b, 16 months after treatment, is excellent. Usually, in the case of ruby laser treatment of the Oriental skin, the ruby laser must be used at under 30 J/cm², or hypertrophic scarring will certainly occur.

3-6-1-(M-2)-(b-9) Hairy Naevus Cell Naevus

Figure 3.71a shows a hairy naevus cell naevus (5 y.o. male), and two areas of ruby laser test treatment. The larger black area is immediately after ruby laser irradiation, and the smaller more normal-coloured circle is the result one month after treatment. In Figure 3.71b the larger area is now 2 months after treatment, and the smaller, 3

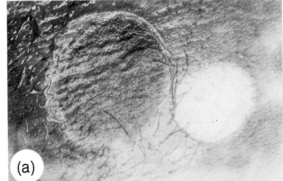

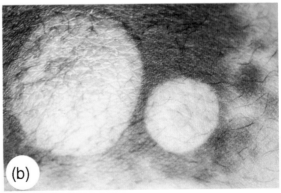

Fig 3.71:
Demonstration of cell-selective ruby laser treatment for hairy naevus cell naevus. **a:** *Test treatment areas: the larger is immediately after ruby laser treatment, and the smaller is one month after.* **b:** *Same areas 2 and 3 months, respectively, after treatment. Good skin colour and texture follows cell-selective laser removal of pigment cells.*

months. Note the good skin texture and selective colour removal in the 3-month area. This indicates that the ruby laser beam selectively damaged only the naevus cell naevus cells in the skin, and so we can refer to this treatment as cell-selective. The black-change area in Figure 3.71a shows how the laser damage can be limited to the pigment cells. The damaged cells in the superficial area will be removed in the wound crust, while those in the deeper area are phagocytosed and removed from the skin that way via the blood and lymphatic system, finally being excreted via the liver.

3-6-1-(M-2)-(b-10) Hairy Naevus Cell Naevus

Figure 3.72a shows a hairy naevus cell naevus on the right side of the face of a 10-year-old male. He was treated 3 times with the ruby laser, and the result can be seen in Figure 3.72b, two years after the initial treatment.

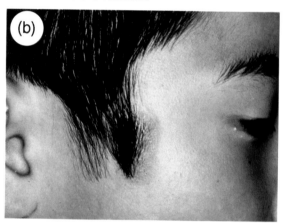

Fig 3.72: a: Hairy naevus cell naevus on right side of the face before treatment. b: Same lesion after 3 ruby laser treatment sessions, two years after first treatment.

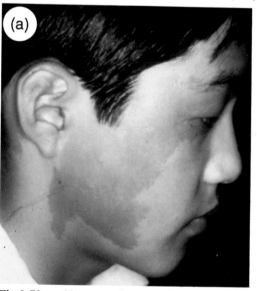
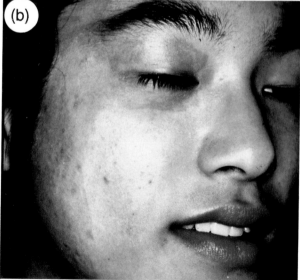

Fig 3.73: a: Naevus spilus on right cheek and forehead, before treatment. Snowy dry ice followed by epithelial peeling was indicated, but there was recurrence: the ruby laser was indicated. b: The result one year after first treatment session.

3-6-1-(M-2)-(b-11) Naevus Spilus

An example of naevus spilus can be seen on the right cheek and forehead of the 15-year-old male in Figure 3.73a. He was treated with snowy dry ice followed by epithelial peeling, but the lesion recurred, and ruby laser was finally used. Figure 3.73b shows the condition one year after the first treatment session.

3-6-1-(M-2)-(b-12) Naevus of Ohta

Figure 3.74a shows the pretreatment finding of a 1-year-old girl with a naevus of Ohta on her right temporal region. She was treated with snowy dry ice followed by epithelial peeling, and then ruby laser. Figure 3.74b shows the condition after three sessions of dry ice and epithelial peeling and one session of ruby laser, 1.5 years after the first dry ice treatment session. This is an example of the author's Combination Treatment Method, where conventional techniques are combined with laser treatment.

3-6-1-(M-2)-(b-13) Naevus of Ohta

Figure 3.75a is the pretreatment condition of Ohta's naevus on the right cheek and temporo-mandibular area of a 37-year-old female. Superficial pigment was removed using application of snowy dry ice followed by epithelial peeling, and the argon laser was applied for the deeper pigment. Figure 3.75b is the condition 15 months after the first dry ice session.

3-6-1-(M-2)-(b-14) Senile Macula

Figure 3.76a shows an example of senile macula or fleck on the left jaw of a 46-year-old female, pretreatment view. The ruby laser was used in a test treatment followed 2 months later by the actual treatment. Topical application of hydroquinone depigmenting ointment was then indicated. Figure 3.76b shows the result 14 months after the initial treatment.

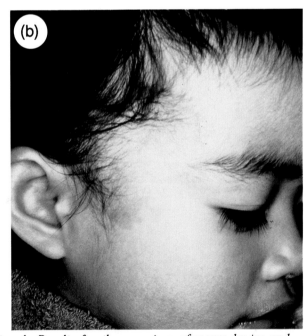

Fig 3.74: *a: Naevus of Ohta on right temporal region. b: Result after three sessions of snowy dry ice and epithelial peeling, and one session of ruby laser, 1.5 years after first treatment.*

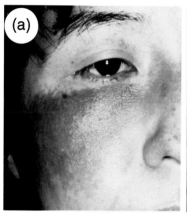
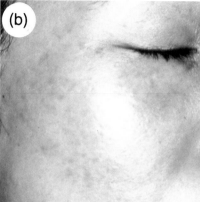

Fig 3.75:
Ohta's naevus on right cheek and temporomandibular region:

a: *Pretreatment finding.*

b: *Condition 15 months after first snowy dry ice and epithelial peeling session, followed by argon laser for the deeper pigment.*

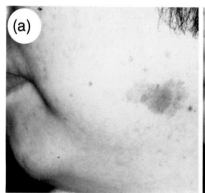
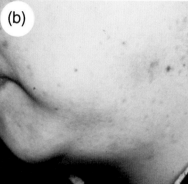

Fig 3.76:
Senile fleck.

a: *Pretreatment.*

b: *Ruby laser and topical application of hydroquinone ointment gave this result, 14 months after initial treatment.*

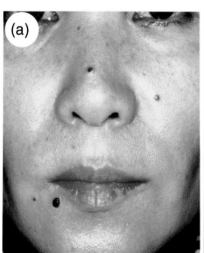
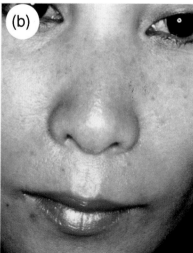

Fig 3.77:
Lentigo

a: *Lentigines on the nose, left cheek and right lower lip, pretreatment.*

b: *Result 1 year after argon laser treatment.*

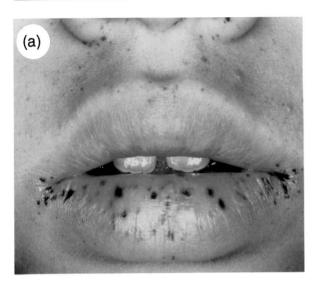

(a)

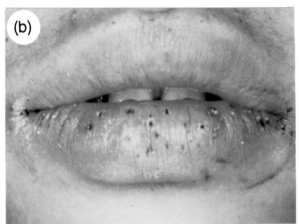

(b)

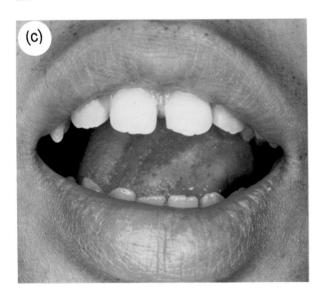

(c)

3-6-1-(M-2)-(b-15) Lentigo

This 44-year-old female (Figure 3.77a, pretreatment finding) has lentigines on her nose, left cheek and near the vermilion margin of her right lower lip. The argon laser was used for the lentigo removal. On the larger lentigines, such as the one near her lip and on the bridge of her nose, the zebra method was used. Figure 3.77b shows the result 1 year after the first argon treatment: she received three treatment sessions in all, and was very satisfied with the result. Because these are elevated lesions, vaporization of the tissue is required, and because of the size of the larger lesions they could not be removed in a single session, taking the concept of damage area, damage volume and intact skin into consideration. The zebra method was therefore applied in this case.

3-6-1-(M-2)-(b-16) Milliary Spots of Peutz-Jeghers Syndrome

(Figure 3.78a, pretreatment) This 13-year-old boy has the milliary black spots of Peutz-Jeghers syndrome on his red lips and upper white lip. He was treated with the ruby laser and argon laser. The argon laser was used at the corners of his mouth, and for the central portion and the mucosa the ruby laser was used. Figure 3.78b shows the immediately postirradiation condition, and Figure 3.78c shows the excellent result 3 months after the treatment.

Fig 3.78:
Peutz-Jeghers syndrome.

a: *Milliary black spots on lip and oral mucosa of Peutz-Jeghers syndrome.*

b: *Immediately after treatment with ruby and argon lasers.*

c: *Result 3 months after treatment.*

3-6-2 Therapeutic Laser treatment (LLLT)

The use of the therapeutic powers of laser energy was first advocated by the late Professor Endre Mester in Budapest in the late 1960's, and has been dealt with in some detail by the author in *"Low Level Laser Therapy: A Practical Introduction"* (Ohshiro T and Calderhead RG, John Wiley & Sons, Chichester, 1988), *"Low reactive-Level Laser Therapy: Practical Application"* (Ohshiro T, John Wiley & Sons, Chichester, 1991), and *"Progress in Laser Therapy, Volume 1"*, Ohshiro T and Calderhead RG, Editors, John Wiley & Sons, Chichester, 1991). A brief overview of the applications of low reactive-level laser therapy (LLLT) will however be given here, but the interested reader is referred to the above publications for an in-depth consideration.

Laser therapy, as the name suggests, involves a therapeutic reaction in the tissue, as distinct to a surgical reaction. The main difference is that the therapeutic reaction is photoactivative in nature, as distinct to the photodestructive reaction seen in HLLT applications.

The rationale behind the use of the terms LLLT and photobioactivation have already been partially covered in Section 2-2-3 above. Briefly, the author would like to remind the reader that as clinicians and researchers, we are concerned with the reaction between the laser energy and the target tissue, and that the laser is therefore only a tool in achieving this reaction. Although there are dedicated LLLT systems, any laser can actually be used for LLLT. A 20 W CO_2 laser, for example, with the correct parameters (20 W, spot size 5 cm in diameter, incident power density approximately 1 W/cm^2) can be used to give an effect which is nonphotothermal and totally therapeutic. It is therefore totally incorrect to talk about low power lasers, or even low level lasers, because we should be looking at the results, not the tool to achieve them.

Despite its nondestructive nature, LLLT has found some applications in the treatment of naevi, both in the direct restoration of normal colour and

configuration, and as an adjunctive therapy together with HLLT. There are two possible methods for the application of LLLT: the contact method and the noncontact method. In addition, two or more LLLT wavelengths may be combined to achieve CLT/LLLT, with effects which may be attributable to a wavelength synergy.

3-6-2-(A) Contact Method

In the contact method, the laser is used in contact with the target tissue. It may be used with or without some degree of pressure. When pressure is applied to the laser probe, the superficial vasculature is compressed, thereby removing a potential absorbing medium, and the probe head is physically placed nearer the target. The combination of these two elements gives a deeper absorption effect in the target tissue. The contact method eliminates any beam power loss due to the gap between the probe and the surface of the target tissue. it also cuts down on beam power loss caused by reflection from the horny layer of the skin. Although any laser can be applied in the contact method, the near infrared wavelengths respond well to this technique.

3-6-2-(B) Noncontact Method

In some cases involving open or infected tissue, or for the therapy of burn wounds, it is not possible to use the contact method. For these examples LLLT can be applied in the noncontact method, with or without some form of scanning mechanism. However, contact technique LLLT can be applied at the wound borders to increase the effect of the noncontact laser therapy. The HeNe or other visible light laser is very effective for these superficial types of treatment, but when used in conjunction with a contact-type LLLT system, usually of a different wavelength, the effect can be enhanced.

3-6-2-(C) Combined LLLT (Multi-Wavelength Synergy)

As mentioned in the previous section, it is possible to use two or more different wavelengths of LLLT simultaneously or more commonly following each other. Visible light and infrared light (IR) energy have different effects in target tissue: the former is mainly photochemical within the cell itself, while the latter is photophysical, being absorbed in specific receptors in the cell membrane. There has been some concern as to how two different photoeffects can end up with the same end reaction, for example the removal of pain. Professor Kendric Smith has put forward a theory for the IR reaction based on Professor Tiina Karu's model for visible light reaction, already proved to occur in the redox reactions within the mitochondria or on other segments of the cell's respiratory chain. Smith suggests that the reaction at the membrane, where the IR energy is specifically absorbed, actually precipitates the same photocascade as the visible light laser causes from within the cell, by activating intra- and extracellular exchange by altering the permeability of the membrane, thereby eventually achieving the same end result. Recent experimental work on the reaction between IR laser energy and neutrophil membranes has pointed to the proof of Smith's theory.

Other aspects of combining laser wavelengths in LLLT to give a synergistic effect have been proposed, but are yet to be scientifically evaluated and demonstrated.

3-6-2-(D) Practical LLLT in the Treatment of Naevi

In addition to its applications in wound healing and pain. LLLT has found applications also in the treatment of naevi. One of the essential basics behind LLLT is its ability to restore normal control to an abnormal situation. In naevus spilus, for example, either the melanocytes in the lesion are producing more melanin than usual, the oxidized melanosomes are not fragmenting into fine granules, or there is a combination of these factors. LLLT appears to restore normal control to the melanocytes, and thus returns normal colour to the skin. This is an example of 'normalizing'. Normalizing can also apply in the opposite situation, such as in a case of vitiligo. In this case LLLT acts as an accelerator, stimulating the melanocytes to return to their normal melanin-secreting function. In the case of naevus spilus, LLLT acts as a brake. The concept of 'accelerator and brake' is also an important one which has applications in HLLT as well as in LLLT.

3-6-2-(D-1) Strawberry Haemangioma

Figure 3.79a shows the pretreatment findings of a strawberry haemangioma (SH) on the right arm of a 6-week-old girl. Diode LLLT (GaAlAs, 60 mW) was applied on its own around the periphery of the lesion and on the lesion itself, twice per week for 4 weeks, once per week for 8 weeks, twice per month for 4 months and once a month for the remaining 12 months, giving the condition seen in Figure 3.79b. Figure 3.79c shows the final result with no further treatment sessions 2 years after the first LLLT session.

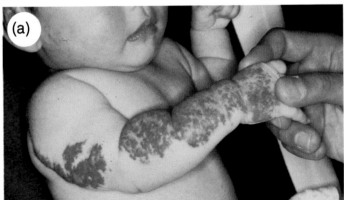

Fig 3.79:
Strawberry haemangioma treated with LLLT alone.
a: *pretreatment findings of large SH of right arm.*

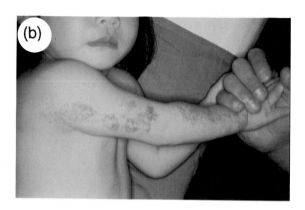

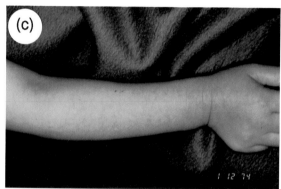

Fig 3.79: (continued)
b: *Result after 19 months.* **c:** *Result after 2 years.*

3-6-2-(D-2) Naevus Spilus

A 14-month-old boy presented with extensive naevus spilus of the left hip, buttock and thigh (Figure 3.80a). LLLT was applied with the GaAlAs diode laser, combined with I depigment-ing ointment. Figure 3.80b shows the result after 11 months, two sessions per week for 4 wks, 1/wk for 8 wks, 2/mnth for 4 mnths and 1/mnth for 4 mnths.

3-6-2-(D-3) Vitiligo

A 44-year-old female developed a case of sys-temic vitiligo on her upper neck at the age of 36 (Figure 3.81a). She had 8 years of PUVA treat-ment, but it was unsuccessful, and left the original lesion together with thinned epidermis. She pre-sented at the author's clinic. The argon laser was used in one treatment session, two irradiations per spot, over the whole lesion, which was stained

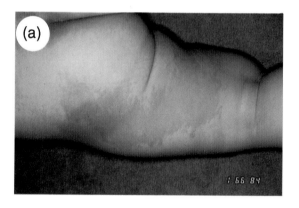

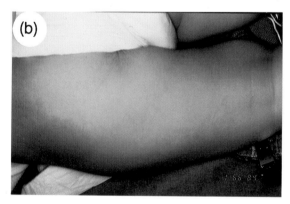

Fig 3.80:
a: *Naevus spilus of left buttock and leg, pretherapy findings.*
b: *Result after 11 months of LLLT and hydroquinone ointment.*

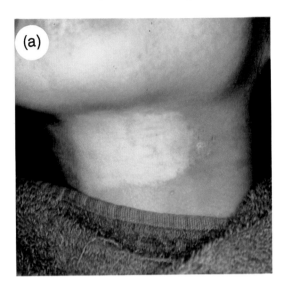

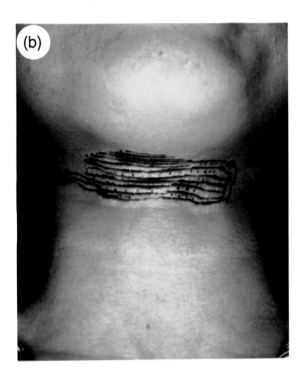

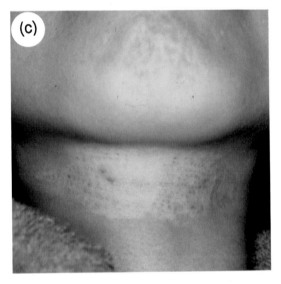

Fig 3.81: Vitiligo.

a: *Systemic vitiligo of upper neck, treated unsuccessfully with 8 years of PUVA.*

b: *Argon laser used in the double impact method using black pigment to enhance thermal effectiveness, followed by diode laser LLLT.*

c: *Result 5 months after single argon laser session.*

with black pigment to enhance laser absorption (Figure 3.81b). GaAlAs diode LLLT was applied immediately after the argon session, and thereafter 1/wk for 2 mon and 2/mon for 3 mon. Figure 81c shows the 5 month posttreatment findings, with good repigmentation and skin texture.

3-6-2-(D-4) Hypertrophic Keloid

In addition to members of the blood vessel and melanin anomaly groups, LLLT has been applied for hypertrophic scar revision and keloids, with considerable success. LLLT has also been indicated in prophylaxis against scar reformation in suspected keloid formers. Figure 3.82a shows the pretreatment condition of a large hypertrophic keloid following a partial hysterectomy on a 20-year-old female. She attended another institution and had the keloid excised twice, but each time it recurred bigger than before. She presented at our clinic. Cut and suture using a W-plasty was indicated, with the CO_2 laser used for the excision. Figure 3.82b is the planned excision, and Figure

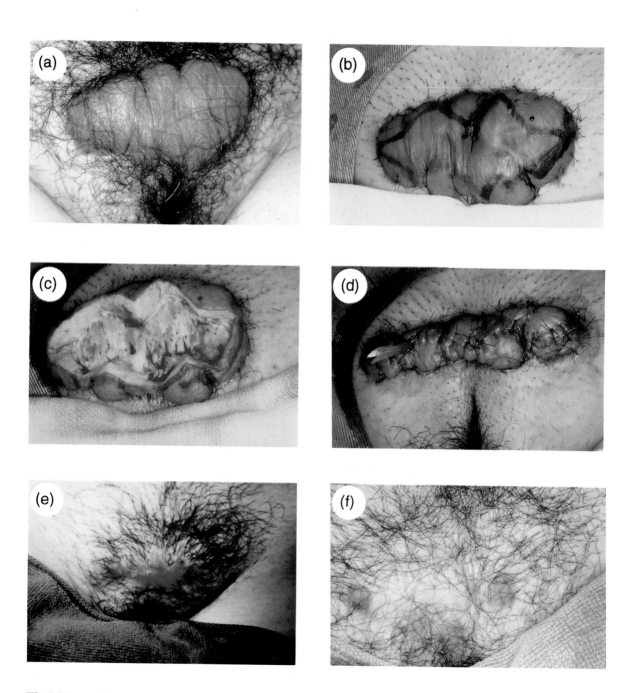

Fig 3.82: **a:** *Recurring hypertrophic keloid in the pubic region following partial hysterectomy.* **b:** *W-plasty design.* **c:** *W-plasty excised with CO_2 laser.* **d:** *Immediately after suturing: note the drain in the corner of the wound.* **e:** *Result 11 months after surgery with LLLT.* **f:** *Result 5 years postoperatively, with no recurrence.*

3.82c shows the W-plasty resection. Figure 3.82d is the immediate postoperative view, with a drain visible in the corner of the sutured wound. LLLT with the GaAlAs diode laser was applied (2/wk - 4 wks, 1/wk - 8wks, 2/mnth - 4 mnths and 1/mnth thereafter). Figure 3.82e is the 11 month postoperative condition, and the final excellent result 5 yrs postoperatively and 150 LLLT sessions is seen in Figure 3.82f.

3-6-2-(D-5) Diseases of the Immune System

As their diets and lifestyles change, patients in Japan are presenting more frequently at dermatologic clinics with outbreaks of atopic dermatitis, presumed to be an immune system-related response to some allergen or allergens as yet not isolated. Normal therapy, including steroids and NS-AIDs (nonsteroidal anti-inflammatory drugs) has little consistent success. Other examples of LLLT indications for skin lesions include treatment of psoriasis and allergy-related ulcerations. Figure 3.83a and b show the pretreatment condition of severe atopic dermatitis in a 22-year-old male. He had immunotherapeutic desensitization sessions in another institute, but they were unsuccessful. LLLT was applied over the whole body, 2/wk - 4 wks, 1/wk - 8 wks, 2/mnth - 4 mnths and 1/mnth till the end of treatment. Figure 3.83c and d show the final result 18 months after the first LLLT session. There has been no recurrence.

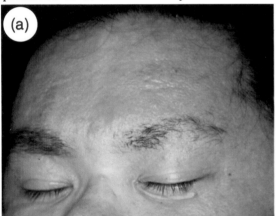

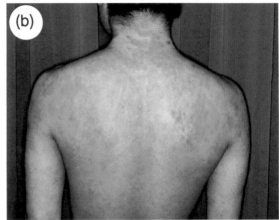

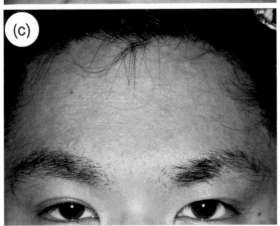

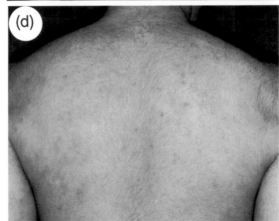

Fig 3.83: **a:** *Atopic dermatitis on forehead, and* **b:** *atopic dermatitis on back of same patient.* **c:** *Result on face and* **d:** *on back 1.5 years after first whole-body LLLT session.*

3-7 CONVENTIONAL TREATMENT

The title of this book is *"Laser Treatment for Naevi"*. However, the laser is not a magic light, and there may well be diseases or conditions for which the laser may not be appropriate. It is also important to understand the advantages and disadvantages of available conventional treatments, so that the best complementary conventional ther-apy can be chosen to use in combination with a laser or lasers. It is equally important to know when not to use a conventional method when in fact the laser offers advantages over that method. Conventional treatment can be classified under surgical, dermatological and other miscellaneous treatments.

3-7-1 Surgical Treatment

Surgical treatment for naevi gives the most basic form of tissue selective treatment, with total excision of the block of tissue containing both normal cells and the naevi cells or materials. The edges of the wound may then be approximated by sutures, or the defect may be filled with a skin graft or a flap (for illustrations and more detials, please refer back to Chapter 1).

3-7-1-(A) Cut and Suture

Cut and suture is a simple surgical technique, by which the tissue containing the naevus cells and materials is excised completely, the edges of the incision undermined, if necessary, and approximated using sutures or some other form of wound closure. Cut and suture is suitable only for small naevi, and considerations such as the stress lines in the tissue must be considered when planning the incision. Compared to tissue transplantation, it has the advantage of simple skin closure, and with good surgical technique the scar will not be too visible, but compared with cell selective or comparatively cell selective laser treatment, it has many disadvantages. Even compared with laser tissue selective treatment, such as CO_2 excision, the scalpel does not have the advantage of laser haemostasis, and there is no simultaneous LLLT.

3-7-1-(B) Tissue Transplantation

Tissue transplantation is necessary for larger surgical defects, which because of their size cannot be closed by approximation and suture, and falls into two main categories: skin graft or flap transplantation.

3-7-1-(B-1) Skin Graft

Skin graft involves removing skin from a donor site somewhere on the patient's body, and using the removed skin to cover the surgical defect on the recipient site. Skin graft is itself divided into thin split thickness, thick split thickness and full thickness grafts. Of these three, from the point of view of final colour and texture of the recipient site, full thickness grafts are preferred, but the damage to the donor site can be bad. The result of skin grafting is often less than satisfactory especially for recipient sites on the face, because it is very difficult to get a good match in colour and texture from skin anywhere else on the body, and there may also be functional irregularity. Of the split thickness grafts, thick split thickness skin grafting (TSTSG) is preferable, because of a better final result in skin colour and texture in the recipient site, but there is inevitable damage to the donor site. Even thin split thickness grafts cause damage to the donor site, and especially in treatment for naevi may not give enough cover in the event of any recurrence. To minimize the size of the donor site, a form of graft known as the mesh graft is available, in which the dermatome harvesting the graft automatically makes a number of carefully placed incisions in the graft, allowing it to be carefully stretched to twice or more its original size. The small holes in the graft then heal by first intention. The final texture, however, is not always particularly good.

3-7-1-(B-2) *The Flap*

For larger and deeper defects of tissue, which cannot be closed by suturing, local or island flaps can be used, and offer the best morphological tissue reconstruction, as tissue from the same area is used for the repair. However, first-class surgical technique is needed, and these methods are used only where the laser cannot be applied, for example because of extensive damage from previous treatment.

When the damage to the recipient site involves more than skin, and goes into the muscle or even bone, then the free flap technique is used to provide tissue for the recipient site. As the name suggests, free flap involves taking a block of tissue from a donor site distant to the recipient site, complete with its feeding and draining vasculature, and using it to fill the defect in the recipient site. Occasionally the vasculature may be left intact, and the flap rotated from the donor

to the recipient site. Otherwise the feeder and draining vessels must be carefully anastomosed to suitable vessels in the recipient site. Apart from the surgical technique called for, the tissue from the donor site may not be a good match at all for the recipient site, and may have to be defatted for example to remove bulk and weight. If there is musculature involved, as in the myocutaneous or fasciomyocutaneous flaps, muscle function may well never be fully regained, and on the face this can give very unfortunate results.

In summary, although skin grafts and flaps can in good surgical hands provide a reasonable repair for a large surgical defect, for the treatment of naevi the laser should be used wherever possible, even for naevi requiring cut and suture. The laser requires no donor site, and can often offer even a partially cell-selective treatment, coupled with the simultaneous LLLT effect already discussed.

3-7-2 Dermatological Treatment

A naevus is nearly always a local phenomenon, and therefore requires local treatment. Local dermatological treatments include phototherapy; cryosurgery; skin abrasion; electrosurgery; ointment or injection therapy.

3-7-2-(A) Phototherapy

Although laser is a form of phototherapy, the 'light' in laser is highly specialized, as discussed in Chapter 2. Phototherapy in naevus treatment includes the use of 'light baths' in conjunction with a photosensitizing drug. A common example is the use of long wavelength ultraviolet light, UVA (320 nm - 400 nm), which is used after the patient has taken usually a psoralen-based drug orally. 8-Methoxypsoralen (8-MOP) is a popular example. The combination of the psoralen with UVA gives the acronym PUVA. The light is usually applied from a bank of specially-coated fluorescent tubes. PUVA is used for the treatment of lesions such as psoriasis, but has the disadvantage of residual photosensitivity, which means the

patient has to remain out of the sun, and in some cases even artificial light, for a 2-3 week period. PUVA has also been used in the treatment of vitiligo, but without too much success. Excessive application can cause thinning of the epidermis with lustred scarring.

Other light sources have been tried in the photocoagulation of blood vessels, for example the xenon lamp. However, they are usually broad waveband lights, and cannot generate enough power selectively to coagulate the target blood vessels.

3-7-2-(B) Cryosurgery

Cryosurgery is treatment applied with some freezing element, such as dry ice, snowy dry ice or liquid helium or nitrogen. The treated tissue is frozen, and selective necrosis occurs if the freezing goes deeply enough. This is at best tissue selective treatment for naevi, as a tissue block is frozen, including the normal tissue surrounding the naevus cells or materials. It has the disadvantage of lack of precision, since the volume damage is not ascertainable from the surface, and will vary depending on patient body temperature, local vasculature and so on.

One area where limited cryosurgery is very useful is to provide a superficial epithelial peel in the treatment of Ohta's naevus, for example. In the author's technique, dry ice spicules, or frost, are gathered and packed in a former to make a snowy dry ice applicator stick. This is then applied to the skin over the naevus. After a few minutes, blisters form in the treated area, with rupture of the dermo-epidermal junction, and the epidermis is peeled intact from the dermis, including the hair sheaths. Care is needed, however, not to overdo the 'freezer burn', otherwise deeper dermal necrosis will occur with a poor result.

3-7-2-(C) Skin Abrasion

Where there is a minor configurational anomaly, for example in a slightly elevated scar, or to disguise the edges of a slightly depressive scar, the skin has to be abraded. This can be done in one of three ways: mechanically, chemically or laser abrasion. Mechanical abrasion requires the use of a high-speed (30,000 - 50,000 rpm) rotating burr or fine wire brush. Care is needed to limit the abrasion to the area of the epidermis above the dermal papillary processes, otherwise some scarring may well occur. In chemical abrasion as the name suggests the skin is abraded using a chemical reagent such as an acid and a neutralizing substance or alkali to halt the reaction. Judging the balance is difficult. Laser abrasion is the best of the three, especially with the CO_2 laser, which can offer precise vaporization with minimal tissue penetration, due to its high absorption in water. It also offers simultaneous LLLT to assist in the healing process. In all of the abrasion techniques, care must be taken not to go too deeply into the dermal papillary processes, or scarring will certainly occur.

3-7-2-(D) Electrosurgery

In electrosurgery, a precisely measured short-wave electric current is applied to the body selectively to destroy the target tissue. Electrosurgery is at best tissue selective only. Electrolysis is a well-recognized method for the removal of unwanted hair, such as in hairy naevus cell naevus. The probe is equipped with a very fine needle, which is carefully inserted into the target hair follicle. The unit is switched on, and a small electric current destroys the hair root by the principle of electrolysis, or the breaking up of water into its component gases by the current passing through it. the dead hair can then be easily removed from the hair sheath, with regrowth retarded because of the damage to the root.

The electroscalpel uses a much more powerful current than the electrolysis probe, and requires a cathode firmly attached to the patient's body, usually on the buttocks, while the cutter acts as the anode. An arc is struck between the cutter and the tissue, and heat is generated at the cutter which vaporizes the tissue. As the 'knife' is drawn across the tissue, the linear vaporization gives a line of incision. Peripheral damage is comparatively high, however, from 3 mm to 5 mm. This tissue will also eventually slough off, so the precision of this device is not very high. Additionally, the cathode must be very firmly attached to the patient tissue, to prevent build up of heat at that point, with possible damage.

Electrocoagulation uses the same principle, with a larger area at the applicator tip and lower output powers than the electroscalpel. electrocoagulation is not highly selective, with the greatest damage being caused near the probe or needle. Accordingly, results in large areas tend to be nonhomogeneous, with small areas of hypertrophic scarring corresponding to the point of contact or insertion.

In electrodessication, a high frequency electric current is applied to the target tissue using a monopolar applicator. The level of heat generated is not enough for full-scale coagulation, but instead 'dries out' the target tissue by protein denaturation and degradation. Electrodessication can be used for the treatment of small naevi such as lentigines or warts.

3-7-2-(E) Ointment

Ointment of any type is usually applied topically, but because of its penetration into the superficial microvasculature the drug can be carried in small doses systemically through the body, including the liver and kidneys. This becomes important in the use of corticosteroid-based ointments. Long-term overuse of these has the possibility of inducing side effects, including thinning of the epidermis with ectatic microvasculature, and more serious effects on the liver or kidneys. In addition, there is the possibility of an allergic reaction to any topical ointment or cream. The necessity for a test patch before prescribing such medication is therefore obvious. Patient education on application and removal is also necessary.

3-7-2-(F) Oral Medicine

Oral medication is designed to have a systemic effect, even although only one area of interest may be the eventual target. Anti-inflammatory steroid or nonsteroid drugs are often prescribed after laser surgery to limit the inflammatory response in the treated area, to enhance wound healing. With any corticosteroid there is the risk of liver or kidney damage with excessive use, so prescriptions should be limited to the minimum

necessary. Large doses of oral vitamins should also be avoided: several times the recommended daily amount (RDA) is what is meant by 'large doses'. Vitamin C is often recommended for the treatment of chloasma, but large doses of vitamin C can also induce a systemic effect on melanin production, not just in the area of the lesion. Large doses of vitamin C, amongst others, over a prolonged period have also been associated with the formation of renal calculi. Patient history should be carefully checked for any other drug-related allergies. For example, antibiotics, allergies to which are not uncommon, are often prescribed phrophylactically against infection following laser treatment.

3-7-2-(G) Injection

One of the former treatments for haemangioma simplex included the injection of a strongly irritating sclerosing agent into the affected vessels, which induced inflammation in the vessel, and eventual thrombosis. Sclerotherapy involved the application of a pressure dressing after the injection to keep the walls of the vessel as close together as possible. This method is also used for the treatment of lower extremity varicosities. In the treatment of haemangioma simplex, the results were less than successful, with the sclerosed vessels clearly visible as dark lines because of haemosiderin deposition from residual red blood cells.

3-7-3 Others

Other treatments for naevi include mainly those which try to camouflage the lesion by covering it with pigment as similar as possible to the surrounding skin. Tattoo camouflage has been tried, but is rarely successful. At best, the colour appears 'flat' and lifeless compared with vital surrounding tissues: no emotional or stress-related colour change, flush or pallor, can be seen. As with any foreign body in the skin, the scavenger cells in the area will try to remove the pigment

particles, and gradually the pigment thins and disappears, usually in a patchy fashion, revealing the lesion again.

Cosmetics camouflage is a safe and often very effective method of covering an abnormally pigmented lesion, especially those with no configurational abnormality. The best-known commercially available range of camouflage cosmetics is 'Covermark'® from the O'Leary Company, USA. Covermark is a well-tried and tested hypoallergenic cosmetic range, and fulfills a number of important functions in addition to simple camouflage. Psychologically, it can help a patient during treatment which may take some years for an extensive lesion, and is particularly effective if there is a resident consultant on the best colours and preparations, and their application, available for consultation, education and advice in the laser clinic. After laser treatment, the immature and newly mature epithelium can be very sensitive to light. The Covermark range includes some good suncut preparations, or a separate suncut preparation can be used, such as French-based Christian Dior ROC® products. A recognized brand of hypoallergenic products should be used, but whatever camouflage cosmet-

ics are applied, it is important that any allergic reaction is tested for beforehand, and also advice and instructions on correct application soon after laser treatment must be included in the patient education programme.

Radiotherapy must also be mentioned under this category of 'other' treatments. A variety of radiotherapeutic modalities are available, from 'soft' x-ray treatment to γ-ray treatment. However, the adverse sequalae following such therapeutic methods well outweigh their possible advantages in the treatment of what are nearly always benign skin lesions. In the case of a malignant change of a naevus, there may be a role for radiotherapy.

3-7-4 Combined Conventional Treatment

Each of the above methods has its own characteristics, some advantages, and (in many cases) moderate to severe disadvantages. Very often the disadvantages can be minimized by using a combination of the conventional techniques. For example, skin graft can often be used to help cover the donor site for a free flap procedure, or the prognosis of a cut and suture procedure for the treatment of hypertrophic scarring can be helped with the injection of steroids, ingestion of non-

steroidal antiinflammatory drugs and the newly-healed wound disguised and protected by camouflage cosmetics. The author refers to this as Combined Conventional Treatment, and it is part of his 'combined' theories, including Combined Laser Therapy, Combined Laser Treatment, and gathered all together in the combination treatment technique: these are all essential elements of the Total Treatment Concept, dealt with in the following section.

3-8 TOTAL TREATMENT CONCEPT (TTC)

Throughout the book, the author has referred in passing to the Total Treatment Concept, or TTC. In this section, he would like to explain what it is, and how it must be applied in order to get a consistently successful result in laser treatment for the large range of disorders which constitute the 'naevi' of the book's title.

Each patient is different, and even on the same patient the one lesion may exhibit different characteristics from site to site. The laser surgeon must therefore have the range of knowledge to enable him or her to select the correct treatment, or combination of treatments, to offer each patient

the best treatment to achieve the best possible result. This range of knowledge must encompass the physiological aspects of the naevus: its type, site and aetiology: these data are contained in Chapter 1. The surgeon must have a thorough grasp of the basic physics of light, the laser beam and its generation, from which the characteristics of the available lasers and the possible range of laser/tissue bioreactions will be known. These data are found in Chapter 2.

The TTC is not confined to physiological knowledge and physical background, however, although these are very important components in the concept. The surgeon must never forget that they are not only treating the naevus, they are also treating the patient. As said already in Chapter 1, looking after the patient's psyche is almost as important as looking after his or her physical disease.

Almost all of the points covered in the following subsections will have already been dealt with in detail in previous sections, so the purpose of this section is not to go over previously discussed ground, but to pull the main kernels of the various separate concepts together, and to show how they must all be considered simultaneously, and their use balanced, as part of the author's Total Treatment Concept.

3-8-1 Single Laser TTC

In some patients, laser treatment for a naevus can be accomplished with a single type of laser. Naturally, this depends on the type, site and distribution or depth of the lesion in the tissue. Photospectrometric analysis [3-2-1-(D) above] will give the surgeon the physical value of the naevus colour over a range of wavelengths compared with the normal skin colour, and will help indicate the 'best' wavelength. The laser nearest that wavelength will thus, in theory, give the best treatment result depending on the degree of colour-dependent absorption. This laser must then be used in a variety of ways in the 'spot, line and area' consideration already discussed, in order to effect the best possible removal of abnormality while achieving the histologically intact skin condition. However, the problem of the site of the lesion may prevent that laser being used. For example, the ruby laser may be ideal for the treatment of a hairy naevus cell naevus, but if the lesion is on an angular body surface, it may be impossible to match the laser beam to that area. In such patients, an alternative laser, or alternative treatment, must be considered for these awkward sites. This flexibility of choice is a consideration of the TTC.

3-8-2 Combined Laser Treatment (CLT)

The simple lesion which can be treated with a single laser type is the ideal. There is in fact no 'ideal laser' despite the claims of laser manufacturers for their particular system or range. Very often, not only the type but the site of the lesion precludes the use of one laser type. The surgeon must possess the knowledge and the ability to apply a number of lasers, using the best characteristics of each in combination to achieve the best result, and this the author calls Combined Laser Treatment, or CLT.

The range of depth of the naevus cells or materials may be such that use of a single laser is not practical, from the point of the intact skin condition. Then two or more lasers must be used, under the volume damage consideration (section 3-6), to remove the colour abnormality in a layered technique, working from the superficial colour down to the deeper-lying cells or materials.

Some lesions consist of an admixture of naevi types, the combined type of naevus with local phacomatosis, covered in section 1-1-4-(D-10). Others may be combined with a configurational abnormality. For these, the use of a single laser is often impossible, if a good treatment result is to be achieved, so the surgeon must apply CLT. It is often beneficial to the final result, as covered previously, to apply a combination of surgical and therapeutic lasers, HLLT and LLLT, which also falls under CLT. The laser surgeon must have full command of both the accelerator and brake of CLT: colour removal must be carefully balanced with colour control. There is no point in removing a blood vessel anomaly group lesion, and leaving in its place an area of postirradiation secondary hyperpigmentation. The patient has then simply traded a red lesion for a brown one. The 'accel-erator and brake' concept is an important component in the TTC.

3-8-3 Combination Treatment Method

The laser, although a unique tool, is not an 'almighty' treatment modality, even when used in Combined Laser Therapy. There are times when the surgeon must use conventional techniques, alone or in combination, combined with the specific advantages of laser treatment. The author refers to this as the Combination Treatment Method. In treatment of Ohta's Naevus, for example, after successful removal of the superficial pigment by snowy dry ice application followed by epithelial peeling, partially defocused laser beams can be used for the intermediate pigment, and focused beams for the remaining deeper visible naevus cell nests. Thus conventional methodology has been combined with laser treatment. Occasionally, visible pigment may remain in the orbicularis orbis muscle, which remains intractable to laser treatment. The surgeon in this case must use conventional plastic and reconstructive surgical techniques to expose the muscle, remove the pigment, and repair the incision with multi-layered closure, to give the intact skin condition. Here there has been a flexible combination of conventional, laser, and again conventional techniques. That is the author's Combination Treatment Method, as part of the Total Treatment Technique, in full action.

3-8-4 Psychosomatic Consideration for TTC

The naevus patient's psyche may well be in a worse state of repair than the physical manifestation of his or her disease, as Dr A.T.J. Squire well knew: "...hideous disfigurement..." were the strong words he used to describe haemangioma simplex (see Chapter 1). Treatment and removal of the lesion is only part of the laser surgeon's task. Restoration of self-esteem to the patient and often to the patient's family, discussed in 1-1-3, is also paramount. The importance of the doctor-patient relationship in all its aspects (3-4 above) has already been covered, but the author would merely like to reinforce its importance under the umbrella of the TTC.

There are a number of ways that the naevus-damaged psyche can be treated. The use of camouflage cosmetics before, during and after treatment is one method. Colour coordination of the patient's clothing and accessories is another.

There are two approaches: one is to try to minimize the impact of the naevus before and during treatment by choosing clothing of the same or a similar colour, in other words of the same value, as the naevus. The other method is to go in the opposite direction, and to use a striking complimentary colour, thereby removing attention from the naevus and attracting it to the clothing. After treatment, the colour of the lesion will have faded to some extent, hopefully to a great extent, but reality often dictates a slow fading of the final remaining lesion colour. In this instance, the patient should be encouraged to use some brilliant colour point, for example a necktie for males or a brooch or scarf for females, to give an accent of colour which will remove the viewer's attention from the fading lesion: this will also make the lesion appear even more faint to the patient.

3-9 PRE- and PERIOPERATIVE MANAGEMENT

Pre- and perioperative management of the patient and his or her naevus are other important points in the TTC, but most of the main topics have already been covered, especially the tenets of good wound management. However, a few remarks on the test treatment, and the best timing of treatment regarding seasonal considerations, are required.

3-9-1 Test Treatment

Just as it is important to assess a patient's possible allergic reaction to drugs, it is equally important to assess the tissue reaction to a laser, and to various doses of that laser, before embarking on the final treatment. The test treatment goes beyond the physical assessment of the laser effect: from past experience, the practising surgeon will have more than a good idea of the possible effect of a variety of wavelengths and doses. The test treatment will also help in a very important way to acclimatize a patient to both the actual laser treatment, and to its sequalae, including wound management and the healing process. For the younger patient and anxious parent, this is almost as important as the actual treatment itself. Thus the test treatment should be approached with the full psychosomatically important support of the doctor-patient relationship, of which this is an important stage.

3-9-2 Preferable Season for Treatment

The season in which a patient undergoes treatment for a naevus can have an important bearing on the timing of that treatment. From a psychological viewpoint, patients will usually prefer to have dressings or crusted and healing wounds as part of the aftermath of laser treatment in the cooler months, as they will be less likely to be out and about, exposing their bodies to the beneficial rays of the sun while on holiday (and thus exposing the wound to the eyes of onlookers). From a clinical viewpoint, summer sunlight contains much more potentially pigmenting UVA and UVB than at the same time in the other seasons, and so the risk of secondary hyperpigmentation in newly-formed epithel is consequently much greater. Firm patient education on the relationship between UV and secondary pigmentation, and on the strict application of a UV suncut, is essential. Tanning is an important consideration, both in patients with depigmented naevi, which will come more obvious, and in increasing the absorption rate of visible light lasers in the extra melanin which accumulates in the granular layer and at the nuclear caps of the ascending skin cells.

The early summer months, especially in Asia, tend to be much more humid than at other times. Humidity is an important factor in wound management (3-3-2), but lack of it can be just as damaging potentially as excess of it. The timing of the treatment and seasonal considerations must also be included in the final treatment decision, as part of the TTC.

3-9-3 Psychosomatic Management

As much has already been written already on the psychosomatic aspects of pre-and perioperative laser treatment for naevi in Chapters 1 and 3, the author merely wishes to remind the reader that these aspects are of at least equal importance to the choice of treatment technique, and would refer the reader back to the appropriate sections in these chapters. Whatever treatment method is chosen, standardization of assessment of the treatment effect is important, so that both the patient and the physician have a realistic and compatible idea of what is happening in the treated areas. The importance of balancing the colour of the naevus with apparel and accessories

during the treatment has already been covered (3-8-4), but the author would like to draw the reader's attention to that again.

3-10 OTHER TYPES OF LASER TREATMENT

There are some other aspects of laser treatment which as yet do not have real applications in the field of treatment for naevi, but they are worth mentioning because of their future potential in this field.

Laser fusion has for some time been an experimental study in a variety of tissue types, as covered above in 3-6-1-(J). Whether the day will come when laser tissue welding will offer a safe alternative to suturing wounds closed depends on the speed of research, and on the final findings in living dermis and, more important for the intact skin condition, epidermis. There are no long-term follow-up studies in the effects of tissue denaturation/renaturation in living human dermal tissue, and until there are, this remains a grey area for dermal tissue laser applications.

Other possible aspects include the individual labelling of naevus cells by a laser-wavelength specific chromophore or receptor, such as is already done in photodynamic therapy (PDT) for superficial cancer lesions. This would enable the use of a deep-penetrating laser beam of the appropriate wavelength, but of very low incident energy doses, which would then selectively destroy the labelled cells only. It has already been shown that the 'speckle phenomenon' of the

HeNe laser is not destroyed after passing through 1.5 cm of packed raw hamburger meat. Because the speckle phenomenon is still visible, it has been argued that coherence is not lost in the first few microns of tissue, a favourite argument of the anti-LLLT critics, since it has also been shown that both coherence and polarization are characteristics of each individual laser speckle. The search for a suitable labelling compound is not yet apparent.

The increasing application of the excimer (EXCited dIMer, see 2-1-4) laser in recanalization of arteriosclerotic blood vessels is an exciting field, with proof that the excimer is capable of the controlled, instant, 'clean' nonthermal photodisruption of living tissue, cell layer by cell layer. Postablational damage in human arteries has been shown to be minimal, presumably because of the nonthermal nature of the photodestructive reaction. This is the same principle now recognized and applied in refractive photokeratoplasty for corneal sculpting. The big question mark still exists as to the possible long-term cytocidal effects of the short UV wavelength of the excimer laser (193 nm - 320 nm), on which its very action in tissue depends.

3-11 FUTURE PROBLEMS OF THE CLINICAL LASER

Some of the problems have already been covered in the previous section: the use of laser tissue welding; specific naevus cell labelling; and possible dermatological applications of the 'cold' excimer laser. The biggest problem is not really a problem of the future, but is with us today. However, as more wavelengths and more sophisti-

cated systems become available, the problem may be intensified. Throughout this book, the author has tried to emphasize that the laser is really only a tool to add to the range of tools available to the plastic and reconstructive surgeon and dermatologist. It is a very sophisticated tool, but it is none-the-less a tool. However, as new and possibly cytocidal wavelengths are explored, the complexity of the tool will also increase, and so will the propensity for serious damage in target tissue.

The author firmly believes that the negative reports on current applications of the laser in the treatment of naevi stem not from poor laser tissue reactions, but from poor understanding on the part of the laser surgeon as to what the actual laser tissue reaction consists of, in both biomedical and biophysical terms. The initial euphoria of the 'new' applications of the laser in dermatology in the late sixties and seventies was replaced in the early and mid eighties with skepticism, and complaints that some of the laser-treated 'afters' were actually worse than the 'befores'. In some cases, it is quite possible that the use of the laser was extremely inappropriate: the precepts of the author's Total Treatment Concept when properly applied should prevent these from happening. In other cases, the laser was correct, with an appropriate wavelength and good laser/tissue interaction potential. The parameters were however totally wrong, and the mode of indication, i.e. the 'spot, line and area' consideration based on maximum repairable damage volume, was totally ig-

nored. The Caucasian skin is known to be much more tolerant of powerful incident doses of laser energy compared with the Oriental skin. But even in the Caucasian skin there are acceptable volume damage limits, and when the maximum damage volume for intact skin condition is ignored [3-6-1-(A)], of course scarring will occur. That is not, however, the fault of the laser treatment, but of the parameters used, which are the eventual responsibility of the laser surgeon. It is the poor workman who blames his tools, provided the tool is appropriate for the job in hand.

In over 18,000 cases, which the author has treated in his clinic over the past 18 years, the success rate has been consistently high. There have of course been failures, but they can be counted on the fingers of both hands. It is based on the sum of that empirical knowledge that the author humbly presents this book as an introductory volume to the exciting field of laser treatment for naevi, and as a possible answer to any future problems of laser application for the treatment of the physically disfiguring and mentally disturbing lesions known collectively as naevi.

3-12 LASER SAFETY

There are many excellent books on safety with lasers or other light sources. Accordingly, the reader interested in detailed information on figures, equations and data related with safety, such as a Laser Safety Officer (LSO) might be required to learn and apply, is referred to such volumes as Sliney & Wolbarsht's *"Safety with Lasers & Other Optical Sources"* (Plenum Press, New York), or to the latest in the ANSI and IEC related publications. This chapter will provide more of a practical overview of laser safety for the practising clinician or health care professional working with the laser in surgery and medicine. However, this is not to play down the importance of laser safety. The fact that a section has been devoted to this subject will, the authors hope, convey the

importance that they place on the subject. It is hoped that by understanding the basic rules of safety with lasers contained hereunder, and then applying them, the laser surgeon, therapist, or other professional will engender a safe environment for themselves, their staff, and of course, the patient. Even well-established and experienced laser users, nurses, paramedical personnel and laser safety officers are encouraged at least to browse through this section: there may be aspects new to you, or approaches which you may not have thought of. For the newcomer to the surgical or therapeutic laser, this section is essential.

Laser safety is an extremely important aspect of any laser therapy programme, whether laser surgery or laser therapy is being applied, and also in the experimental laboratory. Safety criteria must be applied equally to the equipment, the operator, ancillary staff, in a clinical setting to the patient, and in experimental settings to the experimental subject. Laser surgery uses inherently powerful laser energy, and by its very nature is designed to damage the target tissue in a controlled, clinically effective manner. Accordingly, operators and ancillary staff are usually more empirically aware of the damage potential of a stray surgical laser beam. Even though laser therapy, LLLT, is by definition a laser application involving very low output powers, or more accurately, very low levels of incident power densities, laser safety considerations must still be carefully and rigorously applied.

3-12-1 Laser Classification

The American National Standards Institute (ANSI) has, from safety considerations, standardized four classes into which all lasers, including medical lasers, can be grouped. These classes are recognized internationally, with the agreement of other safety bodies such as the World Health Organization (WHO) and the International Electrotechnical Institute (IEC).

3-12-1-(A) Class I Lasers

Class I laser products are essentially safe and are typically very low-powered, enclosed systems which do not emit hazardous levels. Supermarket scanners, laser video players, laser printers, alignment systems, laser theodolites, rangefinders, sighting or aiming systems, communications lasers and some entertainment lasers come into this group. They are deemed safe enough not to cause permanent ocular damage when viewed by an unaccommodated human eye. 'Unaccommodated' means in this context an eye that is not really focused on anything in particular, and is therefore more readily available to seek out and focus on the incident laser energy source.

3-12-1-(B) Class II Lasers

Class II laser products are limited to visible lasers that are safe for momentary viewing but should not be stared into continuously unless the exposure is within the recommended ocular exposure limits (ELs); the dazzle of the brilliant visible light source would normally preclude staring into the source. Even Class II lasers at their upper power limit can be used for only short direct exposures (ANSI recommends a maximum exposure of 0.25 sec). The larger entertainment systems ('laser discos', 'laser light shows') fall into this group, as do many laser pointers used during oral presentations.

3-12-1-(C) Class III Lasers

Class III laser products are not safe even for momentary viewing, and procedural controls and protective equipment are normally required with their use, as they will cause some ocular damage following what the ANSI standard calls 'extended direct viewing', but usually no thermal skin damage from direct irradiation. Class III is divided into IIIa and IIIb lasers, the former being usually limited to visible light systems (HeNe, visible light laser diodes); all infrared lasers within the Class III band are grouped under Class IIIb: Class IIIb lasers have very nearly the same safety requirements as Class IV systems. Protective eyewear is not absolutely required for IIIa systems, but should be worn in situations where direct visualization is a regular occurrence. Class IIIb systems do however require the use of protective eyewear in the area in which they are being applied. Most lasers specifically designed for LLLT fall into Class IIIa or IIIb.

3-12-1-(D) Class IV Lasers

Class IV laser products, into which the majority of the lasers used in medicine and surgery fall, are normally considered much more hazardous than class III devices since they may represent a significant fire hazard or skin hazard and may also produce hazardous diffuse reflections. Hazardous diffuse reflections are of particular concern because the probability of hazardous retinal exposure (if the laser operates between 400 and 1400 nm) is far greater than if the exposure were possible only from specular reflections. Because of this, extremely serious ocular damage will occur from accidental viewing of a direct, or even a reflected, beam. Skin or other tissue damage of a thermal or nonthermal nature may also occur. Protective eyewear is absolutely required. An additional hazard is the possible infective nature of the laser plume associated with laser surgery, and the corresponding need for an efficient evacuator system

3-12-2 Hazards

All lasers, even LLLT systems, are potentially hazardous. Some are naturally more hazardous than others. The main hazards which can be identified when working with lasers in surgery and medicine are:

Ha-1) Electrical, from the system.

Ha-2) Chemical, from contact with laser dye or cryogenic coolant;

Ha-3) Dermal, from accidental exposure to a surgical laser beam;

Ha-4) Optical, from accidental direct or reflected beam exposure, in both HLLT and LLLT systems;

Ha-5) Fire, from ignition of drapes, inappropriate prepping liquids, flammable anaesthetic gas, or potentially explosive biologic gas in rectal procedures.

Ha-6) Side effects, from inappropriate laser parameters, incorrect patient selection or incomplete patient education.

3-12-2-(A) Electrical Hazards

Any piece of equipment which uses electricity as its operating energy source poses potential electrical hazards. This applies equally to a television set, electric drill or a surgical or therapeutic laser system operating from standard household mains supply. The same basic rules therefore apply, specifically:

Ru-1) Make sure all connections are secure.

Ru-2) Use only approved power connectors and sockets.

Ru-3)Do not overload individual sockets.

Ru-4) Do not attempt to carry out unauthorized maintenance, which involves removing any interlock-protected casings or housings, thereby exposing lethally-charged internal components.

Ru-5) Do not pull on the electric connector cord or cable when disconnecting the system from a power socket: grasp the plug firmly and pull it from the socket.

Ru-6) Make absolutely sure the operator's hands, the patient's body and the system itself are dry.

Ru-7) Do not spill or splash water or any other liquid on or into the system console or hand probe. In the event of that happening, turn the system off immediately, and wait until the system is completely dry before continuing.

Provided these basic rules, mostly dictated by good common sense, are followed, no special electrical hazard is present in a standard mains-powered laser system.

Some larger surgical laser systems, however, require a more powerful supply: two- or three-phase power with current requirements and voltages several times higher than standard household supplies are common. Once again, simple and common-sense care and attention in handling the connectors, connecting and disconnecting is sufficient at that end of the system. For these higher-powered systems, in addition to the above standard pointers, the following three points are extremely important:

Po-1) Handle all electrical connectors with dry hands.

Water is a comparatively poor conductor of electricity, but it is better than dry hands. When dealing with 400 volts (V) at 100 amperes (A), dry hands and care in handling become much more important. A healthy human being can stand brief exposure to 220-240 Vac at standard household currents of 15 - 20 A, but even brief contact with higher voltages, and in particular higher currents, can be extremely hazardous to the health!

Po-2) Keep floors dry.

Ensure that the operating room, operating theatre or treatment room floor is dry, at least where the electrical connector or wall socket is located.

Po-3) Turn off system.

To ensure that the system itself is turned off and powered down before disconnecting from or connecting it to the wall receptacle. This will help prevent the unsettling phenomenon of *arcing*, a powerful discharge of electricity in the form of a large and often loud spark between the connector and the wall receptacle.

With some pulsed systems, in particular the ruby laser, power for each pulse is built up in a large bank of capacitors prior to each discharge, giving truly lethal charges. Such capacitor banks must be behind closed, preferably locked doors, with plenty of warning notices around, and a high degree of user education for the staff involved.

As far as electricity is concerned, it is a stable force, which obeys the laws of physics peculiar to it. The laser system will, if properly handled and maintained, also obey these laws. As long as these laws are understood and not abused or even bent slightly by the clinician and his or her ancillary staff, electrical hazards in the clinical use of lasers are minimal.

3-12-2-(B) Chemical Hazards

Certain laser systems rely on a liquid dye as part of the lasing medium. Some of these systems call for the periodic refreshing, or changing of the used dye. In other systems, one dye may be purged from the dye chamber and replaced by another, to give a different wavelength to the laser beam. The problem is that these dyes are messy to handle, at the least, and some of them are possible carcinogens. Once again, common sense and care in handling these materials, and scrupulously following the manufacturer's instructions without 'short cuts' will go a long way to preventing any contact which might be potentially hazardous for the technician, or spills which might have potential hazard for anyone else using that area.

A very few systems have an external or integral cooling system, relying on potentially cryogenic coolants. Contact with unprotected bare coolant pipes could result in freezer burn, during which the tissue of the unfortunate person could be seriously damaged. Proper care and attention around such pipes, clear labelling, and careful lagging of the pipes will prevent this unusual hazard claiming any victims.

3-12-2-(C) Dermal or other Tissue Hazards

Surgical lasers are designed to destroy or selectively damage target tissue using the laser/tissue interaction, be it photothermal or photodisruptive. Because of this, the damage potential from a stray beam to tissue other than the target tissue in the patient, or to accidentally-irradiated skin in the clinician or ancillary staff is very real. Stray beams can happen for a number of reasons:

SB-1) Carelessness

Carelessness on the part of the clinician, such as accidental firing of the laser while moving the footswitch to a more comfortable or convenient position. The new target may be tissue adjacent to the actual target tissue on the patient, exposed skin on ancillary staff, or the hand of the operator him- or herself. This is inexcusable, and can be easily avoided by an established and well-practised routine involving set verbal commands between the clinician and the laser charge nurse, or whoever is looking after the laser console, so that the laser is in the 'ready' state only when the delivery device is properly aimed and the operator is ready to fire it. As soon as each irradiation is complete, the laser must be returned to 'standby'. Request-and-response routines can establish this with great precision, and no real loss of time, compared with leaving the laser continuously in the 'ready' state. The real risks outweigh the advantages.

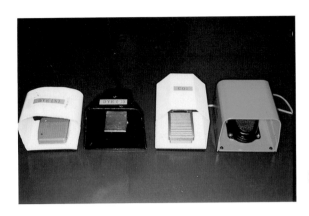

Fig 3.84: *Different design and colour of footswitches will help to avoid accidental firing of the wrong laser.*

Where two or more different lasers are used during a procedure, it is important to ensure that the foot switches are clearly marked, colour coded, and if possible, differently shaped, so that the accidental firing of the incorrect laser is prevented as much as possible (Figure 3.84).

SB-2) Misalignment of the Aiming Beam

Surgical lasers all employ an aiming, pilot or guide beam (the vocabulary varies from country to country). '*Aiming beam*' is used throughout this book as meaning a highly attenuated treatment beam, or a beam from a separate laser or other light system, to allow accurate placement of the surgical beam prior to treatment. In visible light lasers, the aiming beam is usually a highly attenuated treatment beam, so there is no difference in the beam path, or in the aiming beam and treatment beam targets. Infrared lasers, having an invisible treatment beam, usually employ a low-powered HeNe beam using the same optical path as the treatment beam. In some circumstances, the alignment of the two beams may be incorrect, resulting in the highly undesirable event of the aiming beam and the treatment beam striking different targets. This can be prevented by correct and regular main-

tenance. But even with that, it is the responsibility of the surgeon or operator to test the alignment of the beam on an inanimate object, such as a disposable wooden tongue depressor. However, this should be carried out at *low output power*, as it is not uncommon for the higher powered 'superpulsed' laser beams to go straight through the tongue depressor into the leg of the operator, or even worse striking some other second party, including the patient.

SB-3) Accidental Irradiation from Beam Reflection

The laser beam can be accidentally reflected from an instrument or some other apparatus in the operative field. Polished stainless or surgical steel instruments can reflect a laser beam with the accuracy of a mirror. A well-reflected beam has the same damage potential as the actual beam, but with the added hazard that it is not going where the operator thinks it is. Even diffuse reflection of a surgical laser beam has potential for ocular damage. The use of nonreflective and antireflective coated instruments will overcome this to a great extent, but still the number one priority is always care and precision aiming the laser beam on the part of the operator.

Accidental irradiation of tissue other than the target tissue can also be prevented by the use of protective drapes covering all other tissue except the target area. However, the wavelength of the beam will determine the material of these drapes. For visible light lasers, white gauze or other material is adequate protection, dry or damped. For the CO_2 laser, the colour of the material is not important, but it *must be kept wet*, for reasons which will be explained under the section on fire hazards.

SB-4) Diffuse Reflection

Diffuse reflection of the laser beam from the walls of the operating area is potentially hazardous, especially to staff who, having their backs to the operating field, assume they are safe, and have removed their protective

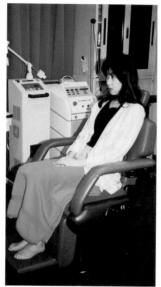

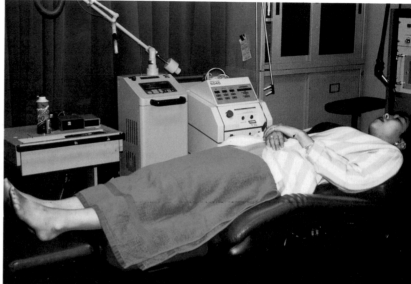

Fig 3.85:
Patient in electrically-operated chair in upright position.

Fig 3.86:
Patient in chair, fully reclined, giving clinical staff good access to patient and also to the other areas of the treatment room.

eyewear. Careful choice of nonreflective wall covering or paint of a neutral blue-gray will help prevent this, as will the design of the treatment area, so that the surgeon is not operating in a cramped space where the possibility of diffuse reflections becomes greater. Good education programmes on the importance of wearing the correct eye protection at all times, as dealt with in detail below, will go one stage further.

Figure 3.85 shows a patient in a well-located fully-adjustable chair, in the centre of the treatment area. Even with the chair fully reclined (Figure 3.86) there is still ample space for the surgeon and his or her staff to move around the table. Note the antireflective drapes on the walls and the nonreflective glass on the instrument storage cupboard seen in the background.

SB-5) Unauthorized Entry to Treatment Area

Someone entering the treatment area might get struck by a stray beam. First of all, no-one should enter a treatment area while the laser is in operation. Signs must be posted on all en-

trances to the effect that potentially hazardous laser radiation is being used in the room, and no unauthorized entry is allowed (Figure 3.87). There are specific sign formats, specifying the laser type, wavelength and powers, approved in each country for this. It is also possible to employ central locking systems to deny access to laser treatment areas, coupled with illuminated warning lights to inform those outside that the laser is in use. Figures 3.88 to 3.91 show a central locking control; an illuminated warning light which will only light when the locks have engaged; a sensor to detect if a door is not properly closed, which will prevent the locks engaging; and the solenoid which actually locks the door. Emergency manual overrides are usually fitted to allow personnel inside a locked room to escape in case of fire or any similar emergency situation.

SB-6) Beam Transmitted outside Treatment Area
Accidental direct or diffuse laser energy (depending on the wavelength) might pass through the windows of the treatment area, and

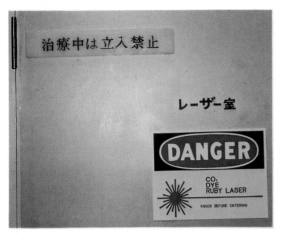

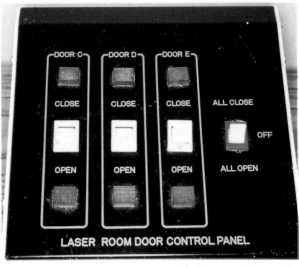

Fig 3.87:
Treatment room door, showing warning signs (in Japanese). The upper sign reads "Entry forbidden when red light is illuminated!" (See fig. 3.89). The lower sign reads "Laser Room".

Fig 3.88: central locking control for treatment room doors. Note colour coded and self-illuminated controls

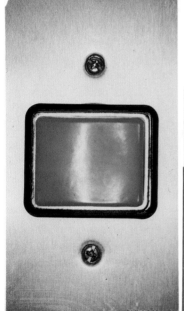

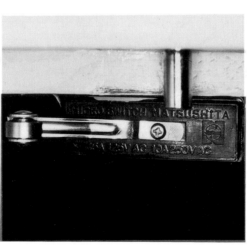

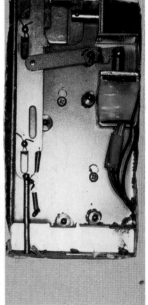

Fig 3.89: (Above, left)
Illuminated warning light, usually mounted beside treatment room door at eye height, showing door locks are activated and that laser treatment is in progress.

Fig 3.90: (Above, Centre)
Sensor to detect if door is completely closed.

Fig 3.91: (Above, right)
Door locking solenoid actuator.

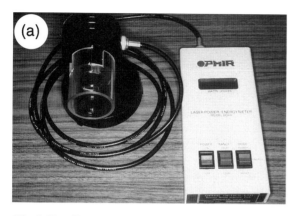 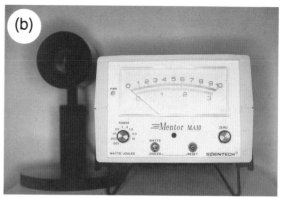

Fig 3.92: *Power meters are essential for calibrating laser output.*
a: *Digital type of power meter.*
b: *Analogue-type master power meter against which other meters can be calibrated. The master meter must itself be calbrated at regular intervals by an external authorized standards laboratory.*

cause damage to someone passing or peering in. All such windows must be curtained off with a suitably thick light-proof material. In addition, warning signs should be hung prominently in the windows between the drapes and the glass, in case anyone is curious enough to try and see what is going on.

SB-7) Defeated Safety Interlocks

During routine maintenance procedures with HLLT systems, some of the interlock-protected panelling which would normally prevent access to laser energy may have to be removed, creating a possible hazard in the area in which the maintenance is being carried out by allowing human access to laser energy even when the laser system is set in the 'standby' mode. If a secure, lockable maintenance room is not available, additional warning signs must be placed at all entrances to prevent unauthorized entry

SB-8) Improperly Calibrated Laser

Lasers are usually set by the operating physician and staff to deliver a specific output power, in order to achieve the desired effect in the target tissue. Because a laser system depends on a number of electro-optical inter-faces, it is possible for a system to deliver less power than it should, or much worse, to deliver more power than the internal power meter on the system indicates. The output power must therefore be checked regularly with an external main calibration meter. The norm in laser clinics is to check the output power before the treatment sessions in the morning and again in the afternoon. If possible, it is good safety practice to check the output before each time the laser is to be used. Figure 3.92a shows an example of an external power meter, and a typical main meter against which the calibration of the other meters may be checked is shown in Figure 3.92b. Current safety regulations demand that the clinic's external main meter is itself calibrated every 6 months against an independent meter, usually at a government-sponsored and approved site, which may be run under the auspices of the national ministry of health or its equivalent.

Laser therapy systems are by their very nature low-powered, and so dermal damage with an LLLT system is not a real hazard, especially given the rapid divergence of the beams. However, with high-powered, potentially harmful surgical sys-

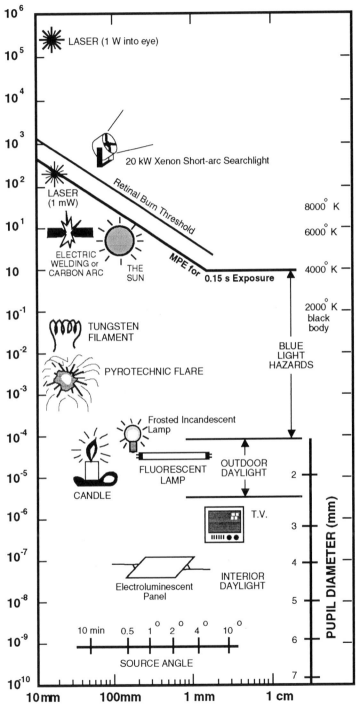

Fig 3.93: *Composite representation of ocular hazards over a variety of wavelengths and devices.*

tems, and even with LLLT systems, it is the responsibility of the clinician in charge to ensure that the laser beam is always aimed precisely where it should be, and only fired when it is in the correct position: and that at all other times the laser is set in the 'standby' state, so that accidental irradiation is prevented.

3-12-2-(D) Optical Hazards

Although accidental laser damage to skin or other connective tissue is unpleasant, it is not usually critical. Laser damage to the eye is another matter entirely. The eye is one of the most efficient light-gathering and focusing devices ever designed. A laser beam, whether a 100 W surgical beam, or a 5 mW laser therapy beam, is still 'laser', and we must never forget that the 'L' in laser stands for light, in HLLT and LLLT both. Laser beams all have certain characteristics in common, as already discussed in earlier chapters, and it is these characteristics which make even a 5 mW laser beam more potentially damaging than a conventional 500 W spotlight beam. The coherence of the beam, which sets it apart from 'normal' light, is what makes a laser beam potentially dangerous to the eye. Even a highly diverging diode laser beam is still generated from a point source, and can be efficiently gathered by the eye, and focused back to a point on the retina at the back of the eye. The damage potential from the less-divergent surgical laser beam is that much greater, since it is first of all intrinsically more powerful, and secondly a greater percentage of the beam energy can be gathered by the eye. Figure 3.93 is a composite representation of ocular hazards at various wavelengths, from a variety of light sources. From this the reader will see that a 1 mW laser has almost the same harmful potential as a 20 kW xenon short-arc searchlight, and a 1 W laser is well in excess of that.

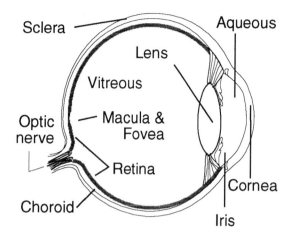

Fig 3.94: *Schematic cross-section of the eye (left eye, seen from above).*

A brief review of the anatomy of the eye is appropriate here. Figure 3.94 shows a schematic cross-section of the left eye, viewed from above. The front of the eye is bounded by the clear cornea (clear, that is, to wavelengths for which it is transparent). Light passing through the cornea is gathered by the lens, the amount reaching the lens governed by the iris surrounding it, as it expands or contracts to allow less or more light in, depending on the intensity. The space between the cornea

and lens, the anterior chamber, is filled with a clear fluid, the aqueous. The lens focuses the incoming light onto the retina, the innermost of the three tunics of the eyeball. To get to the retina, the light has to pass through the clear vitreous body, a jelly-like substance which fills the inner cavity of the eyeball. Next to the retina is the choroid, a richly-vascularized bed which feeds the retina and its components. The tough outer layer of the eye is the sclera, which covers the entire surface of the eyeball except for the cornea at the front. At the back of the eye is the optic disc, or 'blind spot', where the nerve fibres from the retina collect to form the optic nerve. Lateral to, and in towards the centre of the eye from the optic disc is the macula, a yellowish spot in the centre of which is the fovea. The fovea is responsible for visual acuity. Any light damage to the retina is of course potentially serious, but damage to the fovea is irreparable. In order to reach the retina, laser energy has to pass through the cornea, aqueous, lens and vitreous. Only visible and near infrared energy can do this. Ultraviolet and mid infrared (for example the CO_2 laser beam) are absorbed in the corneal epithelium. This is shown diagramatically in Figure 3.95.

Visible and near infrared light however is gathered and focused onto the cornea. Only a very small percentage of the energy from noncoherent light sources is gathered and focused, to produce

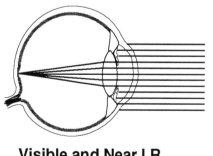

Visible and Near I.R.

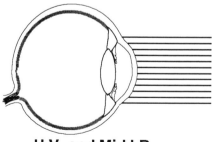

U.V. and Mid I.R.

Fig 3.95: *Wavelength dependent absorption in parts of the eye.*

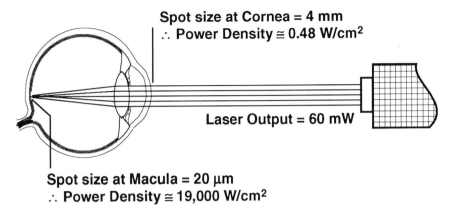

Spot size at Cornea = 4 mm
∴ Power Density ≅ 0.48 W/cm²

Laser Output = 60 mW

Spot size at Macula = 20 µm
∴ Power Density ≅ 19,000 W/cm²

Fig 3.96: *Focusing power of the unaccommodated eye. 60 mW with 20 µm spot on retina can give power densities of over 45,000 W/cm² in the fovea.*

an inverted image of the source. Because of the phase component in even a divergent laser beam, however, the lens can gather a much larger percentage of the energy, and focus it to a very small spot. In the unaccommodated eye, this point of focus might well be in the macula (Figure 3.96). Given the power of the lens to deliver a focused spot of 20 µm on the retina, an incident beam of a seemingly harmless 60 mW at 830 nm from an LLLT diode laser can therefore produce an actual power density of over *45,000 W/cm²*, capable of producing serious photothermal damage. This is for a 60 mW beam, the 'worst-case' instance. Remember however that a 6 W beam of the same or appropriate wavelength to allow transmission through the clear components of the eye is 100 times more powerful than the 60 mW beam, a 60 W beam 1,000 times more powerful, and that surgical laser beams tend to be less divergent than therapeutic laser beams. Also please remember that at power densities in the retina of above 500 W/cm², detectable thermal damage is a real possibility.

Even the 'safe' HeNe laser aiming beams for the CO_2 and the Nd:YAG systems are uncomfortably bright if viewed directly, even though they should only be around the 1.0 mW range: the same applies to laser pointers. Turning to laser therapy briefly, LLLT can be delivered in either the contact or noncontact mode: in non-contact mode, as the name suggests, the delivery device is held at a distance from the target tissue, so non-contact LLLT systems accordingly need more care and attention on the operator's part to avoid possible accidental exposure to the beam. Careful patient education is also necessary to ensure no accidental involuntary movement which might bring the eye into the beam path. In contact systems, as the name suggests, the laser delivery device is placed in direct contact with the tissue: contact systems therefore present less of a hazard, as long as the beam is activated only when the probe is in contact with the target tissue. In some systems this is accomplished by incorporating skin sensor switches in the probe head, thus ensuring the system is active only when in contact with the target tissue, switching off automatically when the probe is removed from the tissue.

Returning to surgical systems, for mid infra-red wavelengths such as the CO_2 laser, damage is limited in the first instance to the outer layers of the cornea, unless the beam is so powerful that it passes through the cornea completely: this is because that wavelength is almost 95% preferentially absorbed in water molecules. Corneal tissue, in common with many of the body's soft tissues, contains a high percentage of water. Such corneal damage will result in varying degrees of opacity in the lesion, and the possibility of corneal ulcer formation. Ultraviolet (UV) energy is totally absorbed in the first few cell layers of the cornea, and at the incident power densities of terrestrial solar UV reflected from snow, for example, is capable of causing cell disruption and photokeratitis with corneal oedema, or snow blindness. This 'limited absorption' of UV energy is used beneficially in excimer laser corneal ablation, refractive keratoplasty, popularly known as corneal sculpting, in one of the most recent advances in vision correction. This is a nonthermal photodisruptive reaction.

It is clearly obvious that the eye is the most vulnerable organ to accidental laser damage. Protection against optical damage naturally involves placing something between the eye and the incident laser radiation. Laser goggles or glasses come in many shapes, sizes and types, but the user must be aware that there is not a pair of 'general purpose' laser goggles available which will afford all-round protection against a wide range of laser wavelengths. Please note especially that the clear goggles used for protective eyewear at the CO_2 laser wavelength will *not* provide any protection at all for most other wavelengths. Also note that, while ordinary eyeglasses do provide protection against a direct frontal incident CO_2 beam, they lack the side shields necessary for complete protection from a stray beam coming in from the side. The capability of the goggles to protect the eyes of the wearer depends on the optical density (OD) of the goggle glass or other lens material at the given wavelength of the laser, and the ability of the lens to withstand a direct laser hit of a given power and duration. An OD of 0 (zero) will allow 100% transmission. For each whole number from 1 upwards, the transmission decreases by an order of magnitude. Thus an OD of 1 for a given wavelength will allow 10% transmission, 2 will allow 1%, 3 will allow 0.1%, and so on. An OD of 4 (0.01% transmission) is usually recommended for surgical laser systems. The best goggles usually have a range of wavelengths and the corresponding OD etched somewhere on the lens. There is a trade-off against visibility and

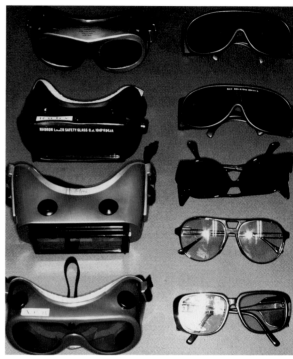

Fig 3.97: *Range of different goggle types.*

protection factor, and comfort, but the higher the OD, the better. Figure 3.97 shows a selection from the range of goggles used in the author's clinic, and Figure 3.98 gives a closer view, showing one set of the lightweight protective glasses, this pair being for the dye laser. Note the side shields on this type to prevent any access to a lateral beam.

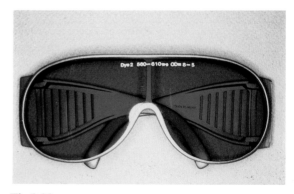

Fig 3.98:
Close-up of goggles designed for use with the dye laser: note details clearly etched on the lens.

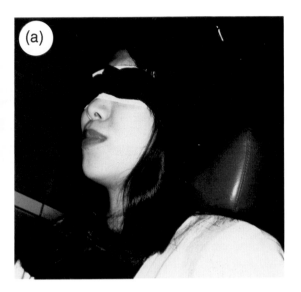

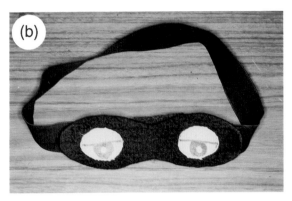

Fig 3.99:
Felt patches designed to protect patient's eyes during laser procedure. These can be used with or without gauze patches.

Note also the wavelengths and corresponding ODs clearly etched on the lenses.

While on the subject of eye protection, the patient also must be considered. For procedures on the body away from the face, on a conscious and alert patient, protective eyewear is sufficient. For an anaesthetized patient, taping the eyes closed, and then taping moist gauze patches over the eyes is acceptable. If the procedure is on or around the face, then dark green or black felt patches can be added over the gauze, even for the conscious patient. Figures 3.99a and b show typi-

cal felt eye patches on and off the patient. Note the 'eyes' drawn on the set in Figure 3.99b, to help put any anxious younger patient more at ease. It is important to ensure that any gauze patches are kept moist, especially for CO_2 procedures. Procedures on the eyelid or around the eye, for full protection, require specially coated contact lenses to be slipped under the eyelids with a little local anaesthetic medium applied to the eye. Figure 3.100a shows a range of contact lenses and applicator, and Figure 3.100b a protective contact lens actually in use during treatment of periocular

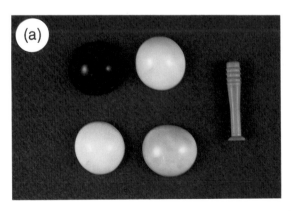

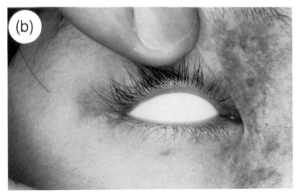

Fig 3.100:   a: *Contact lenses and applicator, designed to protect the eye during periocular laser procedures.*
   b: *Lens in place during a procedure for removal of HS from the eye margin.*

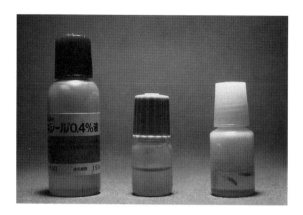

Fig 3.101: *Local anaesthesia for insertion of contact lens, and some postoperative eye drops to eliminate irritation.*

haemagioma simplex. Figure 3.101 shows the local anaesthetic together with some eye drops for postoperative care of any irritation of the eye.

As far as the eye is concerned, as a possible laser target, the laser clinician must always remember that laser energy has the special characteristics which make it more potentially harmful than conventional light sources, and that even LLLT systems are still 'lasers', albeit very low-powered laser energy sources: however even they should be treated with the same respect afforded their higher-powered surgical cousins.

3-12-2-(E) Fire Hazards

Fire hazards with laser surgery are a real problem, as a direct result of the basic thermal laser energy/target material interaction. With certain wavelengths in particular the fire hazard must always be considered in the choice of draping material, for example, or for the material of which the intubation tube is constructed for procedures around the mouth or airway under general anaesthesia. This is one area where dedicated laser therapy systems pose no such hazard because of the low incident power densities and nonthermal tissue reaction associated with LLLT systems.

3-12-2-(E-1) Laser Systems

Fire hazards are very high with the CO_2 laser. CO_2 laser energy at 10,600 nm is preferentially absorbed in water, as said above. Gauze pads, even dry gauze pads, and conventional cotton drapes contain water to a certain extent. If a CO_2 laser beam hits dry gauze or drape material, heat is thus generated, enough certainly to raise the temperature of the material to combustion point, and it can spontaneously ignite. The answer is to give the laser beam an abundance of water, so that the temperature of the drape or gauze is not raised enough to allow combustion, following even an extended laser 'shot'. This is achieved by making sure the protective materials around the target tissue are kept well-moistened. Sterile physiological saline can be used if sterility in the field is to be maintained.

For other lasers, such as the visible light argon, KTP/532, argon dye, pulsed and Q-switched ruby and pulsed flash lamp dye, the use of white gauze is encouraged, to reflect away as much of the beam as possible, but it is still a good idea also to keep these damped. The Nd:YAG beam is not particularly colour-dependent, but whatever colour of drape is used, it too should be kept moist around the target area.

3-12-2-(E-2) Prepping and Anaesthetic Agents

Alcohol-based or any other inflammable prepping agents should not be used, if the time between the preparation of the tissue and the laser radiation is very short. Any surgical laser is capable of igniting flammable prepping agents, and it is disastrous to see the target tissue burst into flames after the first laser impact. Nonflammable agents should be used, to be on the safe side. The same applies to anaesthetic gases, although almost every operating theatre or operating room around the world now prohibits the use of flammable anaesthetic media. However, even with inert anaesthetic agents, oxygen is still passed through the endotracheal tube during anaesthesia. In procedures in or around the oral cavity involving general anaesthesia, the laser surgeon should note that a stray laser impact on the endotracheal tube, cuff or balloon, has the potential to start an airway fire, supported and encouraged by the O_2 flowing through the tube. A small number of fatalities and serious injuries from laser-caused airway fires have been reported in the past 10 years, so careful aiming, and an endotracheal tube material chosen according to the laser wavelength being used are essential. Laser system and endotracheal tube manufacturers have detailed information on this hazard and how best to protect against it.

One final fire hazard which might not appear relevant to this book, but which may become so if any skin lesions are being treated in the perianal region, is the possibility of ignition of an explosive gas emanating from within the patient. Reports have appeared of laser energy igniting pockets of methane gas trapped in the patient's rectum. Enemas should be given as a matter of course if the laser is to be used in the rectum or perianal region.

3-12-2-(F) Laser Plume Hazard

When high powered pulsed or Q-switched lasers impact on tissue, the brief impact of laser energy is absorbed by the target tissue, and a short but very powerful radiant heat reaction is the result which is usually associated with vaporization of the target tissue, cells or materials. This can be seen in high-speed photography as a distinct 'plume' of carbon particles, in which particulate tissue matter can be identified including viable skin cells. An even larger and more pervasive plume is caused by continuous wave laser energy being used to vaporize or excise tissue. The debate as to whether this plume is harmful or not still continues, although viable viral cells have been successfully cultured from the plume when a CO_2 laser was used to vaporize and excise vaginal condyloma. Biologically hazardous or not, the distinctive smell of a laser plume, comprised of smoke and burning flesh, is aesthetically very unpleasant for both clinical staff and the patient. An efficient smoke evacuator is essential for those treatment rooms where the laser is used mostly for vaporization and excision. Some treatment rooms press their fluid aspiration system into use as a smoke evacuator, but the collecting jar soon becomes very unpleasant to look at and in any event the efficiency is low as this system is designed to aspirate fluids, not gases, and the suction tube has a very small bore. In order to deal with both the aesthetic and most probably biologically harmful hazards and effects of laser plume, it is much better to invest in a portable smoke evacuator with a disposable micropore filter, such as the Stackhouse® range. It is a purchase which will be appreciated both by the clinical staff and the patient.

3-12-3 Common Sense in Hazard Prevention

The above hazards, and their prevention, may seem to some readers to have been overstated: they are not. Accidents can, and do happen: occasionally, they have involved severe injury to, or even the death of the patient. The laser, especially the surgical laser, produces a strong beam of potentially hazardous energy: to produce this beam, the laser needs an energy source which has its own inherent hazards. However, as the author hopes to have shown above, these hazards are *all* preventable, and some need ***never*** occur. Com-

placency in the use of any medical tool can lead to carelessness, and carelessness certainly leads to undesirable accidents. Most accidents with HLLT systems are directly attributable to operator carelessness, or to incomplete or incorrect maintenance, which routine preoperative safety check procedures failed to detect, because they were not properly implemented. Accidents with LLLT are by the very nature of laser therapy, much more uncommon. "*A laser, whatever its power, is always a laser.*" this must never be forgotten, and should really be inscribed on the wall of every laser treatment room, along with the principal author's (T.O.) good friend and mentor, Professor Leon Goldman's edict: "If you don't need the laser, don't use it!"

As long as the laser clinician and his or her staff remain aware of the potential hazards, and of why they could happen, sound common sense, respect for the properties and powers of laser energy, and strict adherence to each institute's own safety recommendations will, in almost every single procedure, ensure total safety for the laser system and the treatment area, for the good of all in it, including of course the patient.

REFERENCES,
BIBLIOGRAPHY
&
SUBJECT INDEX

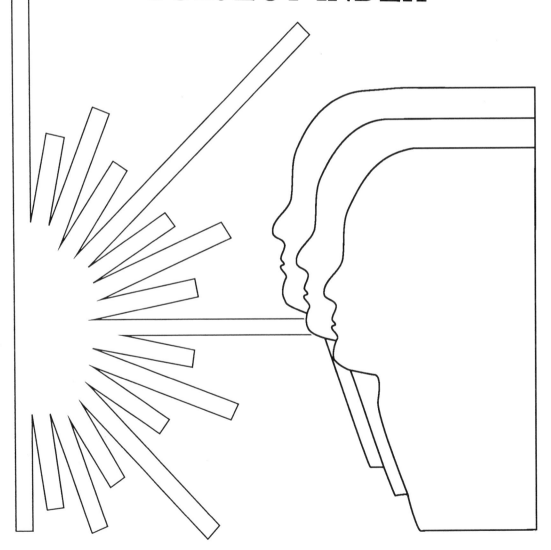

REFERENCES AND BIBLIOGRAPHY

LASER BASIC SCIENCE

Bourgelaise DBC *et al* (1983): The physics of lasers: in Arndt KA *et al* (eds) *Cutaneous Laser Therapy*. John Wiley & Sons, New York: p13.

Calderhead RG (1991): Watt's a joule: on the importance of accurate and correct reporting of laser parameters in low reactive-level laser therapy and photobioactivation research. *Laser Therapy,* **3:** 177 ~ 182.

Carruth JAS, and Mackenzie AL (1986): *Medical Lasers*. Adam Hilger Ltd.

Einstein A (1917): Zur Quantentheorie der Strahlung. *Physiol Z,* **18:** 121.

Fuller AT (1983): Fundamentals of lasers in surgery and medicine: in Dixon JA (ed) *Surgical Applica-*

tions of Lasers, p 11: Year Book Medical Publishers Inc, Chicago.

Gordon JP *et al* (1955): The MASER - A new type of amplifier, frequency standard and spectrometer. *Physiol Rev,* **99:** 1264.

Heitler W (1944): *The Quantum Theory of Radiation*. 2nd edition. Oxford University Press, London & New York.

Lipow M (1986): Laser physics made simple. *Obstet Gynaecol fertil,* **9:** 444 ~ 493.

Maiman TH (1960): Stimulated optical radiation in ruby. *Nature,* **187:** 493.

Siegman AE (1971): *An Introduction to Masers and Lasers*: McGraw-Hill, New York.

LASER SYSTEMS AND COMPONENTS

Beach, AD (1969): A laser manipulator for surgical use. *J Sc Instr,* 2: 931 ~ 932.

Goldman L, *et al* (1965): Radiation from a Q-switched ruby laser: effect of repeated impacts of power output of ten megawatts on a tattoo of man. *J Invest Derm,* **44:** 69.

Goldman L, *et al* (1969): Preliminary investigation of fat embolism from pulsed ruby laser impact on bone. *Nature,* **221:** 361 ~ 363.

Goldman L, *et al* (1973): High-power neodymium-YAG laser surgery. *Acta Derm* (Stockholm) **53:** 45 ~ 49.

Goldman L, Rockwell RJ, jr, Naprstek Z, Silver VE, Hoefer R, Hobeika C, Nishimoto K, Polanyi T, and Bredmeier HC (1970): Some parameters of high output CO_2 laser experimental surgery. *Nature,* **228:** 1344 ~ 1345.

Hall RR, Hill DW, and Beach AD (1971): A carbon dioxide surgical laser. *Ann Royal Coll Surg Engl,* (3): 181 ~ 183.

Hardaway GA (1966): Why lasers fail, and what to do about it. *Microwaves*.

Kaplan I, and Peled I (1975): The carbon dioxide laser in the treatment of superficial telangiectases. *Br J Plas Surg* **28:** 214 ~ 214.

Kaplan I, *et al* (1973): The CO_2 laser in plastic surgery. *Br J Plas Surg,* **26:** 359 ~ 362.

Kaplan I, *et al* (1974): CO_2 laser in head and neck surgery. *Am J Surg,* **128**.

Kato K and Nagasawa A (1991): Imaging technique for near infrared GaAlÀs diode laser beam distribution in tissue. *Laser Therapy,* **3:** 59 ~ 62.

Kott I, *et al* (1976): The surgical knife and the CO_2 laser beam. *Am J Prot,* 27 ~ 23.

Laub DR, Yules RB, Arras M, Murray DE, Crowhey L, and Chase RA (1968): Preliminary histopathological observation of Q-switched ruby laser radiation on dermal tattoo pigment in man. *J Surg Res,* **8:** 220 ~ 224.

Levine N (1974): Use of a CO_2 laser for the debridement of 3rd degree burns. *Ann Surg,* **179:** 246 ~ 252.

Litwin MS (1969): Burn injury after CO_2 laser irradiation. *Arch Surg,* **98:** 219 ~ 223.

Mester E, Tisza S, Csillag L, and Mester A (1977): Laser treatment of coumarin-induced skin necrosis. *Act Chir Sci Acad Hung,* **18:** 141 ~ 148.

Mihashi S (1975): CO_2 laser surgery. *Jap J Otolar,* **78:** 8 ~ 12.

Mihashi S (1977): The change of surface structure of soft tissue induced by CO_2 laser irradiation - observations with the scanning electron microscope. *Jap J Otolar,* **80:** 33 ~ 37.

Mihashi S (1976): Immediate effects of CO_2 laser irradiation on soft tissue. *Jap J Otolar,* **79:** 19 ~ 24.

Ohshiro T (1975): The Korad K2 ruby laser system. *J Jap Soc Plas Recon Surg,* **19:** 164.

Ohshiro T (1980): The GaAlAs semiconductor laser: a new modality in 'laser acupuncture'. *J Jap Soc LaserMed & Surg,* **1:** 47 ~ 50.

LASER SAFETY

Bellina JH, Stjernholm RL, and Kurpel JE (1982): Analysis of plume emissions after papovavirus irradiation with the CO_2 laser. *J Repro Med,* **27:** 268 ~ 270.

Fenner J and Moseley H (1989): Damage thresholds of CO_2 laser protective eyewear. *Lasers Med Sci,* **4:** 33 ~ 40.

Fisher JC (1986): Principles of safety in laser surgery- and therapy. In Baggish MS (ed) *Basic and Advanced Laser Surgery in Gynecology.* Appleton-Century Crofts, Connecticut, pp 85 ~ 130.

Geeraets WJ *et al* (1968): Ocular specular characteristics as related to hazards from lasers and other light sources. *Am J Ophthmol,* **66:**15

Goldman L (1970): Plans and goals of the laser safety conference. *Arch Environ Health,* **20:** 148.

Goldman L (1970): Progress in laser safety in biomedical installations. *Arch Environ Health,* **20:** 193 ~ 196.

Goldman L (1971): Snags ln laser biomedicine. *Biomed Eng,* **6:** 9.

Goldman L (1974): Laser hazards: current and future concerns. *Opt Las Tech,* 3 ~ 4.

Goldman L (1974): Safety programs for current high output lasers and new systems. *Am J Pub Health,* **64:** 812 ~ 813.

Goldman L, *et al (1965):* Personnel protection from high energy lasers. *Am Indust Hyg J,* **26:** 553 ~ 557.

Goldman L, *et al (1969):* lnvestigative laser surgery-safety aspects. *Biomed Eng,* **4:** 415 ~ 418.

Goldman L, *et al (1973):* Studies in laser safety of new high-output systems. *Opt Las Tech,* 11 ~ 13.

Hoye RC (1967): The airborne dissemination of viable tumour by high-power neodimium laser. *Life Sc,* **6:** 119 ~ 125.

lida H (1975): Hazards of and protection against non-ionizing radiation. *J Health Phys Soc,* **10:** 221 ~ 226.

Mallow M and Chabot L (1978): *Laser Safety Handbook.* Van Nostrand Reinhold, New York.

Michaelson SN (1972): Human exposure to non-ionizing radiation energy-potential hazards and safety standards. *I.E.E.E.,* **60.**

Mihashi S, Ueda S, Hirano M, *et al* (1981): Some problems about condensates induced by CO_2 laser irradiation. In Atsumi K (ed) *Laser Tokyo 81.* Intergroup Corp, Tokyo, pp 2 ~ 25 ~ 2-27.

Ohshiro T (1984): Photobiological effects of the dermal laser. In: *The MITI Laser Safety Guidebook.* New Technical Communications, Ltd, Tokyo. pp 150 ~ 156.

Ohshiro T (1985): Laser photobiological effects in the skin. In: *Handbook of Standardization of Safety in Electrooptics of the Japan Institute of Standards.* Ministry of Industry, Trade and Information (MITI), Tokyo. pp 415 ~ 416.

Regulation for the Administration and Enforcement of Radiation Control for Health and Safety Act of 1968: HEW Publ (FDA) 79 ~ 8035.

Sliney D, and Wolbarsht M (1980): *Safety with Lasers and Other Optical Sources:* Plenum Press, New York.

COLOUR AND COLORIMETRY

Birren F (ed) (1975): *AH Munsell - A Grammar of Color.* Van Nostrand Reinhold Company, Nw York.

Birren F (ed) (1975): *W Ostwald - The Color Primer.* Van Nostrand Reinhold Company, Nw York.

Edwards EA, and Duntley SQ (1939): The pigments and color of living human skin. *Am J Anat* **65:** 1

Judd DS, and Wyszecki J (1963): *Colour in Business, Science, and Industry.* pub. John Wiley and Sons, Chichester.

Murakami S: *Instruction Manual of Fast Spectrophotometric Colorimeter CMS-1000.* Murakami Color Research Laboratory.

Ohshiro T (1980): Colorimetry. In: *Laser Treatment for Nevi.* Mel Ltd, Tokyo. pp 27 ~ 34.

SKIN PIGMENTATION SYSTEM

Bernstein IA, Makoto S (1980): *Biochemistry of Normal and Abnormal Epidermal Differentiation.* University of Tokyo Press, Tokyo.

Breathnach, AS (1964): Electron microscopy of melanocytes and melanosomes in freckled human epidermis. *J Invest Dermatol,* **42:** 389 ~ 394.

Fitzpatrick TB, Quevedo WC, Jr, Szabo G, and Seiji M (1971): Biology of the melanin pigmentary system. In *Dermatology in General Medicine* (Fitzpatrick TB, *et al, eds.*), McGraw Hill, New York, pp. 117 ~ 146.

Harrison GA (1973): Differences in human pigmentation: Measurement, geographic variation and causes. *J Invest Dermatol,* **50:** 418 ~ 426.

Kawamura T, Fitzpatrick TB, and Seiji M: *Biology of Normal and Abnormal Melanocytes.* University of Tokyo Press, Tokyo.

Kitano Y, and Hu F (1969): The effects of ultraviolet light on mammalian pigment cells in vitro. *J Invest Dermatol,* **52:** 25 ~ 31.

Lever WF, and Chaumberg-Lever G (1975): *Histopathology of the Skin.* JB Lippincott, Philadelphia.

Loomis WF (1967): Skin-pigment regulation of vitamin-D biosynthesis in man. *Science,* **157:** 490 ~ 501.

Montagna W, and Liu F (1967): *Advances in Biology of the Skin, Vol 8: The Pigmentary System.* Pergamon Press, Oxford.

Ohshiro T (1980): Melanin. In : *Laser Treatment for Nevi.* Mel, Ltd., Tokyo. pp 38 ~ 40.

Pathak MA, Hori Y, Szabo G, and Fitzpatrick TB (1971): The photobiology of melanin pigmentation in human skin. In Kawamura T, Fitzpatrick TB, and Seiji M, (eds.), *Biology of Normal and Abnormal Melanocytes* University of Tokyo Press, Tokyo, pp. 149 ~ 167.

Stern C (1970): Model estimates of the number of gene pairs involved in pigmentation variability of the Negro-American. *Hum Hered,* **20:** 165 ~ 168.

Szabo G (1959): Quantative histological investigations on the melanocytic system: in Gordon M (ed): *Pigment Cell Biology.* Academic Press, New York: p99.

Wolf K, and Konrad K (1971): Melanin pigmentation: An *in vivo* model for studies of melanosome kinetics within keratinocytes. *Science,* **74:** 1034 ~ 1035.

LASER PHOTOBIOLOGY

Anderson RR and Parish JA (1980): Optical properties of the human skin. In *The Science of Photomedicine,* Plenum Press, New York. pp 147 ~ 194.

Barsky S, Rosen S, Geer D, *et al* (1980): The nature and evolution of port wine stains: a computer-assisted study. *J Invest Dermatol,* **74:** 154 ~ 157.

Bayly DJ, Kartha VB and Stevens WH (1963): The absorption spectra of liquid phase H_2O, HDO and D_2O from 0.7 µm to 10 µm. *Infrared Phys,* **3:** 211.

Clark C, Vinegar R, and Hardy, JD (1953): Goniometric spectrometer for the measurement of diffuse reflectance and transmittance of skin in the infrared spectral region. *J Opt Soc Am,* **43:** 993 ~ 998.

Edlow J, Fine S, Vawter GF, Jockin H, and Klein E (1965): Laser irradiation, effect on rat embryo and fetus *in utero. Life Sc,* **4:** 615 ~ 623.

Ehrenberger K, and Innitzer J (1978): The effect of CO_2 laser on skin lymphatics. *Wein Klin Wochen,* (German) **90:** 307 ~ 309.

Finsen NR (1988): *La Phototherapie.* Carre et Naud, Paris.

Fisher JC (1983): The power density of a surgical laser beam: Its meaning and measurement. *Lasers Surg Med,* **2:** 301 ~ 315.

Fubini S (1879): Influenza della luce sulla respirazione del tessuro nervoso. *Archivo per le scienze mediche da G Bizzozero,* **3:** 88.

Fuller TA (1986): Laser tissue interaction: the influence of power density. In Baggish MS (ed) *Basic and Advanced Laser Surgery in Gynecology.* Appleton-Century Crofts, Connecticut, pp 51 ~ 60.

Geise AC (1964): Studies in Photophysiology: in Giese AC (ed) *Photophysiology* Vol 2, p 203: Academic Press, New York.

Geise AC (1974): *Living With Our Sun's Ultraviolet Rays:* Plenum Press, New York.

Giese AC (ed) (1964-1977): *Photophysiology* Vol 1-6, Academic Press, New York.

Jacquez JA, *et al* (1955): Theory of the integrating sphere. *J Opt Soc Am,* **45:** 460 ~ 470.

Jacquez JA. *et al (*1955*):* Spectral Reflectance of human skin in the region 0.7~2.6 µm. *Appl Physiol,* **8:** 212 ~ 274.

Kottler F (1960): Turbid media with plane-parallel surfaces. *J Opt Soc Am,* **50:** 483 ~ 490.

Lever WF (1967): *Histopathology of the Skin:* (4th Edition) JB Lippincott Co, Philadelphia.

Kawamura T (1956): Uber die Herkfunt der Naevuszellen und die genetische werwandtschaft Zwischen Pigmentzellnaevus, blauem Naevus und Recklinghauserscher Phakomatose. *Hautarzt,* **7:** 7.

Kawamura T (1974): Relationship between origin of melanocyte and the naevus cell. *Clin Dermatol (Tokyo),* **16:** 691 ~ 698.

Magnus IA (1976): *Dermatological Photobiology*, Blackwell Scientific, Oxford.

Morison WL (1983): Photoimmunology and humans: in Parrish JA (ed) *The Effects of Ultraviolet Radiation on the Immune System*, Jonson & Jonson, U.S.A., p3.

Ohshiro T (1989): Photoactivation and the Arndt-Schultz law. In: Ohshiro T and Calderhead RG, *Low Level Laser Therapy: A Practical Introduction*. John Wiley & Sons, Chichester. pp 27 ~ 31.

Parrish JA (1982): Photomedicine: potentials for lasers: in Regan JD, Parrish JA (eds) *The Science of Photomedicine*, Springer-Verlag, New York, p147.

Parrish JA (1983): Photobiology and immunology: in Parrish JA (ed) *The Effects of Ultraviolet Radiation on the Immune System*, Jonson & Jonson, New York U.S.A., p3.

Parrish JA (ed) (1983): *The Effects of Ultraviolet Radiation on the Immune System*, Jonson & Jonson, New York, U.S.A.

Patterson MS, Wilson BC, and Wyman DR (1991): The propagation of optical radiation in tissue. I: Models of radiation transport and their application. *Lasers Med Sci*, **6:** 155 ~ 168.

Patterson MS, Wilson BC, and Wyman DR (1991): The propagation of optical radiation in tissue. II: Optical properties of tissues and resulting fluence distributions. *Lasers Med Sci*, **6:** 379 ~ 390.

Regan JD, and Parrish JA (eds) (1982): *The Science of Photomedicine*, Springer-Verlag, New York

Smith K C (ed) (1990): *The Science of Photobiology (2nd Edition)*, Plenum Publishing Co, New York.

Smith KC (1981): Photobiology and photomedicine: the future is bright. *J Invest Dermatol*, **77:** 1.

Smith KC (1991): The photobiological basis of low level laser therapy. *Laser Therapy*, **3:** 19 ~ 24.

Smith KC, and Hanawalt PC (1969): Laws of Photochemistry. In *Molecular Photobiology*. Academic Press, New York.

Stryer L (1981): *Biochemistry*: (2nd Edition), WH Freeman & Co, New York

van Gemert MJC, and Hulsbergen-Hemming JP (1981): A model approach to laser coagulation of dermal vascular lesions. *Arch Dermatol*, **270:** 429 ~ 439.

Walker J, Schwartzwelder HS, and Bondy SC (1989): Suppression of epilieptiform activity *in vitro* after laser exposure. *Laser Therapy*, **1:** 19.

Wolbarsht ML (1977) (ed): *Laser Applications in Medicine & Biology*: Plenum Press, New York & London. Vols 1 - 3, 1971 ~ 1974.

Young S *et al* (1989): Macrophage responsiveness to light therapy. *Las Surg Med*, **9:** p497.

HISTOLOGY & BASIC STUDIES IN LASER /TISSUE INTERACTIONS

Alberts B, Bray D, Lewis J, Raff M, Roberts K, and Watson JD (eds) (1989): *Molecular Biology of the Cell* (2nd Edition). Garland Publishing Inc, New York & London.

Anderson RR and Parish JA (1981): Microvasculature can be selectively damaged using dye lasers: A basic theory and experimental evidence in human skin. *Lasers Surg Med*, **1:** 263 ~ 276.

Apfelberg DP, Maser MR, and Lash H (1979): Histology of port wine stains following argon laser treatment. *Br J Plas Surg*, **32:** 232 ~ 237.

Bayly DJ, Kartha VB, and Stevens WH (1963): The absorption spectra of liquid phase H_2O, HDO and D_2O from 0.7 µm to 10 µm. *Infrared Phys*, **3:** 211.

Ben-Bassat M, and Kaplan I (1976): A study of the ultra-structural features of the cut margin of skin and mucous membrane specimens excised by carbon dioxide laser. *J Surg Res*, **21:** 77 ~ 84.

Bowers RE, Graham EA, and Tomlinson KM (1960): The natural history of the strawberry naevus. *Arch Dermatol*, **82:** 59 ~ 72.

Bozduganov A, and Dragiev M (1973): Histological and histochemical examinations of the skin after irradiation by ruby laser. *Radiobiol Radiotherm*, (German) **14:** 703 ~ 710.

Caro WH (1975): Tumors of the skin. In Moschella S, Pillsbury D and Hurley H, eds: *Dermatology*. WB Saunders Co, Philadelphia. pp 1323 ~ 1406.

Chow JWM, and Flemming AFS (1990): Laser-assisted microvascular anastomoses: a histological study. *Lasers Med Sci*, **5:** 281 ~ 288.

Fine RM, Derbes VJ, and Clark WH, Jr (1961): The Blue rubber bleb nevus. *Arch Dermatol*, **84:** 202 ~ 206.

Goldman L, Blaney DL, Kindel DJ, jr, Richfield D, and Frank EK (1963): Pathology of the effect of the laser beam on the skin. *Nature*, **197:** 912 ~ 914.

Goldman L, *et al* (1971): Orientation of small biopsies. *Arch Derm*, **103:** 407 ~ 408.

Goldman L, Igelman JM, and Richfield DF (1964): Impact of the laser on nevi and melanomas. *Arch Derm*, **40:** 121.

Hardy JD, et al (1956): Spectral Transmittance and Reflection of Excised Human Skin. Appl Physiol, 9: 251 ~ 264.

Hass AF, Isserof RR, Wheeland RG, Rood PA, and Graves PJ (1990): Low energy helium neon laser irradiation increases the motility of cultured human keratinocytes. J Invest Dermatol, 94: 822 ~ 826.

Heiwig EB, et al (1965): Anatomic and histochemical changes in skin after laser irradiation. Fed Am Soc Exp Biol, Fed Suppl, 24: 5483.

Hernandez LC, Santisebastian P, Valle-Sotto ME de, et al (1990): Changes in mRNA of thyroglobulin, cytoskeleton of thyroid cells, and thyroid level of hormones induced by IR-laser irradiation. Laser Therapy, 1: 203 ~ 206.

Hishimoto K (1972): Basic research in liver surgery using laser scalpel. J Jap Surg Soc 73: 1168 ~ 1171.

Hishimoto K (1973): Biophysical study of the incision depth in laser surgery. J Jap Surg Soc, 69: 1066 ~ 1069.

Hoye RC (1967): The airborne dissemination of viable tumour by high-power neodimium laser. Life Sc, 6: 119 ~ 125.

Hughes BF (1962): Preliminary report on the use of a CO_2 surgical laser unit on animals. Invest Urol, 9: 353 ~ 357.

Jacquez JA, et al (1955): Theory of the integrating sphere. J Opt Soc Am, 45: 460 ~ 470.

Jacquez JA. et al (1955): Spectral Reflectance of human skin in the region 0.7~2.6 μm. Appl Physiol, 8: 212 ~ 274.

Jones SG, Shakespeare PG and Carruth JAS (1989): Transcutaneous microscopy and argon laser treatment of port wine stains. Lasers med Sci, 4: 73 ~ 78.

Kaplan I, et al (1974): Excision of subcutaneous fibrosarcoma in mice. Isrl J Med Sc, 10.

Karas', GA (1975): Comparative histochemical analysis of proteins and their functionally active groups in the skin of the neck of albino rats after irradiation with laser beams and electroknife. Zh Ush Nos Gor Bol, (Russian), (4): 35 ~ 41.

Knox C (1966): Holographic microscopy as a technique for recording dynamic microscopic subjects. Science, 153: 989 ~ 990.

Kottler F (1960): Turbid media with plane-parallel surfaces. J Opt Soc Am, 50: 483 ~ 490.

Kovacs IB, et al (1974): Laser-induced stimulation of the vascularisation of the healing wound - an ear chamber experiment. Specialia.

Laub DR, Yules RB, Arras M, Murray DE, Crowhey L, and Chase RA (1968): Preliminary histopathological observation of Q-switched ruby laser radiation on dermal tattoo pigment in man. J Surg Res, 8: 220 ~ 224.

Lever WF, and Chaumberg-Lever G (1975): Histopathology of the Skin. JB Lippincott, Philadelphia.

Iida H (1975): Hazards of and protection against non-ionizing radiation. J Health Phys Soc, 10: 221 ~ 226.

Isenberg G, et al (1976): Cell surgery by laser microdissection - a preparative method. J Micros, 107: 19 ~ 24.

Masson P (1926): Les naeves pigmentaires, tumeures nerveuses. Ann Path et Anat-Chirurg, 3: 657.

Mayao E, Trelles MA, Calderhead RG, et al (1990): Short-term ultrastructural changes in soft tissue (endonysium) after LLLT HeNe laser irradiation. Laser Therapy, 1: 119 ~ 126.

Montgomery H (1967): Dermopathology. Harper & Row, New York.

Moschella S, Pillsbury D, and Hurley H, eds. (1975): Dermatology. WB Saunders Co, Philadelphia.

Mullins JF, Naylor D, and Redetsky J (1962): The Klippel-Trenauny-Weber syndrome. Arch Dermatol, 84: 202 ~ 206.

Nasu F, Tomiyasu K, Inomata K and Calderhead RG (1989): Cytochemical effects of GaAlAs diode laser irradiation on rat saphenous artery calcium ion dependent ATPase activity. Laser Therapy, 1: 89 ~ 92.

Norris CW, Mullarky MB (1982): Experimental skin incision made with the carbon dioxide laser. Laryngoscope, 92: 416 ~ 419.

Nowak WB, et al (1964): The use of thermocouples for temperature measurement during laser irradiation. Life Sci, 3: 1475 ~ 1481.

Ohta K (1951): My conception of cellular naevi. Cancer, 4: 9.

Ohshiro T (1987): Comparative study of argon, Nd:YAG and CO_2 lasers to achieve similar histological changes in ddY mouse skin. Keio J Med, 36: 98 ~ 110.

Parrish JA, Anderson RR, Ying CY, and Pathak MA (1976): Cutaneous effects of pulsed nitrogen gas laser irradiation. J Invest Derm, 67: 603 ~ 608.

Polanyi TG, Bredemeier HC, and Davis TW, jr (1970): Argon laser for surgical research. Med Opt Eng, 8: 541 ~ 548.

Rittor EJ, Goldman L, Richfield D, Rockwell RJ, jr, and Franzen M (1969): The chicken comb and wattle as experimental model for investigative argon laser therapy of angiomas. *Act Derm Vener,* **49:** 304 ~ 308.

Rook A (1968): Naevi and other developmental defects. In Rook A, Wilkinson DS, and Ebling FJG (eds) *Textbook of Dermatology, (Vol I).* pp 73 ~ 111.

Rook A, Wilkinson DS, and Ebling FJG (eds) (1968): *Textbook of Dermatology* (Volumes 1 and 2). Blackwell Scientific Publications, Oxford and Edinburgh.

Rochkind S, Rousso M, Nissan M, Villareal M, Barr-Nea L, and Rees DG (1989): System effects of low-power laser irradiation on the peripheral and central nervous system, cutaneous wounds, and burns. *Lasers Surg Med,* **9:** 147 ~ 182.

Rounds DE, *et al (1967):* Effect of intense light on cellular respiration. *Life Sci,* **6:** 359 ~ 366.

Ryan CB, Cliff WJ, Gabbiani G, *et al* (1974): Myofibroblasts in human granulation tissue. *Hum Path,* **5:** 55.

Shiroto C, Sugawara K, Kumae T *et al* (1990): Effects of diode laser irradiation *in vitro* on activity of human neutrophils. *Laser Therapy,* **1:** 135 ~ 140.

Solomon H, Goldman L, Henderson B, Richfieid D, and Franzen M (1968): Histopathology of the laser treatment of port-wine lesions. Biopsy studies of treated areas observed up to three years after laser impacts. *J Invest Derm,* **50:** 141 ~ 146

Squire AJB (1876): *Essays on the treatment of skin diseases. III. On port-wine mark and its obliteration without scar.* J & A Churchill, London.

Steinlechner CWB, and Dyson M (1993): The effects of low level laser therapy on the proliferation of keratinocytes. *Laser Therapy,* **5:** 65 ~ 74.

Taylor GI, Palmer JH (1987): The vascular territories (angiosomes) of the body: experimental study and clinical applications. *Brit J Plast Surg,* **40:** 113.

Tsai J, and Kao M (1990): The biological effects of low power density laser radiation on cultivated rat glial and gliomal cells. *Laser Therapy,* **1:** 191 ~ 202

Unna PG (1894): *Histologie der Hautkrankeheiten.* Hirschfeld, Berlin.

Wertz RK, *et al (1967):* Ruby laser micro irradiation of single cells vitally stained with Janus green B. *Exp Cell Res,* **45:** 61 ~ 71.

Young S, Bolton P, Dyson M, Harvey W, and Diamantopoulos C (1989): Macrophage responsiveness to light therapy. *Las Surg Med,* **9:** 497.

Yules EB, *et al (1967):* The effect of Q-switched ruby laser radiation on dermal tattoo pigment in man. *Arch Surg,* **95:** 179.

LASER/TISSUE INTERACTIONS

Anderson RR and Parish JA (1981): Microvasculature can be selectively damaged using dye lasers: A basic theory and experimental evidence in human skin. *Lasers Surg Med,* **1:** 263 ~ 276.

Bayly DJ, Kartha VB and Stevens WH (1963): The absorption spectra of liquid phase H_2O, HDO and D_2O from 0.7 μm to 10 μm. *Infrared Phys,* **3:** 211.

Boardon R, Belin JP, and Dana M (1967): The laser. Principle. Dermatologic applications. *Bull Soc Fran Derm Syphil,* (French) **74:** 419 ~ 421.

Fisher JC (1983): The power density of a surgical laser beam: Its meaning and measurement. *Lasers Surg Med,* **2:** 301 ~ 315.

Fuller TA (1986): Laser tissue interaction: the influence of power density. In Baggish MS (ed) *Basic and Advanced Laser Surgery in Gynecology.* Appleton-Century Crofts, Connecticut, pp 51 ~ 60.

Goldman JA, *et al* (1965): Medical intelligence - current concepts (Fibre optics in medicine). *New Engl J Med,* **273:** 1425 ~ 1426.

Goldman L (1965): Biomedical engineering and dermatology. *Arch Derm,* **91:** 493 494.

Goldman L (1969): Biomedical installations. *Arch Environ Health,* **18:** 406 ~ 407.

Lagunova lG, Savchenko ED, Likhovetskaya LL, Garvei NN, and Shamaeva GG (1971): Biological effect of lasers on the skin (preliminary report). *Med Rad (Russian),* **16:** 38 ~ 42.

Moore KC and Calderhead RG (1991): The clinical application of low incident power density 830 nm GaAlAs diode laser radiation in the therapy of chronic intractable pain: A historical and optoelectronic rationale and clinical overview. *Int J Optoelec,* **6:** 503 ~ 520.

Norris CW, Mullarky MB (1982): Experimental skin incision made with thc carbon dioxide laser. *Laryngoscope,* **92:** 416 ~ 419.

Rittor EJ, Goldman L, Richfield D, Rockwell RJ, jr, and Franzen M (1969): The chicken comb and wattle as experimental model for investigative argon Laser Therapy, of angiomas. *Act Derm vener*, **49:** 304 ~ 308.

Shakespeare PG, Hambleton J, and Carruth JAS (1991): Skin surface temperature during argon and

tunable dye laser therapy of port wine stains. *Lasers Med Sci*, **6:** 29 ~ 34.

Wertz RK, *Et al* (1967): Ruby laser micro irradiation of single cells vitally stained with Janus green B. *Exp Cell Res*, **45:** 61 ~ 71.

Yules EB, *et al* (1967): The effect of Q-switched ruby laser radiation on dermal tattoo pigment in man. *Arch Surg*, **95:** 179.

WOUND HEALING

Almquist EE, *et al* (1984): Argon laser in repairing rat and primate nerves. *J Hand Surg*, **9A:** p792.

Baker HJ *et al* (1976): Animal experimentation in wound healing. In Menaker L (ed) *Biologic Basis of Wound Healing*. Harper & Row, Maryland: p311.

Boulnois JL (1986): Photophysical processes in recent medical laser developments. *Lasers med Sci*, **1:** 47 ~ 66.

Diegelmann RF, Cohen IK, and Kaplan AM (1981): The role of the macrophage in wound repair. *Plast Recon Surg*, **68:** 107 ~ 113.

Duance VC, and Bailey AJ (1981): Biosynthesis and degradation of collagen: in Glynn LE (ed) *Tissue Repair & Regeneration*; Elsevier Biomedical Press, Amsterdam: p51.

Dyson M, and Young S (1985): Effect of Laser Therapy, on wound contraction: in Galletti G (ed) *Laser*: Monduzzi Editore, Bologna: p215.

Ferguson MWJ, and Harrison MR (1990): Studies in wound healing, VI. Second and early third trimester fetal wounds demonstrate rapid collagen formation without scar formation. *J Ped Surg*, **25:** 63.

Finsterbush A, Russo M, and Ashur H (1982): Healing and tensile strength of CO_2 laser incisions and scalpel wounds in rabbits. *Plast Reconstr Surg*, **70:** 360 ~ 362.

Foster M (1959): Physiological studies of melanogesis:in Gordon M (ed): *Pigment Cell Biology*: Academic Press, New York: p301.

Glynn LE (ed) 1983: *Tissue Repair & Regeneration*; Elsevier Biomedical Press, Amsterdam

Goslen JB (1988): Wound healing for the dermatological surgeon. *J Dermatol Surg Oncol*, **14:** 959 ~ 972.

Gross J, *et al* (1980): Mode of action and regulation of tissue collagenases: in Wooley DE, Evanson JM (eds) *Collagenase in Normal & Pathological Tissues*, John Wiley & Sons, Chichester; p11.

Hinshaw JR, and Edgar M (1965): Histology of healing of split thickness, full thickness autologous skin grafts and donor sites. *Arch Surg*, **91:** 658 ~ 670.

Horne RSC, Hurley JV, Crowe DM, *et al* (1992): Wound healing in fetal sheep: a histological and electron microscope study. *Br J Plas Surg*, **45:** 333 ~ 344.

Hutschenreiter C, Haina D, Paulini K, and Schumacher G (1980): Wundheilung nach Laser und Rotlichtbestrahlung. *Exp Chir*, **13:** 75 ~ 85.

Lam TS (1983): Biological effects of laser stimulation on collagen production by low energy lasers in human skin fibroblasts. *Lasers Med Surg*, **3:** p285.

Lee P, Kim K, and Kim K (1993): Effects of low incident energy levels of infrared laser irradiation on healing of infected open skin wounds of the rat. *Laser Therapy*, **5:** 59 ~ 64

Lepow IH, and Ward PA *eds*. (1970): *Inflammation: Mechanisms and Control*. Academic Pres, New York.

Lievens PC (1991): The effect of a combined HeNe and IR laser treatment on the regeneration of the lymphatic system during the process of wound healing. *Lasers med Sci*, **6:** 193 ~ 200.

McCaughan J, Bethel B, Johnson T, and Janssen W (1985): Effect of low-dose argon laser irradiation on rate of wound closure. *Lasers Surg Med*, **5:** 607 ~ 614.

Madden JW, and Peacock EE (1981): Studies on the biology of collagen production during wound healing. *Ann Surg*, **174:** 511 ~ 518.

Marin VTW, Corti L, and Velussi C (1988): An experimental study of the healing effect of the HeNe and the IR laser. *Lasers Med Sci*, **3:** 151 ~ 164.

Matsumura C, Murakami F, and Kemmotsu O (1992): Effect of helium neon laser therapy (LLLT) on wound healing in a torpid vasculogenic ulcer on the foot: A case report. *Laser Therapy*, **4:** 101 ~ 106.

Menaker L (1976): Protein synthesis; in Menaker L (ed) *Biologic Basis of Wound Healing:* Harper & Row, Maryland: p192.

Menaker L (ed) (1976): *Biologic Basis of Wound Healing:* Harper & Row, Maryland.

Nicholls JG (ed) (1982): *Repair & Regeneration of the Nervous System:* Springer-Verlag, New York.

Ohshiro T (1980): The essential factors for laser treatment. In: **Laser Treatment for Nevi**. Mel, Ltd., Tokyo. pp 44 ~ 48.

Peacock EE jr, and Van Winkle W jr (1976): *Wound Repair* (2nd Edition), WB Saunders Co, Philadelphia.

Robinson BW, and Goss AN (1981): Intrauterine healing of fetal rat cheek wounds. *Cleft pal J,* **18:** 251.

Roels H (1981): Hyperplasia versus atrophy: in Glynn LE (ed) *Tissue Repair & Regeneration;* Elsevier Biomedical Press, Amsterdam: p243.

Rowsell AR (1984): The intrauterine healing of foetal muscle wounds: experimental study in the rat. *Br J Plas Surg,* **37:** 635.

Ryan CB, Cliff WJ, Gabbiani G, *et al* (1974): Myofibroblasts in human granulation tissue. *Hum Path,* **5:** 55.

Schwartz LW, and Osburn BI (1974): An ontogenic study of the acute inflammatory reaction in the fetal Rhesus monkey. *Lab Invest,* **31:** 441.

Schwartz M *et al* (1987): Effects of low energy HeNe laser irradiation on posttraumatic degeneration of adult rabbit optic nerve. *Laser Surg Med,* **7:** p51.

Stryer L (1981): Introduction to enzymes: in *Biochemistry:* (2nd Edition), WH Freeman & Co, New York, p103.

Stryer L (1981): Protein Synthesis: in *Biochemistry:* (2nd Edition), WH Freeman & Co, New York: p641.

Stryer L (1981): Connective tissue proteins: in Menaker L (ed) *Biologic Basis of Wound Healing:* Harper & Row, Maryland: p192.

Surinchak J *et al* (1983): Effects of low level energy lasers on the healing of full thickness skin defects. *Lasers Surg Med,* **2:** 276.

Trelles MA, *et al* (1985): Low intensity laser irradiation promotes more rapid repair of bone fractures: experimental demonstration: in Galletti G (ed) *Laser,* Monduzzi Editore, Bologna. p395.

Vaes G: (1980): Collagenase, Lysosomes and osteoclastic bone resorption: in Wooley DE, Evanson JM (eds) *Collagenase in Normal & Pathological Tissues;* John Wiley & Sons, Chichester, p185.

Weller EM (1976): Regeneration: in Menaker L (ed) *Biologic Basis of Wound Healing:* Harper & Row, Maryland: p291.

White RA, Abergel RP, Lyons R, Klein SR, *et al* (1986): Biological effects of laser welding on vascular healing. *Lasers Surg Med,* **6:** 137 ~ 141.

Wooley DE, and Evanson JM (eds) (1980): *Collagenase in Normal & Pathological Connective Tissue:* John Wiley & Sons, Chichester.

LLLT AND PHOTOBIOACTIVATION

Abe T (1989): LLLT using a diode laser in successful treatment of herniated lumbar/sacral disc with MRI assessment: a case report. *Laser Therapy,* **1:** 93 ~ 96.

Abergel RP, *et al* (1984): Nonthermal effects of Nd:YAG laser on biological functions of human skin fibroblasts in culture. *Lasers Surg Med,* **3:** p279.

Asada K, Yutani Y and Smiazu A (1990): Diode laser therapy for rheumatoid arthtitis: a clinical evaluation of 102 joints treated with low-reactive level laser therapy (LLLT). *Laser Therapy,* **1:** 147~ 152.

Averbakh MM *et al* (1976): Effect of HeNe laser on the healing of aseptic experimental wounds. *Eksp Khir Anesteziol,* **3:** p56.

Bailes JE *et al* (1984): Fibronolytic activity following laser-assisted vascular anastomosis. *Microsurgery,* **6:** 163.

Bassleer C *et al* (1985): Human articular chondrocytes cultivated in three dimensions: effects of IR laser irradiation: in Galletti G (ed) *Laser,* Monduzzi Editore, Bologna: p381

Bieglio C (1985): A report on experiences of treating pain of spinal origin by low powered laser: in Galletti G (ed) *Laser,* Monduzzi Editore, Bologna: p343:

Bihari I and Mester A (1989): The biostimulative effect of low level Laser Therapy, on long standing crural ulcers using HeNe, HeNe+IR lasers, and noncoherent light: preliminary report of a double-blind randomized comparative studt. Laser Therapy, **1:** 99 ~ 102.

Bischko J (1980): Use of the laser beam in acupuncture. *Acupuncture & Electro-Therapeutic Res, Int J,* **5:** p29.

Buckley WR, Grum MS (1964): Reflection spectrophotometry. *Arch Derm,* **89:** p110.

Calderhead RG *et al* 1981: The Nd:YAG and GaAlAs lasers: a laser comparative analysis in pain therapy: in Atsumi K & Nimsakul N (eds) *Laser Tokyo '81:* Japan Society for Laser Medicine, Tokyo. 21:1.

Castro DJ *et al* (1983): Effects of the Nd:YAG laser on DNA synthesis and collagen production in human skin fibrobalsts. *Ann Plas Surg,* **11:** p214.

Castro DJ *et al* (1983): Wound healing: biological effects of Nd:YAG laser on collagen metabolism in pig skin in comparison to thermal burn. *Ann Plas Surg,* **11:** p131.

Chen Chang-jun *et al* (1984): The preoperative period of the veterinary anesthesia by laser. *Acupuncture Res,* **9:** p16.

Chino N, Noda Y (1985): Efficacy of the laser beam as a pain reliever. *Sogo Riha (Total Rehabilitation),* **13:** p447 (in Japanese).

Dawson JB *et al* (1980): A theoretical and experimental study of light absorption by *in vivo* skin. *Phys Med Biol,* **25:** p695.

De Min L *et al* (1985): Studies on mechanisms of laser acupuncture: Regulation of function:in Galletti G (ed) *Laser,* Monduzzi Editore, Bologna: p225.

De Min L, *et al* (1985): Studies on the mechanisms of laser acupuncture promotion of defence immuno-functions. In Galletti G (ed) *Laser,* Monduzzi Editore, Bologna: p259

Dyson M, and Young S (1985); Effect of Laser Therapy, on wound contraction. In Galletti G (ed) *Laser,* Monduzzi Editore, Bologna: p215

England SM, *et al* (1985): An observed double-blind trial if IR ceb mid *Laser Therapy,* is effective in bicipital tendonitis and supraspinal tendonitis: in Galletti G (ed) *op cit:* p.413.

Fine S, and Klein E (1965): Interaction of laser radiation with biological systems: *Proc. First Annl Conf on Biol Effects of Laser Rad:* Fed Proc **24:** p35.

Galletti G (1989): Deep tissue biostimulation with a low power CO_2 laser beam. *Surgical & Medical Lasers,* **2:** 21~23

Ge Zun-xing, *et al* (1981): Investigations in the effects in human pain threshold and pain tolerance under helium-neon laser acupuncture irradiation. *Sichuan Las J Supplemental issue 2,* p47 (Chinese).

Glynn LE (1981): The pathology of scar tissue formation:in Glynn LE (ed) *Tissue Repair & Regeneration.* Elsevier Biomedical Press, Amsterdam: p285.

Goldman L (1983): Laser diagnostic medicine: in Daheng W *et al* (eds) *Procdings of an International Conference on Lasers,* John Wiley & Sons, New York: p661.

Gregus P (1984): Low Level Laser Therapy: reality or myth? *Opt Las Tech,* p81.

Haas A F, *et al* (1990): Low energy HeNe laser irradiation increases the motility of cultured human keratinicytes. *J Invest Derm ,* **94:** p 822.

Hardy J, *et al* (1956): Spectral transmittance and reflectance of excised human skin. *J Appl Physiol,* **9:** 257.

Hassan P, Rijadi SA, Purnomo S, and Kainama H (1989): The possible application of low reactive level laser therapy (LLLT) in the treatement of male infertility. *Laser Therapy,* **1:** 49~50

He J (1989): The clinical application of HeNe laser in paediatric ailments. A report of 1420 cases treated with low level laser therapy. *Laser Therapy,* 1:2, 75~78.Laser

Hernandez LC, Valle-Sotto ME de, Ayala JM, and Vega JA (1989): Effects of IR laser radiation on the pituitary-thyroid axis. Ultrastructural immuno-histochemical and biochemical studies. *Laser Therapy,* 1:2, 69~74.

Hunter J *et al* (1984): Effects of low energy laser on wound healing in a porcine model. *Laser Surg Med,* **3:** 285.

Inoue K, *et al* (1989): Suppressed tuberclin reaction in guinnea pigs following laser irradiation. *Las Surg Med,* **9:** p271.

Kamikawa K (1985): Double blind experiences with mid-lasers in Japan:in Galletti G (ed) *Laser,* Monduzzi Editore, Bologna: p165.

Kamikawa K *et al* (1981): Development of laser acupuncture system: in Atsumi K & Nimsakul N (eds) *Laser Tokyo 81,* 21:5, Jap Soc for Lasers in Medicine, Tokyo, Japan.

Kana JS, *et al* (1981): Effects of low power density laser irradiation on the healing of open skin wound in rats. *Arch Surg,* **116:** 293.

Karu TI (1985): Biological action of low intensity visible monochromatic light and some of its medical applications:in Galletti G (ed) *Laser,* Monduzzi Editore, Bologna: p381.

Kokino M *et al* (1985): An investigation on the stimulating effect of laser on callus in the treatment of fractures:in Galletti G (ed) *Laser,* Monduzzi Editore, Bologna: p387.

Kokino M *et al* (1985): effect of laser irradiation on tendon healing:in Galletti G (ed) *Laser,* Monduzzi Editore, Bologna: p4054.

Kovacs IB *et al* (1974): Stimulation with wound healing with laser beam in the rat. *Experimentia,* **30:** 1275.

Kovacs L (1981): Experimental investigation of the photostimulative effect of low energy HeNe radiation: in Atsumi K, Nimsakul N (eds) *Laser Tokyo '81*, Japan Socity for Laser Medicine, Tokyo : p22.

Kubota J and Ohshiro T (1990): The effects of diode laser low-reactive level laser therapy (LLLT) on flap survival. *Laser Therapy*, **1**: 127 ~ 134.

Kudoh C, Inomata K, Okajima K *et al* (1989): Effects of 830 nm GaAlAs laser on rat saphenous nerve Na-K-ATPase activity: a possible pain attenuation mechanism examined. *Laser Therapy*, **1**: 63 ~ 68.

Lam TS (1983): Biological effects of laser stimulation of collagen production by low energy lasers in human skin fibroblast cultures. *Lasers Surg Med*, **4**: 381.

Li K, *et al* (1983) Chemical specificity of enzymes and the possibility of laser catalysis: in Daheng W *et al* (eds) *Proceedings of an International Conference on Lasers*, John Wiley & Sons, New York: p661.

Li S, You S, and Zhang S (1989): A new approach in the application of the helium neon laser in acupuncture therapy for prostatitis: a clinical study involving 114 cases. *Laser Therapy*, **1**: 37 ~ 40.

Lievens PC (1991): The effect of a combined HeNe and IR laser treatment on the regeneration of the lymphatic system during the process of wound healing. *Lasers Med Sci*, **6**: 193 ~ 200.

Ma Li, *et al* (1981): The influence of Nalorphene on laser acupuncture analgesic action - experimental animal research: *Sichuan Las J, supplemental issue* **2**: p49 (Chinese)

Ma S, *et al* (1983): Effects of HeNe radiation on the regenerative process of wounded skin of white mice: in Daheng W *et al* (eds) *Procedings of an International Conference on Lasers*, John Wiley & Sons, New York: p583.

Maeda T, *et al* (1989): Morphological demonstration of low reactive leaser therapeutic pain attenuation effect of the GaAlAs laser. *Laser Therapy*, **1**: 23 ~ 26.

Maier M, Haina D, and Landthaler M (1990): Effect of low energy laser on the growth and regeneration of capillaries. *Lasers Med Sci*, **5**: 381 ~ 386.

Marin VTW, Corti L, and Velussi C (1988): An experimental study of the healing effect of the HeNe and the IR laser. *Lasers Med Sci*, **3**: 151 ~ 164.

Marks R (1981): The healing and nonhealing of wounds of the skin and ulcers; in Glynn LE (ed) *Tissue Repair & Regeneration*; Elsevier Biomedical Press, Amsterdam: p309.

Mayordomo M, *et al* (1985): Laser in painful processes of locomoter system: our experiences: in Galletti G (ed) *op cit*: p349.

Mester E, *et al* (1969): Experimentation on the interaction between infrared laser and woundhealing. *Z Exper Chirurgie*, **2**: p94.

Mester E, *et al* (1971): Effect of laser rays on wound healing. *Am J Surg*, **122**: p532.

Mester E, *et al* (1973): The effect of laser radiation on wound healing and collagen synthesis. *Studia Biophys*, **35**: p227.

Mester E, *et al* (1974): *Enzyme histochemistry of wound healing*. VEB G Fischer Vienna.

Mester E, *et al* (1976): Laser stimulation of wound healing. *Acta Chirurgica*, **17**: p49.

Mester E, Mester A, and Mester A (1985): The biomedical effects of laser application. *Lasers Surg Med*, **5**: p31.

Moore K, Hira N, and Kumar PS *et al* (1989): A double-blind corossover trial of LLLT in the treatment of postherpetic neuralgia. *Laser Therapy*, **Pilot Isuue**, 7 ~ 10.

Moore KC (1990): An update on the application of LLLT in the UK. *Laser Therapy*, **1**: 157 ~ 162

Muir VMJ *et al* (1976): Morbidity following dental extraction. *Anes*, **31**: p171.

Nishida N, and Furukawa K (1985): Laser acupuncture treatment for chronic pain. *J Jap Socy Laser Med*, **5**: p243 (in Japanese).

Ohshiro T, and Calderhead RG (1988): *Low Level Laser Therapy: A Practical Introduction*. John Wiley & Sons, Chichester.

Ohshiro T (1989): *In vivo* and *in vitro* low reactive laser therapy experimentation: a possible protocol: 1. The mother computer. *Laser Therapy*, **1**:1, 51 ~ 52.

Ohshiro T (1990): LLLT in dentistry. *Laser Therapy*, **1**:4, 173 ~ 174.

Ohshiro T (1990): Treatment techniques to achieve superficial and intermediate LLLT irradiation. *Laser Therapy*, **1**: 153 ~ 156.

Ohshiro T (1991): *Low Level Laser Therapy: Practical Application*. John Wiley & Sons, Chichester.

Ohshiro T, and Calderhead RG (eds) (1991): *Progress in Laser Therapy*. John Wiley & Sons, Chichester.

Ohshiro T, *et al* (1986): Alleviating sports-related pain by the diode laser: practical considerations and thermographic evaluation. *J Japan Soc Laser Med*, **6**:3 p383.

Ohshiro T, *et al* (1986): Thermographic evaluation of diode laser therapy for lumbago. *J Jap Socy Laser Med*, **6**: p391.

Okada T, and Ohshiro T (1980): Laser acupuncture. *Japan Med Las Soc J*, **1**: p47 (Japanese).

Olson JE (1981): Laser action spectrum of reduced excitability in brain cells. *Brain Res,* **204:** p436.

Oyamada Y (1989): Trials in treatment of RA-related diseases by HeNe laser. *Surgical & Medical Lasers,* **2:** p18.

Persina IS, and Rackcheev AP (1984): *In vitro* fibroblast and dermis fibroblast activation by laser irradiation at low energy. *Allergology,* **95:** 653.

Poon AML, and Yew DT (1980): The effect of low dose laser on the functional activities of the mouse retina. *Anat Anz (Jena)* **148:** p236.

Quiglet MR, *et al* (1985): Microvascular anastomosis using the milliwatt CO_2 laser. *Lasers Surg Med,* **5:** p357.

Robinson JK, *et al* (1978): Wound healing in porcine skin following low output carbon dioxide laser irradiation of the incision. *Ann Plas Surg,* **18:** 499.

Rochkind S, *et al* (1984): HeNe laser stimulation for peripheral nerve regeneration: *Proc Int Cong Derm Surg:* p97.

Rochkind S, *et al* (1989): Systemic effects of low-power laser irradiation on the peripheral and central nervous system, cutaneous wounds, and burns. *Las Surg Med,* **9:** p174.

Scaravilli F, and Duchen LW (1981): Regeneration in the central nervous system: in Glynn LE (ed) *Tissue Repair & Regeneration*; Elsevier Biomedical Press, Amsterdam: p383.

Serure A, *et al* (1988): Comparison of carbon dioxide laser-assisted microvascular anastomosis and conventional microsutured anastomosis. *Surg Forum,* **34:** 634.

Shiroto, C *et al* (1986): The alleviatory effects of the diode laser in treating 1000 cases of pain. *J Jap Soc Laser Med,* **6:** p379 (in Japanese).

Shiroto C, Ono K and Ohshiro T (1989): Retrospective study of diode Laser Therapy, for pain attenuation in 3635 patients: detailed analysis by questionnaire. *Laser Therapy,* **1:** 41 ~ 48.

Tocco G, *et al* (1985): HeNe and infrared laser influence on skin cells in vivo: in Galletti G (ed) *op cit:* p175.

Trelles MA (1981): Laser biostimulative effect for osseous regeneration: *Laser 81 Opto-Elektronik: Proceedings* p 255.

Trelles MA, Mayayo E, Miro J, *et al* (1989): The action of low reactive level laser therapy (LLLT) on mast cells: a possible pain relief mechanism explained. *Laser Therapy,* **1:1,** 27 ~ 30.

Walker J (1983): Relief from chronic pain by low power laser irradiation. *Neurosci Lett,* **43:** p339.

Walker J (1988): Low level Laser Therapy, for pain management: a review of the literature and underlying mechanisms. In Ohshiro T & Calderhead RG, *Low Level Laser Therapy: A Practical Introduction*, John WIley & Sons, 42 ~ 56.

Wang Yun-huo, *et al* (1981): Analgesic effect on various horse nerves under helium-neon laser acupuncture irradiation. *Appl Las,* **1:** p44 (Chinese).

Wang Yun-huo *et al* (1981): Investigation in laser acupuncture anesthesia. *Laser,* **8:** p35 (Chinese).

Wang, Hun-Lo (1987) : Laser acupuncture. *Electro-Optical System Design,* **10:** p21.

Zimmerman DC (1979): Preplanning, surgical, and postoperative considerations in the removal of the difficult impaction. *Dent Clin North Am,* **23:** p451.

PRACTICAL DERMATOLOGICAL LASER APPLICATIONS

Alborova VK, Melnikova AP, Frygin NV, Serebriakov VA, and Gavrilov, NI (1973): Use of optic quantum generators (lasers) for experimental removal of tattooing. *Vest Derm Vener* (Russian) 47: 35 ~ 38.

Anderson RR, *et al* (1982): Lasers in dermatology provide a model for exploring new applications in surgical oncology. *Int Adv Surg Oncol,* **5:** p341.

Apfelberg DB, Maser MR, and Lash H (1976): Argon laser management of cutaneous vascular deformities. A preliminary report. *West J Med,* 124: 99.

Apfelberg DB, Maser MR, and Lash H (1978): Treatment of nevi aranei by means of an argon laser. *J Derm Surg Oncol* 4: 172.

Apfelberg DB. Maser MR, and Lash H (1978): Argon laser treatment of cutaneous vascular abnormalities: progress report. *Ann Plas Surg,* **1:** 14 ~ 18.

Arai K, *et al* (1975): Application of photocoagulation in the field of plastic surgery. *Jap J Plas Recon Surg,* **18:** 702 ~ 708.

Arndt KA, *et al* (eds) 1983: *Cutaneous Laser Therapy* John Wiley & Sons, New York

Atsumi, K (1979): Laser scalpel, the past, present, and future. *J Jap Med Assoc,* **8:** 937 ~ 944.

Atsumi K, and Nimsakul N (eds) (1980): *Laser Tokyo 81* Japan Society for Laser Medicine and Surgery, Tokyo.

Babaiants RD, Rakeheev AP, Konstantinov AV, lvanov OL, and Makeeva NS (1974): Use of low-radiation output lasers in certain dermatoses. *Vest Derm Venerl* (Russian), **48:** 7 ~ 13.

Bailin PL, Ratz JL, and Lutz-Nagey L (1981): CO_2 laser modification of Mohs surgery. *J Dermatol Surg Oncol,* **7:** 621 ~ 623.

Bailin PL, Ratz JR, and Levine HL (1980): Removal of tattoos by CO_2 laser. *J Dermatol Surg Oncol,* **6:** 997 ~ 1001.

Bailin PL, and Wheeland RG (1985): Carbon dioxide (CO_2) laser perforation of exposed cranial bone to stimulate granulation tissue. *Plast Reconstr Surg,* **75:** 898 ~ 902.

Chen J and Zhou Y (1989): Effects of low level carbon dioxide laser radiation on biochemical metabolism of rabbit mandibular bone callus. *Laser Therapy,* **1:** 83 ~ 88.

Cosman B (1980): Argon Laser Therapy, of port wine stains. *J Med Soc NJ,* **77:** 167 ~ 174.

Daheng W, *et al* (eds) 1983: *Proceedings of an International Conference on Lasers,* John Wiley & Sons, New York.

David LM, and Sanders G (1987): CO_2 laser blepharoplasty: A comparison to cold steel and electrocautery. *J Dermatol Surg Oncol,* **13:** 110 ~ 114.

Dittrich H, Druen N, and Schlake W (1975): The use of laser in thoracic, cardiac, and vascular surgery. *Thoraxchirgerie,* **23:** 505 ~ 510.

Fox JL (1969): The use of laser radiation as a surgical 'light knife': *J Surg Res* **9:** 199 ~ 204.

Fruhmorgen P, *et al (1976)*: Laser in der Medizin. *Munch Med Wschr,* **118:** 721 ~ 722.

Fujino T, *et al* (1986): Clinical effect of the diode laser to improve the fair take of grafted skin. *Keio J Med,* **35:** p28.

Galletti G (ed) 1985: *Laser,* Monduzzi Editore, Bologna.

Gamaleja NF, and Polishchuk EI (1974): The experience of skin tumours treatment with laser radiation. *Pan Medica,* **16:** 41 ~ 43.

Goldman L (1965): Dermatological manifestations of laser radiation. *Fed Am Soc Exper Biol, Federation Proceedings Supplement,* **24:** 592.

Goldman L (1969): Laser surgery of angiomas. *Las Electro-Opt Rev,* **4:** 53.

Goldman L (1969): What we plan to do. *Arch Environ Health,* **18:** 390.

Goldman L (1971): Long-term laser exposure of a senile freckle. *Arch envir Health,* **22:** 401.

Goldman L (1973): Recent developments of the laser in medicine. *Proc Soc Photo-Opt Instr Eng,* **41:** 103 ~ 106.

Goldman L (1973): A status report on laser surgery. *Contemp Surg,* **32:** 18 ~ 24.

Goldman L (1973): Effects of new laser systems on the skin. *Arch Derm,* **108:** 385 ~ 390.

Goldman L (1976): Laser surgery in cosmetic dermatology. *Cutis,* **17:** 38.

Goldman L (1977): Laser surgery for skin cancer. *N Y State J Med,* **77:** 1897 ~ 1900.

Goldman L (1979): Surgery by laser for malignant melanoma. *J Derm Surg Oncol,* **5:** 141 ~ 144.

Goldman L (ed) 1981: *The Biomedical Laser. Technology and Clinical Applications,* Springer-Verlag, New York.

Goldman L (ed) 1981: *The Biomedical Laser. Technology and Clinical Applications,* Springer-Verlag, New York.

Goldman L (ed) (1991): *Laser Non-Surgical Medicine.* Technomic Company, Pennsylvania.

Goldman L, and Rockwell RJ Jr. (1972) (eds): *Lasers in Medicine:* Gordon & Breach, New York.

Goldman L, and Wilson RG (1964): Treatment of basal cell epithelioma with laser radiation. *J Am Med Assoc,* **189:** 773 ~ 775.

Goldman L, Dreffer R, Rockwell RJ, jr, and Perry E (1976): Treatment of portwine marks by an argon laser. *J Derm Surg,* **2:** 385 ~ 388.

Goldman L, Rockwell RJ, jr, Meyer R, and Otten R (1968): lnvestigative studies with the laser in the treatment of basal cell epitheliomas. *South Med J,* **61:** 735 ~ 742.

Goldman L, Vahl J, Rockwell RJ, jr, Meyer R, Frazen M, Owens P, and Hyatt S (1969): Replica microscopy and scanning electron microscopy of laser impacts on the skin. *J Invest Derm,* **52:** 18 ~ 24.

Henderson DL, Crowwell TA, and Mes LG (1984): Argon and carbon dioxide laser treatment of hypertrophic and keloid scars. *Lasers Surg Med* **3:** 271 ~ 277.

Hillenkamp F, Pratesi R, and Sacchi CA (eds) (1980): *Lasers in Biology and Medicine.* Plenum Press, New York, London.

Hishimoto K (1962): The laser scalpel and laser surgery - recent and future aspects. *Surg Diag Treat,* **30:** 928.

Hishimoto K (1972): Plasma scalpel and plasma surgery, future prospects and present problems. *Surg Diag Treatment* **943:** 45 ~ 55.

Hishimoto K, *et al (1969)*: Laser radiation of malignancy in man. *J Clin Surg,* **24:** 811 ~ 817.

Hollander A (1974): News in American dermatology. *Hautzart (German)*, **25:** 471 ~ 476.

Jones SG, Shakespeare PG, and Carruth JAS (1989): Transcutaneous microscopy and argon laser treatment of port wine stains. *Lasers Med Sci*, **4:** 73 ~ 78.

Kami T, *et al* (1985): Effects of low-powerd diode lasers on flap survival. *Ann Plast Surg*, **143:** p278.

Kantor GR, Ratz JL, and Wheeland RG (1986): Treatment of acne keloidalis nuchae with carbon dioxide laser. *J Am Acad Dermatol* **14:** 263 ~ 267.

Kantor GR, Wheeland RG, Bailin PL, *et al* (1985): Treatment of earlobe keloids with carbon dioxide laser excision: A report of 16 cases. *J Dermatol Surg Oncol*, **11:** 1063 ~ 1067.

Kaplan I, and Sharon U (1976): Current laser surgery. *Ann NY Acad Sci*, **267:** 247 ~ 253.

Katalinic D (1991): LLLT for postoperative treatment in cosmetic surgery. *Laser Therapy*, **3:** 63 ~ 66.

Kecham AS (1969): A surgeon's appraisal of the laser. *Surg Clin N Am*, **47:** 1249 ~ 1263.

Khromov BM, and Frygin NV (1969): The use of optic quantum generators (lasers) in dermatology (a review of foreign literature). *Vest Derm Vener*, (Russlan) **43:** 14 ~ 21.

Kirschner RA (1984): Cutaneous plastic surgery with the CO_2 laser. *Surg Clin North Am* **64:** 871 ~ 883.

Kitzmilier KW (1970): Laser treatment of tattoos and angiomas. *J Med Assoc Georgia*, **59:** 385 ~ 386.

Kitzmiller KW (1970): Laser treatment of tattoos and angiomas. *J Med Ass Ga*, **59:** 385 ~ 386.

Klein DR (1977): The use of the carbon dioxide laser in plastic surgery. *South Med J*, **70:** 429 ~ 431.

Klein DR (1977): The use of the CO_2 laser In plastic surgery. *S Med J*, **70:** 429 ~ 431.

Koebner HK (1980) (ed): *Lasers in Medicine*: John Wiley & Sons, Chichester, U. K.

Kubota J, and Ohshiro T (1984): Photostimulative effects of the GaAlAs diode laser on flaps: *Proc 27th Cong J Plast Recon Socy*: Japanese Society for Laser Medicine, Tokyo. p156.

Kubota J, and Ohshiro T (1984): The effect of the gallium aluminium arsenide semiconductor laser on flaps. *J Jap Soc Laser Med*, **5:** p97.

Labandter H, and Kaplan I (1977): Experience with a 'continuous' laser in the treatment of suitable cutaneous conditions: preliminary report. *J Derm Surg Oncol* **3:** 527 ~ 530.

Lagunova 1G, Savchenko ED, Likhovetskaya LL, Garvei NN, and Shamaeva GG (1971): Bio-logical effect of lasers on the skin (preliminary report). *Med Rad (Russian)*, **16:** 38 ~ 42.

Lang KR, *et al* (1964): Lasers as tools for embryoiogy and cytology. *Nature*, **201:** 675~ 677, Feb.

Laub DR, Yules RB, Arras M, Murray DE, Crowhey L, and Chase RA (1968): Preliminary histopathological observation of Q-switched ruby laser radiation on dermal tattoo pigment in man. *J Surg Res*, **8:** 220 ~ 224.

McBurney El (1978): Carbon dioxide laser treatment of dermatologic lesions. *S Med J*, **71:** 795 ~ 797.

McCarthy WH, *et al* (1978): Laser surgery for melanoma and superficial malignancies. *Aust New Z J Med*, **48**.

McGuff PE (1966): Laser radiation for basal cell carcinoma. *Dermatologia*, **133:** 379 ~ 383.

Morita H, Kohno J, Tanaka S, Kitano Y, and Sagami S (1993): Clinical Application of GaAlAs 830 nm diode laser for atopic dermatitis. *Laser Therapy*, **5:** 75 ~ 78.

Moskajik KG, and Kozlov AP (1978): Experience in treating skin tumors with pulse laser radiation. *Meditz Radi (Russian)*, **23:** 36 ~ 42.

Mulbauer W, Nath G, and Kreitmair A (1976): Treatment of capillary hemangiomas and nevi fiammei with light. *Lang Arch Chir (German)*, **91** ~ 94.

Nimsakul N (1979): Operations performed from March, 1977 by means of CO_2 surgical laser scalpel. *Tokai University Hosp.*

Ohshiro T (1977): Dermatologic Laser Treatment Successfully Completed in Japan. *Laser Elektro-optik*, **3:** 34 ~ 35.

Ohshiro T (1977): The use of ruby laser beam for the treatment of chromatic maculae - control of irradiated energy and biological response. *2nd Cong Asian-Pacific Section Int Cong Plas Recon Surg*, (abs. p.30).

Ohshiro T (1978): Ohta's Nevus and the Treatment. *Rinsho Derma*, **21:** 681 ~ 687.

Ohshiro T (1978): *Dermatological Appiication of Lasers*. Mainichi Life, Tokyo, Japan. pp. 94 ~ 100.

Ohshiro T (1979): Laser treatment for henangioma simplex - mutual relation between colour sensitivity & colour tone. *Jap J Plas Rec Surg*, **21:** 71.

Ohshiro T (1979): Histologically Selective Treatment for Chromatic Maculae using Ruby & Argon Lasers. *Proc Cong Las Photomed* (Firenze, Italy: Conference Digest No. 19).

Ohshiro T (1979): How to achieve maximum treatment effect with minimum physical damage. *Proc, 3rd Meeting, Jap Soc Las Med:* p. 111.

Ohshiro T (1979): Laser Treatment for Nevi. *J Keio med Soc*, **57:** 100.

Ohshiro T (1979): New Concept of Combined Laser Therapy. *Proc 2nd Cong I.S.L.S.M.*, (Graz, Austria).

Ohshiro T (1979): Ruby & Argon Laser Treatment for Chromatic Maculae. *International Congress of PRS:* (abs. Program p.152).

Ohshiro T (1980): *Laser Treatment For Nevi:* MEL, Tokyo.

Ohshiro T (1980): Treatment of pigmentation of the lips & oral mucosa in Peutz-Jeghers syndrome using ruby & argon lasers. *Br J Plas Surg,* **33:** 2.

Ohshiro T (1981): The color problem in laser treatment of nevi. *Lasers Surg Med,* **1:** 99.

Ohshiro T (1981): The CO2 laser in the treatment of cavernous hemangioma of the lower lip: a case report. *Lasers Surg Med,* **1:** 337.

Ohshiro T (1983): The ruby and argon lasers in the treatment of nevi. *Ann Acad Med,* **12:** 388 ~ 395.

Ohshiro T (1985): The laser in skin surgery. In Harahap M (ed) *Skin Surgery.* Warren H Green, Los Angeles, 891 ~ 933.

Ohshiro T (1986): Clinical salvage of an ischemic flap with the diode laser. *Acta Chirur Plast,* **28:** 4.

Ohshiro T and Chen I (1992): Low reactive-level 830 nm diode laser therapy (LLLT) successfully acelerates regression of strawberry haemangioma in the infant: case reports. *Laser Therapy,* **4:** 127 ~ 132.

Ohshiro T, and Maeda T (1992): Application of 830 nm diode laser as successful adjunctive therapy of hypertrophic scars and keloids. *Laser Therapy,* **4:** 155 ~ 168.

Peled I, *et al* (1976): Excision of epithelial tumours. *Cancer Letters,* **2:** 41 ~ 46.

Reid R, and Muller S (1978): Tattoo removal with laser (letter). *Med J Austral,* **1:** 389.

Rockwell RJ, jr (1970): Designs and functions of laser systems for biomedicai applications. *Ann NY Acad Sci,* **168:** 459 ~ 471.

Sacchini V, Lovo GF, Arioli N, *et al* (1984): Carbon dioxide laser in scalp tumor surgery. *Laser Surg Med,* **4:** 261 ~ 269.

Saks NS (1963): Ruby laser as a microsurgicai instrument. *Science,* **141:** 46 ~ 47.

Sakurai Y (1973): Present and future problems with the laser scalpel. *Surg Ther,* **29:** 569 ~ 578.

Sakurai Y, *et al* (1976): The medical application of the laser scalpel. *Surg Ther,* **35:** 617 ~ 625.

Sakurai Y, *et al,* (1977): Laser operation - utilisation of the coherent light. *Butsuri,* **32:** 146 ~ 154.

Sasaki K, and Ohshiro T (1990): Role of low reactive-level laser therapy in the treatement of acquired and cicatrical vitiligo. *Laser Therapy,* **1:** 3 141 ~ 146.

Schindl L, Kainz A, and Kern H (1992): Effects of low level laser irradiation on indolent ulcers caused by Beurger's disease; literature review and preliminary report. *Laser Therapy,* **4:** 25 ~ 34.

Slutzki S, Shafir R, and Bornstein LA (1977): use of the carbon dioxide laser for large excisions with minimal blood loss. *Plast Reconstr Surg,* **60:** 250 ~ 255.

Stellar S (1983): Surgical applications of lasers: in Daheng W *et al* (eds) *Proceedings of an International Conference on Lasers:* John Wiley & Sons, New York: p 665.

Van Gemert MJC, Carruth JAS, and Shakespeare PG (1991): Has the argon laser ever been used optimally for the treatment of port wine stain birthmarks? *Lasers Med Sci,* **6:** 371 ~ 372.

Vance CA, Fisher J, Wheatly JD, Evans JH, Spyt TJ, Moseley H, and Paul JP (1988): Laser assisted anastomosis of coronary arteries *in vivo:* Optimization of bonding conditions. *Lasers Med Sci,* **3:** 219 ~ 228.

Verschueren RC, Koudstaal J, and Oldhoff J (1975): Surgery with the CO_2 laser. *Pan Med,* **17:** 241 ~ 244.

Wheeland RG, and Bailin PL (1984): Scalp reduction surgery with the carbon dioxide laser. *J Dermatol Surg Oncol,* **10:** 565 ~ 569.

Wolbarsht ML (1977) (ed): *Laser Applications in Medicine & Biology: Plenum Press, New York & London. Vols 1 - 3, 1971 ~ 1974.*

SUBJECT INDEX

Before looking for an entry in the Subject Index, the reader is advised to check first in the Table of Contents, which is extremely comprehensive. Lasers are arranged in the index alphabetically under their name, *e.g.* 'argon laser', 'ruby laser' and so on, rather than under the heading of 'laser'. Eponyms are arranged alphabetically under the person's name, *e.g.* '*Raman-Nas* diffraction', rather than under the phenomenon or condition. In the example given 'diffraction' on its own can be found as a sub-heading in the Table of Contents.